Clinical and Radiological Anatomy of the Lumbar Spine

Commissioning Editor: *Alison Taylor/Claire Wilson*
Development Editor: *Helen Leng*
Project Manager: *Frances Affleck*
Designer/Design Direction: *Stewart Larking*
Illustration Manager: *Bruce Hogarth*

Clinical and Radiological Anatomy of the Lumbar Spine

Fifth Edition

Nikolai Bogduk BSc(Med) MB BS PhD DSc MMed DipAnat FAFMM FAFRM FFPM(ANZCA)

Professor of Pain Medicine, University of Newcastle, and Head, Department of Clinical Research, Royal Newcastle Hospital, Newcastle, New South Wales, Australia

Foreword by Ray M. Baker MD

President, International Spine Intervention Society; Immediate Past President, North American Spine Society; Clinical Professor (adjunct), Department of Anesthesiology, University of Washington, Seattle, WA, USA

ELSEVIER
CHURCHILL
LIVINGSTONE

Edinburgh   London   New York   Oxford   Philadelphia   St Louis   Sydney   Toronto 2012

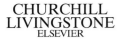

No part of this publication may be reproduced or transmitted in any form or by any means, electronic or mechanical, including photocopying, recording, or any information storage and retrieval system, without permission in writing from the publisher. Details on how to seek permission, further information about the publisher's permissions policies and our arrangements with organizations such as the Copyright Clearance Center and the Copyright Licensing Agency, can be found at our website: www.elsevier.com/permissions.

This book and the individual contributions contained in it are protected under copyright by the Publisher (other than as may be noted herein).

First edition 1987
Second edition 1991
Third edition 1997
Fourth edition 2005
Fifth edition 2012
  Reprinted 2014

ISBN 9780702043420

British Library Cataloguing in Publication Data
A catalogue record for this book is available from the British Library

Library of Congress Cataloging in Publication Data
A catalog record for this book is available from the Library of Congress

Notices
Knowledge and best practice in this field are constantly changing. As new research and experience broaden our understanding, changes in research methods, professional practices, or medical treatment may become necessary.

Practitioners and researchers must always rely on their own experience and knowledge in evaluating and using any information, methods, compounds, or experiments described herein. In using such information or methods they should be mindful of their own safety and the safety of others, including parties for whom they have a professional responsibility.

With respect to any drug or pharmaceutical products identified, readers are advised to check the most current information provided (i) on procedures featured or (ii) by the manufacturer of each product to be administered, to verify the recommended dose or formula, the method and duration of administration, and contraindications. It is the responsibility of practitioners, relying on their own experience and knowledge of their patients, to make diagnoses, to determine dosages and the best treatment for each individual patient, and to take all appropriate safety precautions.

To the fullest extent of the law, neither the publisher nor the authors, contributors, or editors, assume any liability for any injury and/or damage to persons or property as a matter of products liability, negligence or otherwise, or from any use or operation of any methods, products, instructions, or ideas contained in the material herein.

ELSEVIER your source for books, journals and multimedia in the health sciences
www.elsevierhealth.com

Printed in China

Working together to grow libraries in developing countries

www.elsevier.com | www.bookaid.org | www.sabre.org

ELSEVIER   BOOK AID International   Sabre Foundation

The publisher's policy is to use **paper manufactured from sustainable forests**

Contents

Foreword

Since publication of the first edition in 1987, *Clinical Anatomy of the Lumbar Spine and Sacrum* has distinguished itself as the definitive textbook on the subject. It has been hailed internationally for its balance between detail and accessibility, for its clarity and succinctness, and for its clinical relevance. Indeed, the book has become an essential part of the bibliography for a surprisingly diverse group, including practicing and training physicians, chiropractors, physiotherapists, occupational therapists, manual therapists, academicians, and researchers.

Yet, in this time of compressed patient visits, super-specialization, and advanced imaging, is the study of clinical and radiological anatomy of the lumbar spine still relevant? My response is an unqualified yes. For, despite technological advances in the diagnosis and treatment of low back pain, and the logarithmic increases in cost of care, we have not seen a commensurate improvement in outcomes. As the immediate Past President of the North American Spine Society and the current President of the International Spine Intervention Society, I am following with interest (and no small measure of amusement) a return to basics and a questioning of core tenets in the treatment of low back disorders. As we have learned with many other medical disciplines, a thorough understanding of anatomy is the foundation upon which new tests and treatments are developed and outcomes improved.

Sadly, despite its manifest importance, the study of anatomy has been de-emphasized in many medical curricula, including the replacement of hands-on cadaveric labs by DVDs. The unfortunate result is that many practitioners today lack even a basic understanding of anatomic and radiographic relationships and their importance to clinical practice. Too often this translates into perfunctory physical examinations and an over-reliance on imaging and laboratory reports in establishing a diagnosis. This is especially perilous when treating low back pain, a condition defined by its weak evidence base.

For those of us who have dedicated our lives to the diagnosis, treatment, and prevention of low back pain, we understand all too well the dangers of over- or under-estimating the utility of a test or examination finding. We also clearly understand the importance of clinical anatomy in our everyday practices and the lives of our patients. Still, for many, the thought of studying anatomy evokes painful memories of pouring over lists of various anatomic structures without a clear understanding of their day-to-day significance.

Therein lies the strength of *Clinical and Radiological Anatomy of the Lumbar Spine*. Professor Bogduk's mastery of anatomy and clinical science, his decades of lecturing and teaching, his renowned research experience, and his characteristic exactness, are all brought to bear as he breathes life into a subject that would otherwise be relegated to the rote memorization of body parts. His command of the subject and his considerable experience also allows him to render the complex anatomic and radiographic principles accessible to everyone. From the novice medical student to the seasoned practitioner, from the physiotherapist to the orthopaedic surgeon, anyone who treats low back pain would benefit from reading and thoroughly understanding this text.

Building on previous editions, the book maintains a strong logical structure and directly links advanced anatomic concepts to clinical practice. It also remains firmly rooted in evidence with an updated list of references. But Professor Bogduk goes well beyond previous editions by expanding the content considerably.

As connoted by the new title, *Clinical and Radiological Anatomy of the Lumbar Spine,* the fifth edition includes three new chapters devoted to radiological anatomy. Previously placed in the appendix, radiographic anatomy now takes a more central role commensurate with the clinician's reliance on radiographic studies. Additional chapters on sagittal and axial magnetic resonance imaging correlate anatomic knowledge gained in the preceding chapters with various MRI reconstructions.

Bridging the gap between clinical anatomy and radiological anatomy is a chapter on lumbar spine reconstructive anatomy, which introduces the concept of *anatomy by expectation* – the anatomic details that a clinician *expects* to encounter in the lumbar region, even though they might not be visible or palpable. He introduces the topic by having the reader reconstruct the lumbar region one layer at a time, beginning with the basic vertebral body and adding the various muscles, ligaments, nerves, arteries, and other components that make up the region. The exercise is critical in reinforcing the relationship between structures and in developing the *expectation* of what one should observe when viewing plain radiographs or magnetic resonance imaging scans.

In short, my friend and respected colleague, Professor Nikolai Bogduk, has once again demonstrated his considerable talent as a scholar, clinician, writer, and teacher with this fifth edition of *Clinical and Radiological Anatomy of the Lumbar Spine.* What is more, he has produced a text worthy of his reputation, which will undoubtedly hold a prominent place in the list of reference books owned by every spine care provider.

RMB
2011

Preface
to the fifth edition

When asked to produce a new edition, authors are subject to various pressures. The publisher wants a new edition, and they want something different that distinguishes it from previous editions. Meanwhile, there may or may not have been developments in the material covered by the book. On top of these concerns there are the demands of continuing clinical practice and research.

I apologise to those authors of new research papers whose work I have not cited in this fifth edition. It would have been appropriate to have added their new observations, but practically I have not had the time to reconcile what is in the text and what is in my collection of recent findings. However, it is the nature of anatomy that big things do not change. Therefore, the message of this fifth edition is not seriously compromised by the lack of newly discovered detail.

What I have done in this fifth edition is expanded the book to embrace medical imaging. Clinical practitioners rarely get the opportunity to visit anatomy in cadavers, but they are likely to encounter images of their patients. Yet to many practitioners, images of the lumbar spine can be overwhelming, mysterious or threatening. In the course of conducting programmes of continuing professional development, I have encountered practitioners who have difficulty finding a pedicle on radiographs, or finding a transverse process on lateral radiographs of the lumbar spine.

So, the new feature of this fifth edition is a strategic elaboration of the regional anatomy of the lumbar spine. It starts with a chapter on reconstructive anatomy, which provides an algorithm for how to put the entire lumbar spine back together. The emphasis is *anatomy by expectation*. Readers are shown how to expect what should be present, rather than being required to identify what is evident in a medical image. Subsequent, new chapters apply these principles to the reconstruction of the lumbar spine on plain radiographs and the reconstruction of sagittal and axial magnetic resonance images. The reconstruction of coronal views is an exercise for the future.

Nikolai Bogduk

Preface
to the first edition

Low back pain is a major problem in medicine and can constitute more than 60% of consultations in private physiotherapy practice. Yet, the emphasis given to spinal anatomy in conventional courses in anatomy for medical students and physiotherapists is not commensurate with the magnitude of the problem of spinal pain in clinical practice. The anatomy of the lumbar spine usually constitutes only a small component of such courses.

Having been involved in spinal research and in teaching medical students and physiotherapists both at undergraduate and postgraduate levels, we have become conscious of how little of the basic sciences relating to the lumbar spine is taught to students, and how difficult it can be to obtain information which is available but scattered through a diversity of textbooks and journal articles. Therefore, we have composed this textbook in order to collate that material which we consider fundamental to the understanding of the structure, function and common disorders of the lumbar spine.

We see the text as one which can be used as a companion to other textbooks in introductory courses in anatomy, and which can also remain as a resource throughout later years of undergraduate and postgraduate education in physiotherapy and physical medicine. In this regard, references are made throughout the text to contemporary and major earlier research papers so that the reader may consult the original literature upon which descriptions, interpretations and points of view are based. Moreover, the reference list has been made extensive in order to provide students seeking to undertake research projects on some aspect of the lumbar spine with a suitable starting point in their search through the literature.

Chapters 1–4 outline the structure of the individual components of the lumbar spine, and the intact spine is described in Chapter 5. In describing the lumbar vertebrae and their joints, we have gone beyond the usual scope of textbooks of anatomy by endeavouring to explain why the vertebrae and their components are constructed the way they are.

Chapter 6 summarises some basic principles of biomechanics in preparation for the study of the movements of the lumbar spine which is dealt with in Chapter 7. Chapter 8 provides an account of the lumbar back muscles which are described in exhaustive detail because of the increasing contemporary interest amongst physiotherapists and others in physical medicine in the biomechanical functions and so-called dysfunctional states of the back muscles.

Chapters 9 and 10 describe the nerves and blood supply of the lumbar spine, and its embryology and development is described in Chapter 11. This leads to a description of the age-changes of the lumbar spine in Chapter 12. The theme developed through Chapters 11 and 12 is that the lumbar spine is not a constant stereotyped structure as described in conventional textbooks, but one that continually changes in form and functional capacity throughout life. Any concept of normality must be modified according to the age of the patient or subject.

The final two chapters provide a bridge between basic anatomy and the clinical problem of lumbar pain syndromes. Chapter 13 outlines the possible mechanisms of lumbar pain in terms of the innervation of the lumbar spine and the relations of the lumbar spinal nerves and nerve roots, thereby providing an anatomical foundation for the appreciation of pathological conditions that can cause spinal pain.

Chapter 14 deals with pathological anatomy. Traditional topics like congenital disorders, fractures, dislocations and tumours are not covered, although the reader is directed to the pertinent literature on these topics. Instead, the scope is restricted to conditions which clinically are interpreted as mechanical disorders. The aetiology and pathology of these conditions are described in terms of the structural and biomechanical principles developed in earlier chapters, with the view to providing a rational basis for the interpretation and treatment of a group of otherwise poorly understood conditions which account for the majority of presentations of low back pain syndromes.

We anticipate that the detail and extent of our account of the clinical anatomy of the lumbar spine will be perceived as far in excess of what is conventionally taught. However, we believe that our text is not simply an expression of a personal interest of the authors, but rather is an embodiment of what we consider the essential knowledge of basic sciences for anyone seeking to be trained to deal with disorders of the lumbar spine.

Nikolai Bogduk
Lance Twomey

Chapter | 1 |

The lumbar vertebrae

The lumbar vertebral column consists of five separate vertebrae, which are named according to their location in the intact column. From above downwards they are named as the first, second, third, fourth and fifth lumbar vertebrae (Fig. 1.1). Although there are certain features that typify each lumbar vertebra, and enable each to be individually identified and numbered, at an early stage of study it is not necessary for students to be able to do so. Indeed, to learn to do so would be impractical, burdensome and educationally unsound. Many of the distinguishing features are better appreciated and more easily understood once the whole structure of the lumbar vertebral column and its mechanics have been studied. To this end, a description of the features of individual lumbar vertebrae is provided in the Appendix and it is recommended that this be studied after Chapter 7.

What is appropriate at this stage is to consider those features common to all lumbar vertebrae and to appreciate how typical lumbar vertebrae are designed to subserve their functional roles. Accordingly, the following description is divided into parts. In the first part, the features of a typical lumbar vertebra are described. This section serves either as an introduction for students commencing their study of the lumbar vertebral column or as a revision for students already familiar with the essentials of vertebral anatomy. The second section deals with particular details relevant to the appreciation of the function of the lumbar vertebrae, and provides a foundation for later chapters.

It is strongly recommended that these sections be read with specimens of the lumbar vertebrae at the reader's disposal, for not only will visual inspection reinforce the written information but tactile examination of a specimen will enhance the three-dimensional perception of structure.

A TYPICAL LUMBAR VERTEBRA

The lumbar vertebrae are irregular bones consisting of various named parts (Fig. 1.2). The anterior part of each vertebra is a large block of bone called the **vertebral body**. The vertebral body is more or less box shaped, with essentially flat top and bottom surfaces, and slightly concave anterior and lateral surfaces. Viewed from above or below the vertebral body has a curved perimeter that is more or less kidney shaped. The posterior surface of the body is essentially flat but is obscured from thorough inspection by the posterior elements of the vertebra.

The greater part of the top and bottom surfaces of each vertebral body is smooth and perforated by tiny holes. However, the perimeter of each surface is marked by a narrow rim of smoother, less perforated bone, which is slightly raised from the surface. This rim represents the fused **ring apophysis**, which is a secondary ossification centre of the vertebral body (see Ch. 12).

The posterior surface of the vertebral body is marked by one or more large holes known as the **nutrient foramina**. These foramina transmit the nutrient arteries of the vertebral body and the basivertebral veins (see Ch. 11). The

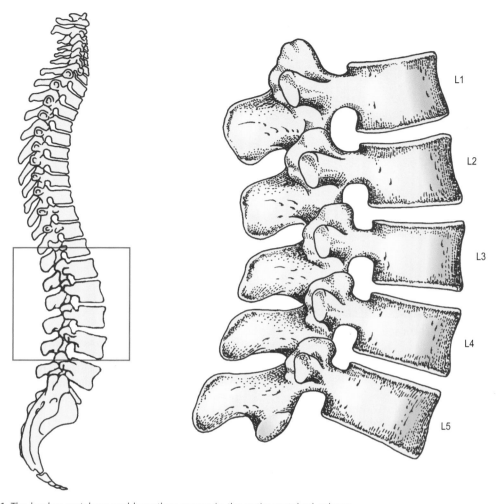

Figure 1.1 The lumbar vertebrae and how they appear in the entire vertebral column.

anterolateral surfaces of the vertebral body are marked by similar but smaller foramina which transmit additional intra-osseous arteries.

Projecting from the back of the vertebral body are two stout pillars of bone. Each of these is called a **pedicle**. The pedicles attach to the upper part of the back of the vertebral body; this is one feature that allows the superior and inferior aspects of the vertebral body to be identified. To orientate a vertebra correctly, view it from the side. That end of the posterior surface of the body to which the pedicles are more closely attached is the superior end (Fig. 1.2A, B).

The word 'pedicle' is derived from the Latin *pediculus* meaning little foot; the reason for this nomenclature is apparent when the vertebra is viewed from above (Fig. 1.2E). It can be seen that attached to the back of the

vertebral body is an arch of bone, the **neural arch**, so called because it surrounds the neural elements that pass through the vertebral column. The neural arch has several parts and several projections but the pedicles are those parts that look like short legs with which it appears to 'stand' on the back of the vertebral body (see Fig. 1.2E), hence the derivation from the Latin.

Projecting from each pedicle towards the midline is a sheet of bone called the **lamina**. The name is derived from the Latin *lamina* meaning leaf or plate. The two laminae meet and fuse with one another in the midline so that in a top view, the laminae look like the roof of a tent, and indeed form the so-called 'roof' of the neural arch. (Strictly speaking, there are two laminae in each vertebra, one on the left and one on the right, and the two meet posteriorly in the midline, but in some circles the term 'lamina' is

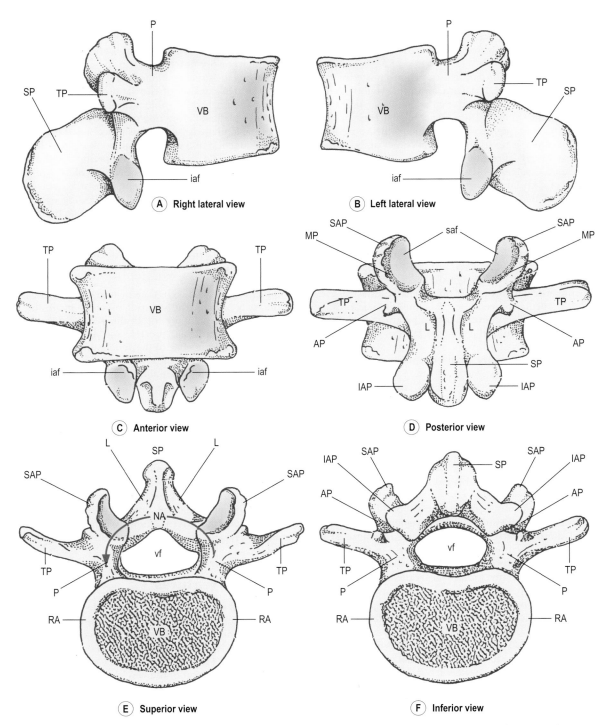

Figure 1.2 The parts of a typical lumbar vertebra: AP, accessory process; iaf, inferior articular facet; IAP, inferior articular process; L, lamina; MP, mamillary process; NA, neural arch; P, pedicle; RA, ring apophysis; saf, superior articular facet; SAP, superior articular process; SP, spinous process; TP, transverse process; VB, vertebral body; vf, vertebral foramen.

used incorrectly to refer to both laminae collectively. When this is the usage, the term 'hemilamina' is used to refer to what has been described above as a true lamina.)

The full extent of the laminae is seen in a posterior view of the vertebra (Fig. 1.2D). Each lamina has slightly irregular and perhaps sharp superior edges but its lateral edge is rounded and smooth. There is no medial edge of each lamina because the two laminae blend in the midline. Similarly, there is no superior lateral corner of the lamina because in this direction the lamina blends with the pedicle on that side. The inferolateral corner and inferior border of each lamina are extended and enlarged into a specialised mass of bone called the **inferior articular process**. A similar mass of bone extends upwards from the junction of the lamina with the pedicle, to form the **superior articular process**.

Each vertebra thus presents four articular processes: a right and left inferior articular process; and a right and left superior articular process. On the medial surface of each superior articular process and on the lateral surface of each inferior articular process there is a smooth area of bone which in the intact spine is covered by articular cartilage. This area is known as the articular **facet** of each articular process.

Projecting posteriorly from the junction of the two laminae is a narrow blade of bone (readily gripped between the thumb and index finger), which in a side view resembles the blade of an axe. This is the **spinous process**, so named because in other regions of the vertebral column these processes form projections under the skin that are reminiscent of the dorsal spines of fish and other animals. The base of the spinous process blends imperceptibly with the two laminae but otherwise the spinous process presents free superior and inferior edges and a broader posterior edge.

Extending laterally from the junction of the pedicle and the lamina, on each side, is a flat, rectangular bar of bone called the **transverse process**, so named because of its transverse orientation. Near its attachment to the pedicle, each transverse process bears on its posterior surface a small, irregular bony prominence called the **accessory process**. Accessory processes vary in form and size from a simple bump on the back of the transverse process to a more pronounced mass of bone, or a definitive pointed projection of variable length.[1,2] Regardless of its actual form, the accessory process is identifiable as the only bony projection from the back of the proximal end of the transverse process. It is most evident if the vertebra is viewed from behind and from below (Fig. 1.2D, F).

Close inspection of the posterior edge of each of the superior articular processes reveals another small bump, distinguishable from its surroundings by its smoothness. Apparently, because this structure reminded early anatomists of the shape of breasts, it was called the **mamillary process**, derived from the Latin *mamilla* meaning little

breast. It lies just above and slightly medial to the accessory process, and the two processes are separated by a notch, of variable depth, that may be referred to as the **mamillo-accessory notch**.

Reviewing the structure of the neural arch, it can be seen that each arch consists of two laminae, meeting in the midline and anchored to the back of the vertebral body by the two pedicles. Projecting posteriorly from the junction of the laminae is the spinous process, and projecting from the junction of the lamina and pedicle, on each side, are the transverse processes. The superior and inferior articular processes project from the corners of the laminae.

The other named features of the lumbar vertebrae are not bony parts but spaces and notches. Viewing a vertebra from above, it can be seen that the neural arch and the back of the vertebral body surround a space that is just about large enough to admit an examining finger. This space is the **vertebral foramen**, which amongst other things transmits the nervous structures enclosed by the vertebral column.

In a side view, two notches can be recognised above and below each pedicle. The superior notch is small and is bounded inferiorly by the top of the pedicle, posteriorly by the superior articular process, and anteriorly by the uppermost posterior edge of the vertebral body. The inferior notch is deeper and more pronounced. It lies behind the lower part of the vertebral body, below the lower edge of the pedicle and in front of the lamina and the inferior articular process. The difference in size of these notches can be used to correctly identify the upper and lower ends of a lumbar vertebra. The deeper, more obvious notch will always be the inferior.

Apart from providing this aid in orientating a lumbar vertebra, these notches have no intrinsic significance and have not been given a formal name. However, when consecutive lumbar vertebrae are articulated (see Fig. 1.7), the superior and inferior notches face one another and form most of what is known as the **intervertebral foramen**, whose anatomy is described in further detail in Chapter 5.

Particular features

Conceptually, a lumbar vertebra may be divided into three functional components (Fig. 1.3). These are the vertebral body, the pedicles and the posterior elements consisting of the laminae and their processes. Each of these components subserves a unique function but each contributes to the integrated function of the whole vertebra.

Vertebral body

The vertebral body subserves the weight-bearing function of the vertebra and is perfectly designed for this purpose. Its flat superior and inferior surfaces are dedicated to supporting longitudinally applied loads.

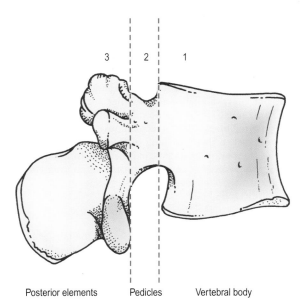

Figure 1.3 The division of a lumbar vertebra into its three functional components.

Posterior elements   Pedicles   Vertebral body

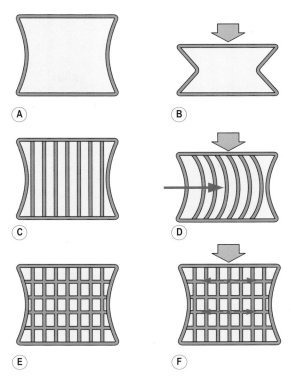

Figure 1.4 Reconstruction of the internal architecture of the vertebral body. (A) With just a shell of cortical bone, a vertebral body is like a box and collapses when a load is applied (B). (C) Internal vertical struts brace the box (D). (E) Transverse connections prevent the vertical struts from bowing and increase the load-bearing capacity of the box. Loads are resisted by tension in the transverse connections (F).

Take two lumbar vertebrae and fit them together so that the inferior surface of one body rests on the superior surface of the other. Now squeeze them together, as strongly as you can. Feel how well they resist the applied longitudinal compression. The experiment can be repeated by placing the pair of vertebrae upright on a table (near the edge so that the inferior articular processes can hang down over the edge). Now press down on the upper vertebra and feel how the pair of vertebrae sustains the pressure, even up to taking your whole body weight. These experiments illustrate how the flatness of the vertebral bodies confers stability to an intervertebral joint, in the longitudinal direction. Even without intervening and other supporting structures, two articulated vertebrae can stably sustain immense longitudinal loads.

The load-bearing design of the vertebral body is also reflected in its internal structure. The vertebral body is not a solid block of bone but a shell of cortical bone surrounding a cancellous cavity. The advantages of this design are several. Consider the problems of a solid block of bone: although strong, a solid block of bone is heavy. (Compare the weight of five lumbar vertebrae with that of five similarly sized stones.) More significantly, although solid blocks are suitable for maintaining static loads, solid structures are not ideal for dynamic load-bearing. Their crystalline structure tends to fracture along cleavage planes when sudden forces are applied. The reason for this is that crystalline structures cannot absorb and dissipate loads suddenly applied to them. They lack resilience, and the energy goes into breaking the bonds between the constituent

crystals. The manner in which vertebral bodies overcome these physical problems can be appreciated if the internal structure of the vertebral body is reconstructed.

With just an outer layer of cortical bone, a vertebral body would be merely a shell (Fig. 1.4A). This shell is not strong enough to sustain longitudinal compression and would collapse like a cardboard box (Fig. 1.4B). It needs to be reinforced. This can be achieved by introducing some vertical struts between the superior and inferior surfaces (Fig. 1.4C). A strut acts like a solid but narrow block of bone and, provided it is kept straight, it can sustain immense longitudinal loads. The problem with a strut, however, is that it tends to bend or bow when subjected to a longitudinal force. Nevertheless, a box with vertical struts, even if they bend, is still somewhat stronger than an empty box (Fig. 1.4D). The load-bearing capacity of a vertical strut can be preserved, however, if it is prevented from bowing. By introducing a series of cross-beams, connecting the struts, the strength of a box can be further enhanced (Fig. 1.4E). Now, when a load is applied, the

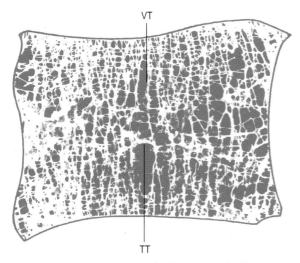

VT

TT

Figure 1.5 A sagittal section of a lumbar vertebral body showing its vertical (VT) and transverse (TT) trabeculae. *(Courtesy of Professor Lance Twomey.)*

cross-beams hold the struts in place, preventing them from deforming and preventing the box from collapsing (Fig. 1.4F).

The internal architecture of the vertebral body follows this same design. The struts and cross-beams are formed by thin rods of bone, respectively called vertical and transverse **trabeculae** (Fig. 1.5). The trabeculae endow the vertebral body with weight-bearing strength and resilience. Any applied load is first borne by the vertical trabeculae, and when these attempt to bow they are restrained from doing so by the horizontal trabeculae. Consequently, the load is sustained by a combination of vertical pressure and transverse tension in the trabeculae. It is the transfer of load from vertical pressure to transverse tension that endows the vertebra with resilience. The advantage of this design is that a strong but lightweight load-bearing structure is constructed with the minimum use of material (bone).

A further benefit is that the space between the trabeculae can be profitably used as convenient channels for the blood supply and venous drainage of the vertebral body, and under certain conditions as an accessory site for hae-mopoiesis (making blood cells). Indeed, the presence of blood in the intertrabecular spaces acts as a further useful element for transmitting the loads of weight-bearing and absorbing force.[3] When filled with blood, the trabeculated cavity of the vertebral body appears like a sponge, and for this reason it is sometimes referred to as the **vertebral spongiosa**.

The vertebral body is thus ideally designed, externally and internally, to sustain longitudinally applied loads.

However, it is virtually exclusively dedicated to this function and there are no features of the vertebral body that confer stability to the intervertebral joint in any other direction.

Taking two vertebral bodies, attempt to slide one over the other, backwards, forwards and sideways. Twist one vertebral body in relation to the other. Feel how easily the vertebrae move. There are no hooks, bumps or ridges on the vertebral bodies that prevent gliding or twisting movements between them. Lacking such features, the vertebral bodies are totally dependent on other structures for stability in the horizontal plane, and foremost amongst these are the posterior elements of the vertebrae.

Posterior elements

The posterior elements of a vertebra are the laminae, the articular processes and the spinous processes (see Fig. 1.3). The transverse processes are not customarily regarded as part of the posterior elements because they have a slightly different embryological origin (see Ch. 12), but for present purposes they can be considered together with them.

Collectively, the posterior elements form a very irregular mass of bone, with various bars of bone projecting in all directions. This is because the various posterior elements are specially adapted to receive the different forces that act on a vertebra.

The inferior articular processes form obvious hooks that project downwards. In the intact lumbar vertebral column, these processes will lock into the superior articular processes of the vertebra below, forming synovial joints whose principal function is to provide a locking mechanism that resists forward sliding and twisting of the vertebral bodies. This action can be illustrated by the following experiment.

Place two consecutive vertebrae together so that their bodies rest on one another and the inferior articular processes of the upper vertebra lock behind the superior articular processes of the lower vertebra. Slide the upper vertebra forwards and feel how the locked articular processes resist this movement. Next, holding the vertebral bodies slightly pressed together, attempt to twist them. Note how one of the inferior articular processes rams into its apposed superior articular process, and realise that further twisting can occur only if the vertebral bodies slide off one another.

The spinous, transverse, accessory and mamillary processes provide areas for muscle attachments. Moreover, the longer processes (the transverse and spinous processes) form substantial levers, which enhance the action of the muscles that attach to them. The details of the attachments of muscles are described in Chapter 9 but it is worth noting at this stage that every muscle that acts on the lumbar vertebral column is attached somewhere on the posterior elements. Only the crura of the diaphragm and parts of the psoas muscles attach to the vertebral bodies but these muscles have no primary action on the lumbar vertebrae. Every other muscle attaches to either the transverse, spinous, accessory or mamillary processes or laminae. This emphasises how all the muscular forces acting on a vertebra are delivered first to the posterior elements.

Traditionally, the function of the laminae has been dismissed simply as a protective one. The laminae are described as forming a bony protective covering over the neural contents of the vertebral canal. While this is a worthwhile function, it is not an essential function as demonstrated by patients who suffer no ill-effects to their nervous systems when laminae have been removed at operation. In such patients, it is only under unusual circumstances that the neural contents of the vertebral canal can be injured.

The laminae serve a more significant, but subtle and therefore overlooked, function. Amongst the posterior elements, they are centrally placed, and the various forces that act on the spinous and articular processes are ultimately transmitted to the laminae. By inspecting a vertebra, note how any force acting on the spinous process or the inferior articular processes must next be transmitted to the laminae. This concept is most important for appreciating how the stability of the lumbar spine can be compromised when a lamina is destroyed or weakened by disease, injury or surgery. Without a lamina to transmit the forces from the spinous and inferior articular processes, a vertebral body would be denied the benefit of these forces that either execute movement or provide stability.

That part of the lamina that intervenes between the superior and inferior articular process on each side is given a special name, the **pars interarticularis**, meaning 'interarticular part'. The pars interarticularis runs obliquely from the lateral border of the lamina to its upper border. The biomechanical significance of the pars interarticularis is that it lies at the junction of the vertically orientated lamina and the horizontally projecting pedicle. It is therefore subjected to considerable bending forces as the forces transmitted by the lamina undergo a change of direction into the pedicle. To withstand these forces, the cortical bone in the pars interarticularis is generally thicker than anywhere else in the lamina.[4] However, in some individuals the cortical bone is insufficiently thick to withstand excessive or sudden forces applied to the pars interarticularis,[5] and such individuals are susceptible to fatigue fractures, or stress fractures to the pars interarticularis.[5-7]

Pedicles

Customarily, the pedicles are parts of the lumbar vertebrae that are simply named, and no particular function is ascribed to them. However, as with the laminae, their function is so subtle (or so obvious) that it is overlooked or neglected.

The pedicles are the only connection between the posterior elements and the vertebral bodies. As described above, the bodies are designed for weight-bearing but cannot resist sliding or twisting movements, while the posterior elements are adapted to receive various forces, the articular processes locking against rotations and forward slides, and the other processes receiving the action of muscles. All forces sustained by any of the posterior elements are ultimately channelled towards the pedicles, which then transmit the benefit of these forces to the vertebral bodies.

The pedicles transmit both tension and bending forces. If a vertebral body slides forwards, the inferior articular processes of that vertebra will lock against the superior articular processes of the next lower vertebra and resist the slide. This resistance is transmitted to the vertebral body as tension along the pedicles. Bending forces are exerted by the muscles attached to the posterior elements. Conspicuously (see Ch. 9), all the muscles that act on a lumbar vertebra pull downwards. Therefore, muscular action is transmitted to the vertebral body through the pedicles, which act as levers and thereby are subjected to a certain amount of bending.

The pedicles are superbly designed to sustain these forces. Externally, they are stout pillars of bone. In cross-section they are found to be cylinders with thick walls. This structure enables them to resist bending in any direction. When a pedicle is bent downwards its upper wall is tensed while its lower wall is compressed. Similarly, if it is bent medially its outer wall is tensed while its inner wall is compressed. Through such combinations of tension and compression along opposite walls, the pedicle can resist bending forces applied to it. In accordance with engineering principles, a beam when bent resists deformation with its peripheral surfaces; towards its centre, forces reduce to zero. Consequently, there is no need for bone in the centre of a pedicle, which explains why the pedicle is hollow but surrounded by thick walls of bone.

Internal structure

The trabecular structure of the vertebral body (Fig. 1.6A) extends into the posterior elements. Bundles of trabeculae sweep out of the vertebral body, through the pedicles, and into the articular processes, laminae and transverse processes. They reinforce these processes like internal buttresses, and are orientated to resist the forces and deformations that the processes habitually sustain.[8] From the superior and inferior surfaces of the vertebral body, longitudinal trabeculae sweep into the inferior and articular processes (Fig. 1.6B). From opposite sides of the vertebral body, horizontal trabeculae sweep into the laminae and transverse processes (Fig. 1.6C). Within each process the

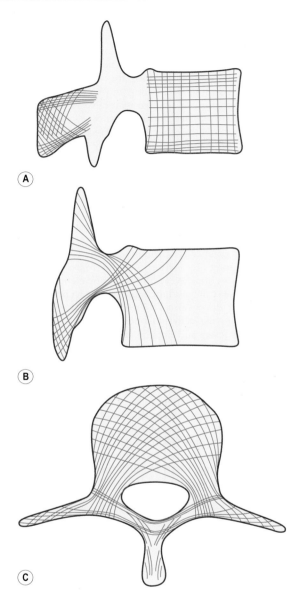

Figure 1.6 Internal architecture of a lumbar vertebra. (A) A midsagittal section showing the vertical and horizontal trabeculae of the vertebral body, and the trabeculae of the spinous process. (B) A lateral sagittal section showing the trabeculae passing through the pedicle into the articular processes. (C) A transverse section showing the trabeculae sweeping out of the vertebral body into the laminae and transverse processes. *(Based on Gallois and Japiot.[8])*

extrinsic trabeculae from the vertebral body intersect with intrinsic trabeculae from the opposite surface of the process. The trabeculae of the spinous process are difficult to discern in detail, but seem to be anchored in the lamina and along the borders of the process.[8]

THE INTERVERTEBRAL JOINTS

When any two consecutive lumbar vertebrae are articulated, they form three joints. One is formed between the two vertebral bodies. The other two are formed by the articulation of the superior articular process of one vertebra with the inferior articular processes of the vertebra above (Fig. 1.7). The nomenclature of these joints is varied, irregular and confusing.

The joints between the articular processes have an 'official' name. Each is known as a **zygapophysial joint**.[9] Individual zygapophysial joints can be specified by using the adjectives 'left' or 'right' and the numbers of the vertebrae involved in the formation of the joint. For example, the left L3–4 zygapophysial joint refers to the joint on the left, formed between the third and fourth lumbar vertebrae.

The term 'zygapophysial', is derived from the Greek words *apophysis*, meaning outgrowth, and *zygos*, meaning yoke or bridge. The term 'zygapophysis', therefore, means 'a bridging outgrowth' and refers to any articular process. The derivation relates to how, when two articulated vertebrae are viewed from the side, the articular processes appear to arch towards one another to form a bridge between the two vertebrae.

Other names used for the zygapophysial joints are 'apophysial' joints and 'facet' joints. 'Apophysial' predominates in the British literature and is simply a contraction of 'zygapophysial', which is the correct term. 'Facet' joint is a lazy and deplorable term. It is popularised in the American literature, probably because it is conveniently short but it carries no formal endorsement and is essentially ambiguous. The term stems from the fact that the joints are formed by the articular facets of the articular processes but the term 'facet' applies to any such structure in the skeleton. Every small joint has a facet. For example, in the thoracic spine, there are facets not only for the zygapophysial joints but also for the costovertebral joints and the costotransverse joints. Facets are not restricted to zygapophysial articular processes and strictly the term 'facet' joint does not imply only zygapophysial joints.

Because the zygapophysial joints are located posteriorly, they are also known as the posterior intervertebral joints. This nomenclature implies that the joint between the vertebral bodies is known as the anterior intervertebral joint (Table 1.1) but this latter term is rarely, if ever, used. In fact, there is no formal name for the joint between the vertebral bodies, and difficulties arise if one seeks to refer

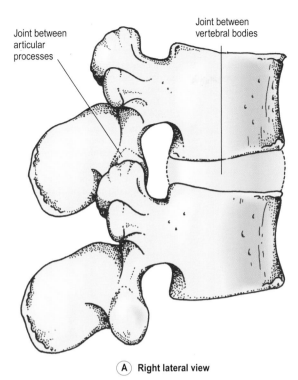

A Right lateral view

Table 1.1 Systematic nomenclature of the intervertebral joints

Joints between articular process	Joints between vertebral bodies
Zygapophysial joints	(No equivalent term)
(No equivalent term)	Interbody joints
Posterior intervertebral joints	Anterior intervertebral joints
Intervertebral diarthroses	Intervertebral amphiarthroses or intervertebral symphyses

to this joint. The term '**interbody joint**' is descriptive and usable but carries no formal endorsement and is not conventional. The term 'anterior intervertebral joint' is equally descriptive but is too unwieldy for convenient usage.

The only formal technical term for the joints between the vertebral bodies is the classification to which the joints belong. These joints are symphyses, and so can be called intervertebral symphyses[9] or intervertebral amphiarthroses, but again these are unwieldy terms. Moreover, if this system of nomenclature were adopted, to maintain consistency the zygapophysial joints would have to be known as the intervertebral diarthroses (see Table 1.1), which would compound the complexity of nomenclature of the intervertebral joints.

In this text, the terms 'zygapophysial joint' and 'interbody joint' will be used, and the details of the structure of these joints is described in the following chapters.

Spelling

Some editors of journals and books have deferred to dictionaries that spell the word 'zygapophysial' as 'zygapophyseal'. It has been argued that this fashion is not consistent with the derivation of the word.[10]

The English word is derived from the singular: zygapophysis. Consequently the adjective 'zygapophysial' is also derived from the singular and is spelled with an 'i'. This is the interpretation adopted by the International Anatomical Nomenclature Committee in the latest edition of the *Nomina Anatomica*.[9]

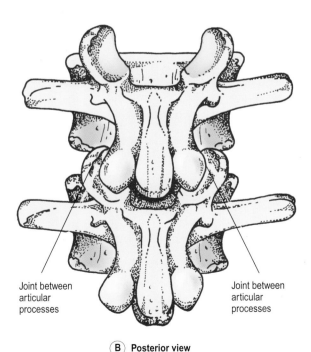

B Posterior view

Figure 1.7 The joints between two lumbar vertebrae.

REFERENCES

1. Le Double AF. *Traité des Variations de la Colonne Vertébral de l'Homme.* Paris: Vigot; 1912:271–274.

2. Louyot P. Propos sur le tubercle accessoire de l'apophyse costiforme lombaire. *J Radiol Electrol.* 1976;57:905–906.

3. White AA, Panjabi MM. *Clinical Biomechanics of the Spine.* Philadelphia: Lippincott; 1978.

4. Krenz J, Troup JDG. The structure of the pars interarticularis of the lower lumbar vertebrae and its relation to the etiology of spondylolysis. *J Bone Joint Surg.* 1973;55B:735–741.

5. Cyron BM, Hutton WC. Variations in the amount and distribution of cortical bone across the partes interarticulares of L5. A predisposing factor in spondylolysis? *Spine.* 1979;4:163–167.

6. Hutton WC, Stott JRR, Cyron BM. Is spondylolysis a fatigue fracture? *Spine.* 1977;2:202–209.

7. Troup JDG. The etiology of spondylolysis. *Orthop Clin North Am.* 1977;8:57–64.

8. Gallois M, Japiot M. Architecture intérieure des vertébrés (statique et physiologie de la colonne vertébrale). *Rev Chirurgie.* 1925;63:687–708.

9. International Anatomical Nomenclature Committee. *Nomina Anatomica.* 6th edn. Edinburgh: Churchill Livingstone; 1989.

10. Bogduk N. On the spelling of zygapophysial and of anulus. *Spine.* 1994;19:1771.

Chapter | 2 |

The interbody joint and the intervertebral discs

A joint could be formed simply by resting two consecutive vertebral bodies on top of one another (Fig. 2.1A). Such a joint could adequately bear weight and would allow gliding movements between the two bodies. However, because of the flatness of the vertebral surfaces, the joint would not allow the rocking movements that are necessary if flexion and extension or lateral bending are to occur at the joint. Rocking movements could occur only if one of two modifications were made. The first could be to introduce a curvature to the surfaces of the vertebral bodies. For example, the lower surface of a vertebral body could be curved (like the condyles of a femur). The upper vertebral body in an interbody joint could then roll forwards on the flat upper surface of the body below (Fig. 2.1B). However, this adaptation would compromise the weight-bearing capacity and stability of the interbody joint. The bony surface in contact with the lower vertebra would be reduced, and there would be a strong tendency for the upper vertebra to roll backwards or forwards whenever a weight was applied to it. This adaptation, therefore, would be inappropriate if the weight-bearing capacity and stability of the interbody joint are to be preserved. It is noteworthy, however, that in some species where weight-bearing is not important, for example in fish, a form of ball-and-socket joint is formed between vertebral bodies to provide mobility of the vertebral column.[1]

An alternative modification, and the one that occurs in humans and most mammals, is to interpose between the vertebral bodies a layer of strong but deformable soft tissue. This soft tissue is provided in the form of the **intervertebral disc**. The foremost effect of an intervertebral disc is to separate two vertebral bodies. The space between the vertebral bodies allows the upper vertebra to tilt forwards without its lower edge coming into contact with the lower vertebral body (Fig. 2.1C).

The consequent biomechanical requirements of an intervertebral disc are threefold. In the first instance, it must be strong enough to sustain weight, i.e. transfer the load from one vertebra to the next, without collapsing (being squashed). Secondly, without unduly compromising its strength, the disc must be deformable to accommodate the rocking movements of the vertebrae. Thirdly, it must be sufficiently strong so as not to be injured during movement. The structure of the intervertebral discs, therefore, should be studied with these requirements in mind.

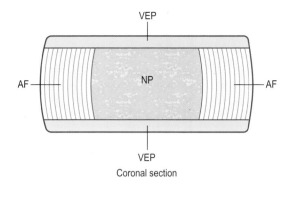

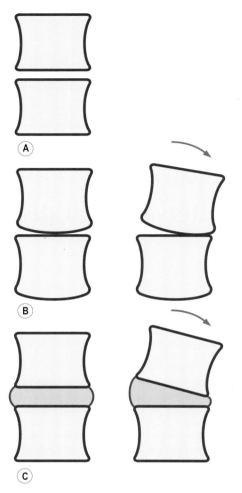

Coronal section

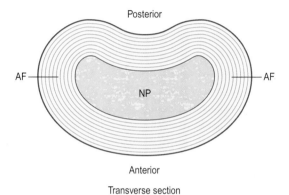

Transverse section

Figure 2.2 The basic structure of a lumbar intervertebral disc. The disc consists of a nucleus pulposus (NP) surrounded by an anulus fibrosus (AF), both sandwiched between two cartilaginous vertebral endplates (VEP).

Figure 2.1 Possible designs of an interbody joint. (A) The vertebral bodies rest directly on one another. (B) Adding a curvature to the bottom of a vertebra allows rocking movements to occur. (C) Interposing soft tissue between the vertebral bodies separates them and allows rocking movements to occur.

STRUCTURE OF THE INTERVERTEBRAL DISC

Each intervertebral disc consists of two basic components: a central **nucleus pulposus** surrounded by a peripheral **anulus fibrosus**. Although the nucleus pulposus is quite distinct in the centre of the disc, and the anulus fibrosus is distinct at its periphery, there is no clear boundary between the nucleus and the anulus within the disc. Rather, the peripheral parts of the nucleus pulposus merge with the deeper parts of the anulus fibrosus.

A third component of the intervertebral disc comprises two layers of cartilage which cover the top and bottom aspects of each disc. Each is called a **vertebral endplate** (Fig. 2.2). The vertebral endplates separate the disc from the adjacent vertebral bodies, and it is debatable whether the endplates are strictly components of the disc or whether they actually belong to the respective vertebral bodies. The interpretation used here is that the endplates are components of the intervertebral disc.

Nucleus pulposus

In typical, healthy, intervertebral discs of young adults, the nucleus pulposus is a semifluid mass of mucoid material (with the consistency, more or less, of toothpaste). Embryologically, the nucleus pulposus is a remnant of the notochord (see Ch. 12). Histologically, it consists of a few cartilage cells and some irregularly arranged collagen fibres, dispersed in a medium of semifluid ground substance (see below). Biomechanically, the fluid nature of the nucleus pulposus allows it to be deformed under pressure, but as a fluid its volume cannot be compressed. If subjected to pressure from any direction, the nucleus will attempt to deform and will thereby transmit the applied pressure in all directions. A suitable analogy is a balloon filled with water. Compression of the balloon deforms it; pressure in the balloon rises and stretches the walls of the balloon in all directions.

Anulus fibrosus

The anulus fibrosus consists of collagen fibres arranged in a highly ordered pattern. Foremost, the collagen fibres are arranged in between 10 and 20 sheets[2,3] called **lamellae** (from the Latin *lamella* meaning little leaf). The lamellae are arranged in concentric rings which surround the nucleus pulposus (Figs 2.2 and 2.3). The lamellae are thicker towards the centre of the disc;[4] they are thick in the anterior and lateral portions of the anulus but posteriorly they are finer and more tightly packed. Consequently the posterior portion of the anulus fibrosus is thinner than the rest of the anulus.[2,5,6]

Within each lamella, the collagen fibres lie parallel to one another, passing from the vertebra above to the vertebra below. The orientation of all the fibres in any given lamella is therefore the same and measures about 65–70° from the vertical.[7,8] However, while the angle is the same, the direction of this inclination alternates with each lamella. Viewed from the front, the fibres in one lamella may be orientated 65° to the right but those in the next deeper lamella will be orientated 65° to the left. The fibres in the next lamella will again lie 65° to the right, and

so on (see Fig. 2.3). Every second lamella, therefore, has exactly the same orientation. These figures, however, constitute an average orientation of fibres in the mid-portion of any lamella. Near their attachments, fibres may be orientated more steeply or less steeply with respect to the sagittal plane.[4]

The implication of the classic description of the anulus fibrosus is that the lamellae of the anulus form complete rings around the circumference of the disc. However, this proves not to be the case. In any given quadrant of the anulus, some 40% of the lamellae are incomplete, and in the posterolateral quadrant some 50% are incomplete.[4] An incomplete lamella is one that ceases to pass around the circumference of the disc. Around its terminal edge the lamellae superficial and deep to it either approximate or fuse (Fig. 2.4). Incomplete lamellae seem to be more frequent in the middle portion of the anulus.[9]

Vertebral endplates

Each vertebral endplate is a layer of cartilage about 0.6–1 mm thick[10-12] that covers the area on the vertebral body encircled by the ring apophysis. The two endplates of each disc, therefore, cover the nucleus pulposus in its entirety, but peripherally they fail to cover the entire extent of the anulus fibrosus (Fig. 2.5). Histologically, the endplate consists of both hyaline cartilage and fibrocartilage. Hyaline cartilage occurs towards the vertebral body and is most evident in neonatal and young discs (see Ch. 12). Fibrocartilage occurs towards the nucleus pulposus; in older discs the endplates are virtually entirely fibrocartilage (see Ch. 13). The fibrocartilage is formed by the insertion into the endplate of collagen fibres of the anulus fibrosus.[6]

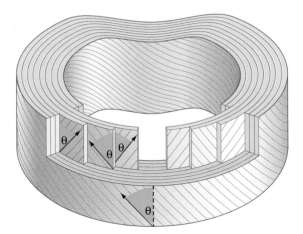

Figure 2.3 The detailed structure of the anulus fibrosus. Collagen fibres are arranged in 10–20 concentric circumferential lamellae. The orientation of fibres alternates in successive lamellae but their orientation with respect to the vertical (θ) is always the same and measures about 65°.

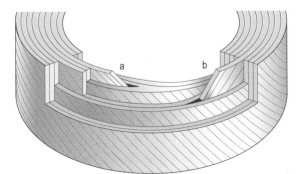

Figure 2.4 The appearance of incomplete lamellae of the anulus fibrosus. At 'a', two subconsecutive lamellae fuse around the terminal end of an incomplete lamella. At 'b', two subconsecutive lamellae become apposed, without fusing, around the end of another incomplete lamella.

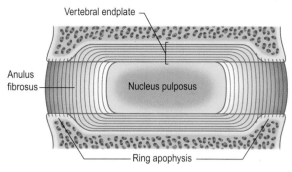

Figure 2.5 Detailed structure of the vertebral endplate. The collagen fibres of the inner two-thirds of the anulus fibrosus sweep around into the vertebral endplate, forming its fibrocartilaginous component. The peripheral fibres of the anulus are anchored into the bone of the ring apophysis.

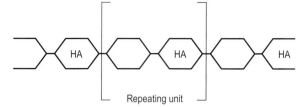

Figure 2.6 The molecular structure of a mucopolysaccharide. The molecule consists of a chain of sugar molecules, each being a six-carbon ring (hexose). Every second sugar is a hexose-amine (HA). The chain is a repetition of identical pairs of hexose, hexose-amine units, called the repeating unit.

The collagen fibres of the inner lamellae of the anulus enter the endplate and swing centrally within it.[3,13,14] By tracing these fibres along their entire length it can be seen that the nucleus pulposus is enclosed by a sphere of collagen fibres, more or less like a capsule. Anteriorly, posteriorly and laterally, this capsule is apparent as the innermost lamellae of the anulus fibrosus, but superiorly and inferiorly the 'capsule' is absorbed into the vertebral endplates (see Fig. 2.5).

Where the endplate is deficient, over the ring apophysis, the collagen fibres of the most superficial lamellae of the anulus insert directly into the bone of the vertebral body (see Fig. 2.5).[14] In their original form, in younger discs, these fibres attach to the vertebral endplate which fully covers the vertebral bodies in the developing lumbar spine, but they are absorbed secondarily into bone when the ring apophysis ossifies (see Ch. 12).

Because of the attachment of the anulus fibrosus to the vertebral endplates, the endplates are strongly bound to the intervertebral disc. In contrast, the endplates are only weakly attached to the vertebral bodies[13,14] and can be wholly torn from the vertebral bodies in certain forms of spinal trauma.[15] It is for this and other morphological reasons that the endplates are regarded as constituents of the intervertebral disc rather than as parts of the vertebral bodies.[10,12,13,16–18]

Over some of the surface area of the vertebral endplate (about 10%) the subchondral bone of the vertebral body is deficient and pockets of the marrow cavity touch the surface of the endplate or penetrate a short distance into it.[11,19] These pockets facilitate the diffusion of nutrients from blood vessels in the marrow space and are important for the nutrition of the endplate and intervertebral disc (see Ch. 11).

DETAILED STRUCTURE OF THE INTERVERTEBRAL DISC

Constituents

Glycosaminoglycans

As a class of chemicals **glycosaminoglycans** (GAGs) are present in most forms of connective tissue. They are found in skin, bone, cartilage, tendon, heart valves, arterial walls, synovial fluid and the aqueous humour of the eye. Chemically, they are long chains of polysaccharides, each chain consisting of a repeated sequence of two molecules called the **repeating unit** (Fig. 2.6).[20,21] These repeating units consist of a sugar molecule and a sugar molecule with an amine attached, and the nomenclature 'glycosaminoglycan' is designed to reflect the sequence of 'sugar amine–sugar– …' in their structure.

The length of individual GAGs varies but is characteristically about 20 repeating units.[21] Each different GAG is characterised by the particular molecules that make up its repeating unit. The GAGs predominantly found in human intervertebral discs are chondroitin-6-sulphate, chondroitin-4-sulphate, keratan sulphate and hyaluronic acid.[22,23] The structures of the repeating units of these molecules are shown in Figure 2.7.

Proteoglycans

Proteoglycans are very large molecules consisting of many GAGs linked to proteins. They occur in two basic forms: proteoglycan **units** and proteoglycan **aggregates**. Proteoglycan units are formed when several GAGs are linked to a polypeptide chain known as a core protein (Fig. 2.8).[22,24] A single core protein may carry as few as six or as many as 60 polysaccharide chains.[21] The GAGs are joined to the core protein by covalent bonds involving special sugar molecules.[22,23] Proteoglycan aggregates are formed when several proteoglycan units are linked to a chain of

Hyaluronic Acid

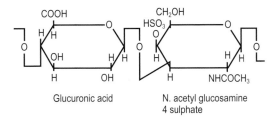

Glucuronic acid   N. acetyl glucosamine

Chondroitin 4 Sulphate

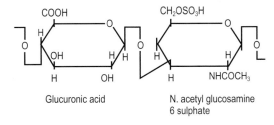

Glucuronic acid   N. acetyl glucosamine
4 sulphate

Chondroitin 6 Sulphate

Glucuronic acid   N. acetyl glucosamine
6 sulphate

Keratan Sulphate

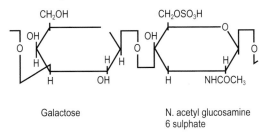

Galactose   N. acetyl glucosamine
6 sulphate

Figure 2.7 The chemical structure of the repeating units of the glycosaminoglycans.

hyaluronic acid. A single hyaluronic chain may bind 20 to 100 proteoglycan units.[22] The linkage between the proteoglycan units and the hyaluronic acid is stabilised by a relatively small mass of protein known as the **link protein** (see Fig. 2.8).[22]

The cardinal proteoglycan of the intervertebral disc resembles that of articular cartilage and is known as

aggrecan.[25] Its detailed structure is shown in Figure 2.9. Its core protein exhibits three coiled regions called globular domains (G1, G2 and G3) and two relatively straight regions called extended domains (E1 and E2).[26] GAGs are bound principally and most densely to the E1 domain. Chondroitin sulphate binds to the terminal three-quarters or so of the E2 domain (i.e. towards the carboxyl end, or C-terminal, of the core protein).[22–24,26] Keratan sulphate binds predominantly towards the N-terminal of the E2 domain but also occurs amongst the chondroitin chains.[22–24,26,27] Some keratan sulphate chains also bind to the E1 domain.

The N-terminal of the core protein bears the G1 domain, which is folded like an immunoglobulin; a similar structure is exhibited by the link protein. It is these coiled structures that bind hyaluronic acid and allow the aggrecan molecules to aggregate.[26] The G1 domain does not assume its structure until after a newly synthesised molecule of aggrecan has left the cell that produces it.[25] This ensures that aggregation occurs only in the extracellular matrix.

Details of the G3 domain are still being determined but it seems to have a carbohydrate-binding capacity, which might enable aggrecan molecules to attach to cell surfaces. The functions of the G2 domain remain unclear. Functionally, the E2 domain is the important one, for it is this region that is responsible for the water-binding properties of the molecule.

Large proteoglycans that aggregate with hyaluronic acid are characteristic of hyaline cartilage and they occur in immature intervertebral discs.[23] They are rich in chondroitin sulphate, carrying about 100 of these chains, each with an average molecular weight of about 20 000. They carry 30–60 keratan sulphate chains, each with a molecular weight of 4000 to 8000.[23] Large and moderately sized proteoglycans that do not aggregate with hyaluronic acid are the major proteoglycans that occur in the mature nucleus pulposus.[23]

In vivo, proteoglycan units and aggregates are convoluted to form complex, three-dimensional molecules, like large and small tangles of cotton wool (Fig. 2.10). Physicochemically, these molecules have the property of attracting and retaining water (compare this with the water-absorbing properties of a ball of cotton wool). The volume enclosed by a proteoglycan molecule, and into which it can attract water, is known as its **domain**.[21]

The water-binding capacity of a proteoglycan molecule is partially a property of its size and physical shape, but the main force that holds water to the molecule stems from the ionic, carboxyl (COOH) and sulphate (SO_4) radicals of the GAG chains (see Fig. 2.7). These radicals attract water electrically, and the water-binding capacity of a proteoglycan can be shown to be proportional to the density of these ionic radicals in its structure. In this respect, sulphated GAGs attract water more strongly than other mucopolysaccharides of similar size that lack sulphate radicals.

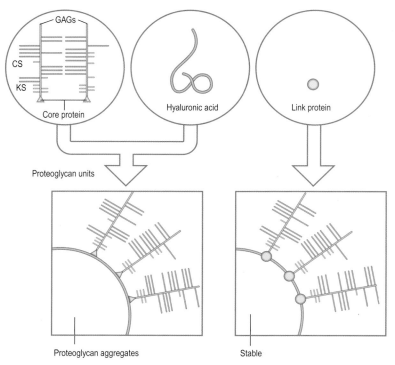

Figure 2.8 The structure of proteoglycans. Proteoglycan units are formed by many GAGs linked to a core protein. Keratan sulphate chains (KS) tend to occur closer to the head of the core protein. Longer chains of chondroitin sulphate (CS) are attached along the entire length of the core protein. Proteoglycan aggregates are formed when several protein units are linked to a chain of hyaluronic acid. Their linkage is stabilised by a link protein.

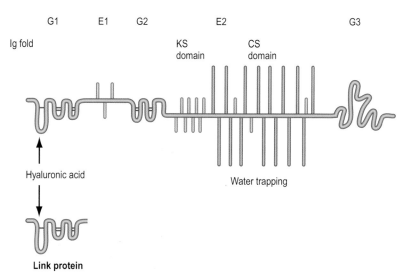

Figure 2.9 The structure of aggrecan. The core protein exhibits three globular domains (G1, G2 and G3) and two extended domains (E1 and E2). The E2 domain binds keratan sulphate (KS) and chondroitin sulphate (CS). The G1 domain is coiled like an immunoglobulin (Ig), as is the link protein, and is the site of the aggrecan molecule that binds with hyaluronic acid.

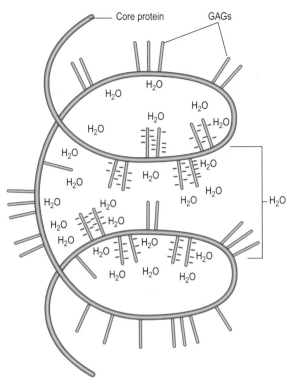

Figure 2.10 A coiled proteoglycan unit, illustrating how the ionic radicals on its GAGs attract water into its 'domain'.

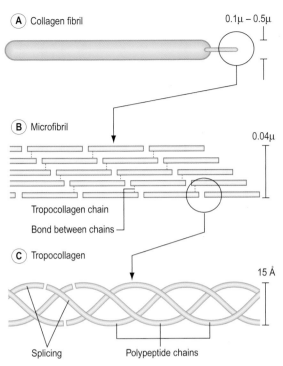

Figure 2.11 The structure of collagen. A collagen fibril (A) is made up of several microfibrils (B). Each microfibril consists of several chains of tropocollagen (C) held together side to side by covalent bonds involving hydroxylysine molecules (…). Tropocollagen consists of three polypeptide chains wound around one another in a helical fashion. Tropocollagen chains are formed by the peptide chains in consecutive molecules splicing and being held together by electrostatic bonds between their ends.

Furthermore, it is readily apparent that because the chondroitin sulphates have both sulphate and carboxyl radicals in their repeating units (see Fig. 2.7), they will have twice the water-binding capacity of keratan sulphate, which, although carrying a sulphate radical, lacks a carboxyl radical. The water-binding capacity of any proteoglycan will therefore be largely dependent on the concentration of chondroitin sulphate within its structure.[24]

Collagen

Fundamentally, collagen consists of strands of protein molecules. The fundamental unit of collagen is the **tropocollagen** molecule, which itself consists of three polypeptide chains wound around one another in a helical fashion and held together end to end by hydrogen bonds (Fig. 2.11). Collagen is formed when many tropocollagen molecules are arrayed end-on and side by side. When only a few tropocollagen chains are arrayed side by side, the structure formed is known as a small collagen **fibril**. When the structure is made thicker, by the addition of further layers of tropocollagen chains, it becomes a **large fibril**. The aggregation of several large fibrils forms a collagen **fibre**. The tropocollagen chains within a collagen fibre are

held together, side by side, by covalent bonds involving a molecule of hydroxylysine (see Fig. 2.11).[28–30]

There are 11 types of collagen found in connective tissue.[31] Each type is genetically determined and differs in the chemical nature of the polypeptide chains that form the tropocollagen molecules found in the collagen fibre and in the microstructure of the fibre. The different types of collagen are denoted by Roman numerals as types I, II, III up to type XI.

Types I, II, III, V and XI exhibit the typical triple helical structure described above. Types IV and VII are long-chain molecules that bear a globular extension at one end and whose triple helix is interrupted periodically by non-helical segments. Types VI, VIII, IX and X are much shorter molecules with interrupted or uniform helical segments that bear globular extensions at one or both ends.[31]

Type I, II and III molecules form most of the collagen fibres of the body; types I and II are typical of musculo-skeletal tissues. Their distribution is shown in Table 2.1.

Table 2.1 Genetic types of collagen and their distribution in connective tissues

Type	Distribution
I	Skin, bone, tendon, meniscus, dentine, anulus fibrosus
II	Cartilage, vitreous humour, nucleus pulposus
III	Dermis, heart, blood vessels, synovium
IV	Basement membrane
V	Co-distributed with type I
VI	Blood vessels, viscera, muscle
VII	Ectodermal basement membranes
VIII	Descemet's membrane
IX	Cartilage, vitreous humour
X	Epiphysial plates
XI	Co-distributed with type II

Type I collagen is essentially tensile in nature and is found in tissues that are typically subjected to tension and compression. Type II collagen is more elastic in nature and is typically found in tissues habitually exposed to pressure.

Type III collagen is typical of the dermis, blood vessels and synovium. Type IV collagen occurs only in basement membranes; type VII is found in basement membranes of ectodermal origin; and type VIII is found in Descemet's membrane of the cornea; type X has been found only in epiphysial plates; type VI is characteristically found in blood vessels, viscera and muscles while type IX occurs in cartilage.[31]

The principal types of collagen found in the intervertebral disc are types I and II. Other types of collagen occur in much lesser amounts. Type V collagen is regularly associated with type I collagen and is co-distributed with it, but its concentration is only about 3% of that of type I. Similarly, type XI coexists with type II but at only about 3% of its concentration.[31] Type IX collagen occurs in discs at about 2% of the concentration of type II; its function appears to be to link proteoglycans to collagen fibres and to control the size of type II fibrils.[31] Small amounts of type VI collagen occur in both the nucleus pulposus and anulus fibrosus, and traces of type III collagen occur within the nucleus pulposus and inner anulus fibrosus; these collagens are located in the immediate pericellular regions of the matrix,[32] but their functions are still unknown.[31]

Both type I and type II collagen are present in the anulus fibrosus but type I is the predominant form.[28,29,33–37] Type II collagen predominates in the nucleus pulposus and is located between cells in the interterritorial matrix.[32] Type I collagen is absent from the central portions of the nucleus or is present only in small amounts. This difference in distribution within the intervertebral disc correlates with the different biomechanical roles of the anulus fibrosus and the nucleus pulposus. From a knowledge of the biochemistry of the collagen in the intervertebral disc, it can be anticipated that the nucleus pulposus, with only type II collagen, will be involved more in processes involving pressure, while the anulus fibrosus, containing both type I and type II collagen, will be involved in both tension-related and pressure-related processes.

An important property of collagen and proteoglycans is that they can bind together. The binding involves both electrostatic and covalent bonds,[20,28,37–40] and these bonds contribute to the strength of structures whose principal constituents are proteoglycans and collagen. Bonds are formed directly between proteoglycans and type I and type II collagen, or indirectly through type IX collagen.

Other proteoglycans

Like articular cartilage, the intervertebral disc contains small quantities of two small proteoglycans – decorin and biglycan[41] – whose core proteins bear chains of the glycosaminoglycan dermatan sulphate, one chain in the case of decorin, two in the case of biglycan. These proteoglycans interact with collagen, fibronectin and growth factors in the matrix of the disc, and are therefore critical factors in the homeostasis and repair of the matrix.[42]

Enzymes

The intervertebral disc, like articular cartilage, contains proteolytic enzymes.[43–45] These enzymes are known as **matrix metalloproteinases** (MMPs). The three main types are MMP-1 (or **collagenase**), MMP-2 (or **gelatinase**) and MMP-3 (or **stromelysin**). Collagenase and gelatinase have very selective substrates. Collagenase can cleave type II collagen; gelatinase cannot but it can cleave the fragments of type II collagen produced by collagenase. Stromelysin is the most destructive of the enzymes. It can cleave types II, XI and IX collagen as well as fibronectin but it also has an aggressive action on proteoglycans, cleaving aggrecan molecules between their E1 and G2 domains.

Under normal circumstances, these enzymes function to remove old components of the matrix, allowing them to be replaced with fresh components. The enzymes are secreted as inactive forms, which are subsequently activated by agents such as plasmin, and are inhibited by proteins known as tissue inhibitors of metalloproteinases, which prevent excessive enzyme activity.[43,44] If the balance between activators and inhibitors is disturbed, excessive action of stromelysin may result in degradation of the matrix, at a rate that normal repair processes cannot keep up with.

Microstructure

Nucleus pulposus

The nucleus pulposus is 70–90% water[17,30,46–49] although the exact proportion varies with age (see Ch. 13). Proteoglycans are the next major component, and they constitute about 65% of the dry weight of the nucleus.[46,47] The water of the nucleus is contained within the domains of these proteoglycans. Only about 25% of the proteoglycans occur in an aggregated form.[24] The majority are in the form of freely dispersed proteoglycan units that lack a functional binding site that would enable them to aggregate with hyaluronic acid.[23]

About two-thirds of the proteoglycan aggregates in the nucleus pulposus are smaller than those typically found in articular cartilage.[27] Each consists of about 8 to 18 proteoglycan units closely spaced on a short chain of hyaluronic acid.[27]

Interspersed through the proteoglycan medium are thin fibrils of type II collagen, which serve to hold proteoglycan aggregates together.[50,51] The mixture of proteoglycan units, aggregates and collagen fibres within the nucleus pulposus is referred to collectively as the **matrix** of the nucleus.

Collagen constitutes 15–20% of the dry weight of the nucleus[22,46] and the remainder of the nucleus consists of some elastic fibres and small quantities of various other proteins known as non-collagenous proteins.[30,44,46,48,52,53] These include the link proteins of the proteoglycans[37,44] and other proteins involved in stabilising the structure of large collagen fibrils[37] and other components of the nuclear matrix;[44] however, the function of many of these non-collagenous proteins remains unknown.[44]

Embedded in the proteoglycan medium of the nucleus are cartilage cells (chondrocytes), and in the newborn there are also some remnant cells of the notochord (see Ch. 12).[38] The cartilage cells are located predominantly in the regions of the vertebral endplates and are responsible for the synthesis of the proteoglycans and collagen of the nucleus pulposus.[19,24] The type III collagen that occurs in the intervertebral disc is characteristically located around the cells of the nucleus pulposus and the inner anulus fibrosus.[31]

It is the presence of water, in large volumes, that endows the nucleus pulposus with its fluid properties, and the proteoglycans and collagen fibrils account for its 'thickness' and viscosity ('stickiness').

Anulus fibrosus

Water is also the principal structural component of the anulus fibrosus, amounting to 60–70% of its weight.[17,30,46–49] Collagen makes up 50–60% of the dry weight of the anulus,[30,33,46,52] and the tight spaces between collagen fibres and between separate lamellae are filled with a proteoglycan gel that binds the collagen fibres and lamellae together to prevent them from buckling or fraying.[24] Proteoglycans make up about 20% of the dry weight of the anulus,[46] and it is this gel that binds the water of the anulus. About 50–60% of the proteoglycans of the anulus fibrosus are aggregated, principally in the form of large aggregates.[27] The concentration of proteoglycans and water is somewhat greater in the anterior anulus than in the posterior anulus, and in both regions increases from the outer to the inner anulus; conversely, there is progressively less collagen from the outer to the inner anulus.[54]

Interspersed among the collagen fibres and lamellae are chondrocytes and fibroblasts that are responsible for synthesising the collagen and the proteoglycan gel of the anulus fibrosus. The fibroblasts are located predominantly towards the periphery of the anulus while the chondrocytes occur in the deeper anulus, towards the nucleus.[19,24]

From a biochemical standpoint, it can be seen that the nucleus pulposus and anulus fibrosus are similar. Both consist of water, collagen and proteoglycans. The differences lie only in the relative concentrations of these components, and in the particular type of collagen that predominates in each part. The nucleus pulposus consists predominantly of proteoglycans and water, with some type II collagen. The anulus fibrosus also consists of proteoglycans and a large amount of water but is essentially 'thickened' by a high concentration of collagen, type II collagen being found throughout the anulus and type I concentrated largely in the outer anulus.[32]

The anulus fibrosus also contains a notable quantity of elastic fibres.[55–58] Elastic fibres constitute about 10% of the anulus fibrosus and are arranged circularly, obliquely and vertically within the lamellae of the anulus.[58] They appear to be concentrated towards the attachment sites of the anulus with the vertebral endplate.[59]

Vertebral endplates

The chemical structure of the vertebral endplate resembles and parallels that of the rest of the disc. It consists of proteoglycans and collagen fibres, with cartilage cells aligned along the collagen fibres.[11] It resembles the rest of the disc by having a higher concentration of water and proteoglycans and a lower collagen content towards its central region, which covers the nucleus pulposus, with a reciprocal pattern over the anulus fibrosus. Across the thickness of the endplate the tissue nearer bone contains more collagen while that nearer the nucleus pulposus contains more proteoglycans and water.[11] This resemblance to the rest of the disc means that at a chemical level the

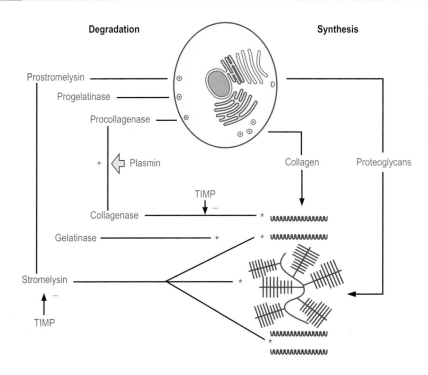

Degradation   **Synthesis**

Figure 2.12 Metabolism of the matrix of an intervertebral disc. Chondrocytes synthesise collagen and proteoglycans, which form the matrix and retain water. They also produce enzymes that can degrade the collagens and proteoglycans. The enzymes, in turn, are controlled by activators such as plasmin, and inhibitors such as tissue inhibitors of metalloproteinases (TIMP).

endplate does not constitute an additional barrier to diffusion. Small molecules pass through an essentially uniform, chemical environment to move from the vertebral body to the centre of the disc.

Metabolism

The proteoglycans and collagen of the intervertebral disc are synthesised and maintained by the chondrocytes and fibroblasts of the nucleus and anulus (Fig. 2.12). In fetal and newborn discs, cells in the nucleus exhibit far greater synthetic activity than those in the anulus, but in mature discs the greatest activity occurs in the mid-portion of the anulus, there being progressively less activity exhibited towards the outer anulus and towards the nucleus.[60]

Once synthesised and delivered out of the cell, the proteoglycans aggregate and bind to the collagen fibres, thereby establishing the solid phase of the matrix. Water is then retained in the domains of the proteoglycans. This matrix, however, undergoes a slow turnover. Systematically, old proteoglycans and collagen are constantly removed and replaced. Removal is achieved by the metalloproteinases. Collagenase degrades type II collagen whereas stromelysin degrades both collagen and proteoglycans (see Fig. 2.12).

All these activities require the cells to be metabolically active; they require oxygen, glucose, the substrates for the products they produce, and cofactors involved in their production. However, the disc essentially lacks a blood supply and the cells therefore rely on diffusion for their nutrition (see Ch. 11). Because of this low blood supply, the oxygen concentrations in the centre of a disc are only 2–5% of those at its periphery,[61] and the cells of the disc must rely on anaerobic metabolism. As a result, the cells produce large amounts of lactic acid, which makes the environment of the disc acidic[61,62] with a pH in the range of 6.9–7.1.[61,62]

The metabolism of cells in the nucleus is very sensitive to changes in pH. They are maximally active in pH ranges of 6.9–7.2, but below 6.8 their activity falls steeply. Below 6.3 their activity is only about 15% maximum.[62]

The status of the matrix relies on a critical balance between the synthetic and degradative activities of the cells, and this balance can be disturbed by any number of factors such as impaired nutrition, inflammatory mediators or changes in pH. Seemingly trivial changes in these factors can lead to major changes in the status of the matrix.

FUNCTIONS OF THE DISC

The principal functions of the disc are to allow movement between vertebral bodies and to transmit loads from one vertebral body to the next. Having reviewed the detailed structure of the intervertebral disc, it is possible to appreciate how this structure accommodates these functions.

Weight-bearing

Both the nucleus pulposus and the anulus fibrosus are involved in weight-bearing. The anulus participates in two ways: independently; and in concert with the nucleus pulposus. Its independent role will be considered first.

Although the anulus is 60–70% water, its densely packed collagen lamellae make it a turgid, relatively stiff body. In a sense, the collagen lamellae endow the anulus with 'bulk'. As long as the lamellae remain healthy and intact and are held together by their proteoglycan gel, the anulus will resist buckling and will be capable of sustaining weight in a passive way, simply on the basis of its bulk.

A suitable analogy for this phenomenon is a thick book like a telephone directory. If the book is wrapped into a semicylindrical form and stood on its end, its weight-bearing capacity can be tested and appreciated. So long as the pages of the book do not buckle, the book standing on end can sustain large weights.

The compression stiffness of the anulus fibrosus is essentially uniform across the thickness of the anulus, although there is a tendency for the inner anulus to be less stiff than the middle and outer anuli.[54] The compression stiffness of the anulus correlates inversely but weakly with its water content but not with its proteoglycan content.[54]

It has been shown experimentally that, under briefly applied loads, a disc with its nucleus removed maintains virtually the same axial load-bearing capacity as an intact disc.[63] These observations demonstrate that the anulus fibrosus is able to act as a passive space filler and to act alone in transmitting weights from one vertebra to the next. The disc does not necessarily need a nucleus pulposus to do this – the anulus alone can be sufficient.

The liability of an isolated anulus fibrosus, however, is that if subjected to prolonged weight-bearing, it will tend to deform, i.e. it will be slowly squashed by any sustained weight. Sustained pressure will buckle the collagen lamellae and water will be squeezed out of the anulus. Both processes will lessen the height of the anulus. The binding of the collagen by proteoglycan gel will not be enough to prevent this prolonged deformation. Some form of additional bracing mechanism is required. This is provided by the nucleus pulposus.

As a ball of fluid, the nucleus pulposus may be deformed but its volume cannot be compressed. Thus, when a weight is applied to a nucleus from above it tends to reduce the height of the nucleus, and the nucleus tries to expand radially, i.e. outwards towards the anulus fibrosus. This radial expansion exerts a pressure on the anulus that tends to stretch its collagen lamellae outwards; however, the tensile properties of the collagen resist this stretch, and the collagen lamellae of the anulus oppose the outward pressure exerted on them by the nucleus (Fig. 2.13).

For any given load applied to the disc, an equilibrium will eventually be attained in which the radial pressure exerted by the nucleus will be exactly balanced by the tension developed in the anulus. In a healthy disc with intact collagen lamellae, this equilibrium is attained with minimum radial expansion of the nucleus. The anulus fibrosus is normally so thick and strong that, during weight-bearing, it resists any tendency for the disc to bulge radially. Application of a 40 kg load to an intervertebral disc causes only 1 mm of vertical compression and only 0.5 mm of radial expansion of the disc.[64]

The other direction in which the nucleus exerts its pressure is towards the vertebral endplates (see Fig. 2.13) but because the endplates are applied to the vertebral bodies they too will resist deformation. The situation that arises, therefore, is that when subjected to a load, the nucleus attempts to deform but it is prevented from doing so. Radially it is constrained by the anulus fibrosus, and upwards and downwards it is constrained by the vertebral endplates and vertebral bodies. All that the nucleus can do is exert its raised pressure against the anulus and the endplates.

This achieves two things. The pressure exerted on the endplates serves to transmit part of the applied load from one vertebra to the next, thereby lessening the load borne by the anulus fibrosus. Secondly, the radial pressure on the anulus fibrosus braces it and prevents the anulus from buckling. This aids the anulus in its own capacity to transmit weight.

The advantage of the cooperative action of the nucleus and the anulus is that the disc can sustain loads that otherwise might tend to buckle an anulus fibrosus acting alone.[65] The essence of the combined mechanism is the fluid property of the nucleus pulposus. The water content of the nucleus makes the disc a turgid body that resists compression, and the water content of the nucleus is therefore of critical importance to the disc. Because the water content of the nucleus is, in turn, a function of its proteoglycan content, the normal mechanics of the disc will ultimately depend on a normal proteoglycan content of the nucleus pulposus. Any change in the proteoglycan and water content of the nucleus will inevitably alter the mechanical properties of the disc (see Ch. 13).

A further property of the disc is its capacity to absorb and store energy. As the nucleus tries to expand radially, energy is used to stretch the collagen of the anulus fibrosus. The collagen fibres are elastic and stretch like springs, and as such they store the energy that went into stretching them. If the load applied to the disc is released, the elastic recoil of the collagen fibres causes the energy stored in them to be exerted back onto the nucleus pulposus, where it is used to restore any deformation that the nucleus may have undergone. This combined action of the nucleus and anulus endows the disc with a resilience or 'springiness'.

In essence, the fluid nature of the nucleus enables it to translate vertically applied pressure into circumferential tension in the anulus. In a static situation this tension balances the pressure in the nucleus, but if the applied load is released the tension is used to restore any

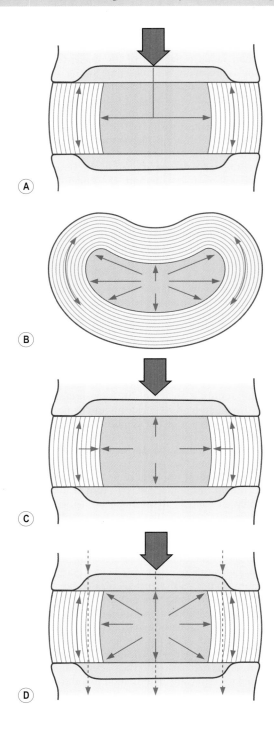

Figure 2.13 The mechanism of weight transmission in an intervertebral disc. (A) Compression raises the pressure in the nucleus pulposus. This is exerted radially onto the anulus fibrosus and the tension in the anulus rises. (B) The tension in the anulus is exerted on the nucleus preventing it from expanding radially. Nuclear pressure is then exerted on the vertebral endplates. (C) Weight is borne, in part, by the anulus fibrosus and by the nucleus pulposus. The radial pressure in the nucleus braces the anulus, and the pressure on the endplates transmits the load from one vertebra to the next.

deformation of the disc that may have occurred. Biochemically, this mechanical property of the disc is due to the presence of proteoglycans and water in the nucleus, and the tensile properties of the type I collagen in the anulus fibrosus.

In a more global sense, the resilience of the intervertebral disc enables it to act as a shock absorber. If a force is rapidly applied to a disc, it will be diverted momentarily into stretching the anulus fibrosus. This brief diversion attenuates the speed at which a force is transmitted from one vertebra to the next; the size of the force is not lessened. Ultimately, it is fully transmitted to the next vertebra. However, by temporarily diverting the force into the anulus fibrosus, a disc can protect its underlying vertebra by slowing the rate at which the applied force is transmitted to that vertebra.

Movements

It is somewhat artificial to consider the movements of an interbody joint, as in-vivo movement of any lumbar vertebra always involves movement not only at the interbody joint but at the zygapophysial joints as well. However, in order to establish principles relevant to the appreciation of the role played by interbody joints in the movements of the intact lumbar spine, it is worth while to consider the interbody joints separately, as if they were capable of independent movement.

If unrestricted by any of the posterior elements of the vertebrae, two vertebral bodies united by an intervertebral disc can move in virtually any direction. In weight-bearing they can press together. Conversely, if distracted, they can separate. They can slide forwards, backwards or sideways; they can rock forwards, backwards and sideways, or in any direction in between; and they can twist. Deformation of the disc accommodates all of these movements but at the same time the disc confers varying degrees of stability to the interbody joint during these movements. The mechanics of the disc during compression (weight-bearing) has already been described but a study of each of the other movements of the interbody joint illustrates how well the disc is designed to also accommodate and stabilise these movements.

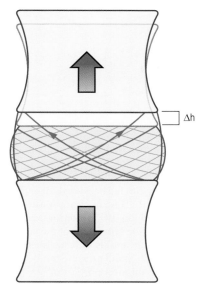

Figure 2.14 Distraction of the interbody joint. Separation of the vertebral bodies increases the height of the intervertebral disc (Δh), and all the collagen fibres in the anulus fibrosus are lengthened and tensed, regardless of their orientation.

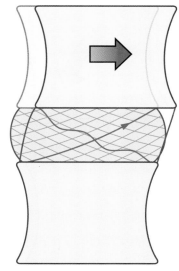

Figure 2.15 Sliding movements of an interbody joint. Those fibres of the anulus that are orientated in the direction of movement have their points of attachment separated, and therefore they are stretched. Fibres in every second lamella of the anulus have their points of attachment approximated, and these fibres are relaxed.

During distraction, all points on one vertebral body move an equal distance perpendicularly from the upper surface of the other vertebral body (Fig. 2.14). Consequently, the attachments of every collagen fibre in the anulus fibrosus are separated an equal distance. Every fibre is therefore strained and every fibre in the anulus resists distraction. Because of the density of collagen fibres in the anulus fibrosus, distraction is strongly resisted by the anulus. The capacity of the discs in this regard is illustrated by how well they sustain the load of the trunk and lower limbs in activities like hanging by the hands. Hanging by the hands, however, is not a common activity of daily living, and vertebral distraction is not a particularly common event. On the other hand, distraction is induced clinically, in the form of traction. A further description of the mechanics of traction, however, is deferred until Chapter 8, when it is considered in the context of the whole lumbar spine.

In pure sliding movements of the interbody joint, all points on one vertebra move an equal distance parallel to the upper surface of the next vertebra (Fig. 2.15). This movement is resisted by the anulus fibrosus but the fibres of the anulus act differently according to their location within the anulus and in relation to the direction of movement. In forward sliding, the fibres at the sides of the disc lie in a plane more or less parallel to the direction of movement and run obliquely between the vertebral bodies but in opposite directions in each successive lamella. Consequently, during forward sliding, only half of the fibres in the lateral anulus will be strained, for only half of the fibres have their points of attachment separated by the movement. The other half have their points approximated (see Fig. 2.15). Therefore, only half the fibres in the lateral anulus contribute to resisting forward sliding.

Fibres in the anterior and posterior anuli also contribute resistance but not to as great an extent as the lateral fibres. Although the movement separates the points of attachment of all the fibres in the anterior and posterior anuli, the separation is not in the principal direction of orientation of the fibres. These fibres run either to the left or to the right, whereas the movement is forwards. The effect of forward sliding is simply to incline the planes of the lamellae in the anterior and posterior anuli anteriorly. Under these circumstances, the degree of stretch imparted to the anterior and posterior anuli is less than that imparted to the lateral anulus, whose fibres are stretched principally longitudinally.

Bending or rocking movements involve the lowering of one end of the vertebral body and the raising of the opposite end. This necessarily causes distortion of the anulus fibrosus and the nucleus pulposus, and it is the fluid content of the nucleus and anulus that permits this deformation. In forward bending, the anterior end of the vertebral body lowers, while the posterior end rises. Consequently, the anterior anulus will be compressed and will

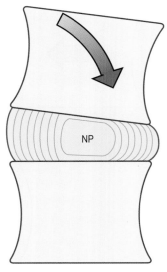

Figure 2.16 Rocking movement of the interbody joint. Rocking causes compression of the anulus fibrosus in the direction of movement, and stretching of the anulus on the opposite side. NP, nucleus pulposus.

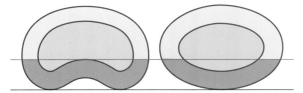

Figure 2.17 Discs that are concave posteriorly have a greater portion of anulus fibrosus located posteriorly. Therefore, concave discs have more anulus available to resist the posterior stretch that occurs in flexion.

tend to buckle[66–69] (Fig. 2.16). The nucleus pulposus will also be compressed but mainly anteriorly. The elevation of the posterior end of the vertebral body relieves pressure on the nucleus pulposus posteriorly but at the same time stretches the posterior anulus.

The anterior anulus buckles because it is directly and selectively compressed by the tilting vertebral body, and because it is not braced internally by the nucleus pulposus. Although the nucleus is compressed anteriorly, it is relieved posteriorly and is able to deform posteriorly.

Mathematical analyses indicate that if the disc is not otherwise loaded (e.g. also bearing weight), there should be no rise in nuclear pressure during bending of an interbody joint as the volume of the nucleus pulposus remains unchanged.[8] Experimental studies, however, show that in cadaveric discs, 5° of bending is associated with a rise in nuclear pressure of about 0.7 kPa cm^{-2}.[70] This rise is the same regardless of the load carried by the disc, therefore the relative increase in disc pressure caused by bending decreases as greater external loads are applied. The increase in disc pressure amounts to about 22% of the total disc pressure for loads of 2 kPa cm^{-2} but is only 5% for loads of 10 kPa cm^{-2}.[70]

The large increases in disc pressure seen in vivo during bending of the lumbar spine are not intrinsically due to the bending but are the result of the additional compressive loads applied to the discs by the action of the back muscles that control the bending (see Ch. 9).

When an interbody joint bends, the anterior compression deforms the nucleus pulposus, which tries to 'escape'

the compression by moving backwards. If at the same time a load is applied to the disc, nuclear pressure will rise and this will be exerted on the posterior anulus which is already stretched by the separation of the vertebral bodies posteriorly. A normal anulus will adequately resist this combination of tension and pressure but because the posterior anulus is the thinnest portion of the entire anulus, its capacity to resist is readily compromised.

Previous injury, or erosion as a result of disc disease, may weaken some of the lamellae of the posterior anulus, and the remaining lamellae may be insufficient to resist the tension and posterior pressure that occurs in loaded forward bending. Consequently, the pressure of the nucleus may rupture the remaining lamellae, and extrusion, or herniation, of the nucleus pulposus may result (see Ch. 15). The resistance to this type of injury is proportional to the density of collagen fibres in the posterior anulus. Thicker anuli afford more protection than thinner ones but the shape of the posterior anulus also plays a role.

Discs that are concave posteriorly have a greater cross-sectional area of anulus posteriorly than do discs with an elliptical shape, even if the anulus is the same thickness (Fig. 2.17). Thus, concave discs are better designed than posteriorly convex discs to withstand forward bending and injury during this movement,[8] and this difference has a bearing on the pattern of injuries seen in intervertebral discs (see Ch. 15).

During twisting movements of the interbody joint, all points on the lower surface of one vertebra will move circumferentially in the direction of the twist; this has a unique effect on the anulus fibrosus. Because of the alternating direction of orientation of the collagen fibres in the anulus, only those fibres inclined in the direction of movement will have their points of attachment separated. Those inclined in the opposite direction will have their points of attachment approximated (Fig. 2.18). Thus, at any time, the anulus resists twisting movements with only half of its complement of collagen fibres. Half of the number of lamellae in the anulus will be stretched, while the other half will be relaxed. This is one of the reasons why twisting movements of an interbody joint are the most likely to injure the anulus (see Chs 8 and 15).

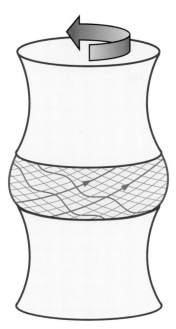

Figure 2.18 Twisting movements of the interbody joint. Those fibres of the anulus that are orientated in the direction of the twist have their points of attachment separated, and are therefore stretched. Fibres in every second lamella of the anulus have their points of attachment approximated and these fibres are relaxed.

SUMMARY

From the preceding accounts, it is evident that the different components of an intervertebral disc act in different ways, both independently and cooperatively, during the various functions of the disc. The nucleus pulposus is designed to sustain and transmit pressure. It is principally involved in weight-bearing, when it transmits loads and braces the anulus fibrosus. During bending it deforms in a passive manner, unless the joint is additionally loaded, in which case its weight-bearing function is superimposed on the mechanics of bending. The nucleus pulposus does not participate in the other movements of the interbody joint. These are resisted by the anulus fibrosus.

In all movements, the anulus fibrosus acts like a ligament to restrain movements and to stabilise the joint to some degree. Whenever the attachments of individual collagen fibres are separated, these fibres will be stretched and will resist the movement. All fibres resist distraction, and all are involved in weight-bearing. In other movements, the participation of individual collagen fibres will depend on their orientation with respect to the movement. In this way, the alternating oblique orientation of the collagen fibres of the anulus fibrosus optimises the capacity of the anulus to restrain various movements in various directions.

If the fibres of the anulus were arranged perpendicular to the vertebral bodies, they would be optimally orientated to resist distraction. However, they would afford virtually no resistance to sliding movements of the joint. The advantage of the oblique orientation is that each fibre can offer a component of resistance both vertically and horizontally, and therefore the anulus fibrosus can participate in resisting movements in all directions. The degree of obliquity governs the extent to which a fibre resists horizontal movement, versus vertical movement, and it can be shown mathematically that the orientation of 65° is optimal for the various strains that an anulus is called upon to sustain.[8] A steeper orientation would enhance resistance to distraction but would compromise resistance to sliding and twisting. Conversely, a flatter orientation would enhance resistance to twisting, but would compromise resistance to distraction and bending. The alternation of the direction of fibres in alternate lamellae of the anulus fibrosus is integral to the capacity of the disc to resist twisting. Half of the lamellae are dedicated to resisting twisting to the right, the other half resist twisting to the left. For a more detailed analysis of the mechanics of the anulus fibrosus, the reader is referred to the papers of Hickey and Hukins,[8] Hukins,[71] Broberg[72] and Farfan and Gracovetsky.[73]

REFERENCES

1. Kingsley JS. *The Vertebrate Skeleton*. London: Murray; 1925:22.

2. Armstrong JR. *Lumbar Disc Lesions*. 3rd edn. Edinburgh: Churchill Livingstone; 1965:13.

3. Taylor JR. The development and adult structure of lumbar intervertebral discs. *J Man Med.* 1990;5:43–47.

4. Marchand F, Ahmed AM. Investigation of the laminate structure of lumbar disc anulus fibrosus. *Spine.* 1990;15:402–410.

5. Jayson MIV, Barks JS. Structural changes in the intervertebral disc. *Ann Rheum Dis.* 1973;32:10–15.

6. Peacock A. Observations on the pre-natal development of the intervertebral disc in man. *J Anat.* 1951;85:260–274.

7. Hickey DS, Hukins DWL. X-ray diffraction studies of the arrangement of collagen fibres in human fetal intervertebral disc. *J Anat.* 1980;131:81–90.

8. Hickey DS, Hukins DWL. Relation between the structure of the

annulus fibrosus and the function and failure of the intervertebral disc. *Spine*. 1980;5:100–116.

9. Tsuji H, Hirano N, Ohshima H, et al. Structural variation of the anterior and posterior anulus fibrosus in the development of human lumbar intervertebral disc: a risk factor for intervertebral disc rupture. *Spine*. 1993;18:204–210.

10. Eyring EJ. The biochemistry and physiology of the intervertebral disk. *Clin Orthop*. 1969;67:16–28.

11. Roberts S, Menage J, Urban JP. Biochemical and structural properties of the cartilage end-plate and its relation to the intervertebral disc. *Spine*. 1989;14:166–174.

12. Saunders JB, de CM, Inman VT. Pathology of the intervertebral disk. *Arch Surg*. 1940;40:380–416.

13. Coventry MB, Ghormley RK, Kernohan JW. The intervertebral disc: its microscopic anatomy and pathology. Part I. Anatomy, development and physiology. *J Bone Joint Surg*. 1945;27:105–112.

14. Inoue H. Three-dimensional architecture of lumbar intervertebral discs. *Spine*. 1981;6:138–146.

15. MacNab I. *Backache*. Baltimore: Williams & Wilkins; 1977:4–7.

16. Coventry MB. Anatomy of the intervertebral disk. *Clin Orthop*. 1969;67:9–15.

17. Schmorl G, Junghanns H. *The Human Spine in Health and Disease*. 2nd American edn. New York: Grune & Stratton; 1971:18.

18. Taylor JR. Growth of the human intervertebral discs and vertebral bodies. *J Anat*. 1975;120:49–68.

19. Maroudas A, Nachemson A, Stockwell R, et al. Some factors involved in the nutrition of the intervertebral disc. *J Anat*. 1975;120:113–130.

20. Comper WD, Laurent TC. Physiological function of connective tissue polysaccharides. *Physiol Rev*. 1978;58:255–315.

21. White A, Handler P, Smith EL. *Principles of Biochemistry*. 4th edn. New York: McGraw-Hill; 1968:871–886.

22. Bushell GR, Ghosh P, Taylor TKF, et al. Proteoglycan chemistry of the intervertebral disks. *Clin Orthop*. 1977;129:115–123.

23. McDevitt CA. Proteoglycans of the intervertebral disc. In: Ghosh P, ed. *The Biology of the Intervertebral Disc*. Vol. 1. Boca Raton: CRC Press; 1988:Ch. 6, 151–170.

24. Urban JP, Maroudas A. The chemistry of the intervertebral disc in relation to its physiological function. *Clin Rheum Dis*. 1980;6:51–76.

25. Johnstone B, Bayliss MT. The large proteoglycans of the human intervertebral disc. *Spine*. 1995;20:674–684.

26. Hardingham T, Bayliss M. Proteoglycans of articular cartilage: changes in aging and in joint disease. *Semin Arthritis Rheum*. 1990;20S:12–33.

27. Buckwalter JA, Pedrini-Mille A, Pedrini V, et al. Proteoglycans of human infant intervertebral discs. *J Bone Joint Surg*. 1985;67A:284–294.

28. Bailey AJ, Herbert CM, Jayson MIV. Collagen of the intervertebral disc. In: Jayson MIV, ed. *The Lumbar Spine and Backache*. New York: Grune & Stratton; 1976:Ch. 12, 327–340.

29. Herbert CM, Lindberg KA, Jayson MIV, et al. Changes in the collagen of human intervertebral discs during ageing and degenerative disc disease. *J Mol Med*. 1975;1:79–91.

30. Naylor A, Shental R. Biochemical aspects of intervertebral discs in ageing and disease. In: Jayson MIV, ed. *The Lumbar Spine and Backache*. New York: Grune & Stratton; 1976:Ch. 4, 317–326.

31. Eyre D. Collagens of the disc. In: Ghosh P, ed. *The Biology of the Intervertebral Disc*. Vol. I. Boca Raton: CRC Press; 1988:171–188.

32. Roberts S, Menage J, Duance V, et al. Collagen types around the cells of the intervertebral disc and cartilage end plate: an immunolocalization study. *Spine*. 1991;16:1030–1038.

33. Adams P, Eyre DR, Muir H. Biochemical aspects of development and ageing of human lumbar intervertebral discs. *Rheumatol Rehab*. 1977;16:22–29.

34. Brickley-Parsons D, Glimcher MJ. Is the chemistry of collagen in intervertebral discs an expression of Wolff's law? A study of the human lumbar spine. *Spine*. 1984;9:148–163.

35. Eyre D, Muir H. Type I and Type II collagen in intervertebral disk. Interchanging radial distribution in annulus fibrosus. *Biochem J*. 1976;157:267–270.

36. Eyre D, Muir H. Quantitative analysis of types I and II collagen in human intervertebral discs at various ages. *Biochimica et Biophysica Acta*. 1977;492:29–42.

37. Ghosh P, Bushell GK, Taylor TFK, et al. Collagen, elastin, and non-collagenous protein of the intervertebral disk. *Clin Orthop*. 1977;129:123–132.

38. Meachim G, Cornah MS. Fine structure of juvenile human nucleus pulposus. *J Anat*. 1970;107:337–350.

39. Pearson CH, Happey F, Naylor A, et al. Collagens and associated glycoproteins in the human intervertebral disc. *Ann Rheum Dis*. 1972;31:45–53.

40. Stevens FS, Jackson DS, Broady K. Protein of the human intervertebral disc. The association of collagen with a protein fraction having an unusual amino acid composition. *Biochim Biophys Acta*. 1968;160:435–446.

41. Johnstone B, Markopoulous M, Neame P, et al. Identification and characterization of glycanated and non-glycanated forms of biglycan and decorin in the human intervertebral disc. *Biochem J*. 1993;292:661–666.

42. Kuettner KE. Cartilage integrity and homeostasis. In: Klippel JH, Dieppe PA, eds. *Rheumatology*. St Louis: Mosby; 1994:7.6.1–7.6.16.

43. Kanemoto M, Hukuda S, Komiya Y, et al. Immunohistochemical study of matrix metalloproteinase-3 and tissue inhibitor of metalloproteinase-1 in human intervertebral discs. *Spine*. 1996;21:1–8.

44. Melrose J, Ghosh P. The noncollagenous proteins of the intervertebral disc. In: Ghosh P, ed. *The Biology of the Intervertebral Disc*. Vol. I. Boca Raton: CRC Press; 1988:Ch. 8, 189–237.

45. Sedowfia KA, Tomlinson IW, Weiss JB, et al. Collagenolytic enzyme

systems in human intervertebral disc. *Spine*. 1982;7:213–222.

46. Beard HK, Stevens RL. Biochemical changes in the intervertebral disc. In: Jayson MIV, ed. *The Lumbar Spine and Backache*. 2nd edn. London: Pitman; 1980:407–436.

47. Gower WE, Pedrini V. Age-related variation in protein polysaccharides from human nucleus pulposus, annulus fibrosus and costal cartilage. *J Bone Joint Surg*. 1969;51A:1154–1162.

48. Naylor A. Intervertebral disc prolapse and degeneration. The biochemical and biophysical approach. *Spine*. 1976;1:108–114.

49. Puschel J. Der Wassergehalt normaler und degenerierter Zwischenwirbelscheiben. *Beitr path Anat* 1930;84:123–130.

50. Inoue H, Takeda T. Three-dimensional observation of collagen framework of lumbar intervertebral discs. *Acta Orthop Scand*. 1975;46:949–956.

51. Sylven B, Paulson S, Hirsch C, et al. Biophysical and physiological investigations on cartilage and other mesenchymal tissues. *J Bone Joint Surg*. 1951;33A:333–340.

52. Dickson IR, Happey F, Pearson CH, et al. Variations in the protein components of human intervertebral disk with age. *Nature*. 1967;215:52–53.

53. Taylor TKF, Little K. Intercellular matrix of the intervertebral disk in ageing and in prolapse. *Nature*. 1965;208:384–386.

54. Best BA, Guilak F, Setton LA, et al. Compressive mechanical properties of the human anulus fibrosus and their relationship to biochemical composition. *Spine*. 1994;19:212–221.

55. Buckwalter JA, Cooper RR, Maynard JA. Elastic fibers in human intervertebral disks. *J Bone Joint Surg*. 1976;58A:73–76.

56. Hickey DS, Hukins DWL. Collagen fibril diameters and elastic fibres in the annulus fibrosus of human fetal intervertebral disc. *J Anat*. 1981;133:351–357.

57. Hickey DS, Hukins DWL. Aging changes in the macromolecular organization of the intervertebral disc. An X-ray diffraction and electron microscopic study. *Spine*. 1982;7:234–242.

58. Johnson EF, Berryman H, Mitchell R, et al. Elastic fibres in the anulus fibrosus of the human lumbar intervertebral disc. A preliminary report. *J Anat*. 1985;143:57–63.

59. Johnson EF, Chetty K, Moore IM, et al. The distribution and arrangement of elastic fibres in the IVD of the adult human. *J Anat*. 1982;135:301–309.

60. Bayliss MT, Johnstone B, O'Brien JP. Proteoglycan synthesis in the human intervertebral disc: variation with age, region and pathology. *Spine*. 1988;13:972–981.

61. Holm S, Maroudas A, Urban JP, et al. Nutrition of the intervertebral disc: solute transport and metabolism. *Connect Tissue Res*. 1981;8:101–119.

62. Ohshima H, Urban JP. The effect of lactate and pH on proteoglycan and protein synthesis rates in the intervertebral disc. *Spine*. 1992;17:1079–1082.

63. Markolf KL, Morris JM. The structural components of the intervertebral disc. *J Bone Joint Surg*. 1974;56A:675–687.

64. Hirsch C, Nachemson A. New observations on mechanical behaviour of lumbar discs. *Acta Orthop Scand*. 1954;23:254–283.

65. Roaf R. A study of the mechanics of spinal injuries. *J Bone Joint Surg*. 1960;42B:810–823.

66. Brown T, Hansen RJ, Yorra AJ. Some mechanical tests on the lumbosacral spine with particular reference to the intervertebral discs. *J Bone Joint Surg*. 1957;39A:1135–1164.

67. Shah JS. Structure, morphology and mechanics of the lumbar spine. In: Jayson MIV, ed. *The Lumbar Spine and Backache*. 2nd edn. London: Pitman; 1980:Ch. 13, 359–405.

68. Shah JS, Hampson WGJ, Jayson MIV. The distribution of surface strain in the cadaveric lumbar spine. *J Bone Joint Surg*. 1978;60B:246–251.

69. White AA, Panjabi MM. *Clinical Biomechanics of the Spine*. Philadelphia: Lippincott; 1978.

70. Nachemson A. The influence of spinal movements on the lumbar intradiscal pressure and on the tensile stresses in the annulus fibrosus. *Acta Orthop Scand*. 1963;33:183–207.

71. Hukins DWL. Disc structure and function. In: Ghosh P, ed. *The Biology of the Intervertebral Disc*. Vol. I. Boca Raton: CRC Press; 1988:Ch. 1, 1–37.

72. Broberg KB. On the mechanical behaviour of intervertebral discs. *Spine*. 1983;8:151–165.

73. Farfan HF, Gracovetsky S. The nature of instability. *Spine*. 1984;9:714–719.

The zygapophysial joints – detailed structure

The lumbar zygapophysial joints are formed by the articulation of the inferior articular processes of one lumbar vertebra with the superior articular processes of the next vertebra. The joints exhibit the features typical of synovial joints. The articular facets are covered by articular cartilage, and a synovial membrane bridges the margins of the articular cartilages of the two facets in each joint. Surrounding the synovial membrane is a joint capsule which attaches to the articular processes a short distance beyond the margin of the articular cartilage (Fig. 3.1).

ARTICULAR FACETS

The articular facets of the lumbar vertebrae are ovoid in shape, measuring some 16 mm in height and 14 mm in width, and having a surface area of about 160 mm². The facets of upper vertebrae are slightly smaller than these values indicate; those of the lower vertebrae are slightly smaller.[1]

Viewed from behind (see Fig. 3.1), the articular facets of the lumbar zygapophysial joints appear as straight surfaces, suggesting that the joints are planar. However,

viewed from above (Fig. 3.2), the articular facets vary both in the shape of their articular surfaces and in the general direction they face. Both of these features have significant ramifications in the biomechanics of these joints and, consequently, of the lumbar spine, and should be understood and appreciated.

In the transverse plane, the articular facets may be flat or planar, or may be curved to varying extents (Fig. 3.3).[2] The curvature may be little different from a flat plane (Fig. 3.3D) or may be more pronounced, with the superior articular facets depicting a C shape (Fig. 3.3E) or a J shape (Fig. 3.3F). The relative incidence of flat and curved facets at various vertebral levels is shown in Table 3.1.

The orientation of a lumbar zygapophysial joint is, by convention, defined by the angle made by the average plane of the joint with respect to the sagittal plane (see Fig. 3.3). In the case of joints with flat articular facets, the plane of the joint is readily depicted as a line parallel to the facets. The average plane of joints with curved facets is usually depicted as a line passing through the anteromedial and posterolateral ends of the joint cavity (see Fig. 3.3). The incidence of various orientations at different levels is shown in Figure 3.4.

The variations in the shape and orientation of the lumbar zygapophysial joints govern the role of these joints in preventing forward displacement and rotatory dislocation of the intervertebral joint. The extent to which a given joint can resist forward displacement depends on the extent to which its superior articular facets face backwards. Conversely, the extent to which the joint can resist rotation is related to the extent to which its superior articular facets face medially.

In the case of planar zygapophysial joints, the analysis is straightforward. In a joint with an oblique orientation,

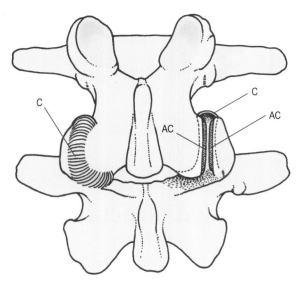

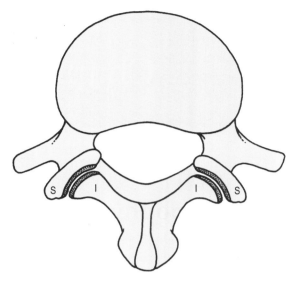

Figure 3.1 A posterior view of the L3–4 zygapophysial joints. On the left, the capsule of the joint (C) is intact. On the right, the posterior capsule has been resected to reveal the joint cavity, the articular cartilages (AC) and the line of attachment of the joint capsule (- - -). The upper joint capsule (C) attaches further from the articular margin than the posterior capsule.

Figure 3.2 A top view of an L3–4 zygapophysial joint showing how the joint space and articular facets are curved in the transverse plane. I, inferior articular process L3; S, superior articular process L4.

Table 3.1 The incidence of flat and curved lumbar zygapophysial joints at different segmental levels. (Based on Horwitz and Smith 1940.[3])

	Joint level and percentage incidence of feature				
	L1–2	L2–3	L3–4	L4–5	L5–S1
Flat	44	21	19	51	86
Curved	56	79	81	49	14
Number of specimens	11	40	73	80	80

the superior articular facets face backwards and medially (Fig. 3.5A). Because of their backward orientation, these facets can resist forward displacement. If the upper vertebra in a joint attempts to move forwards, its inferior articular processes will impact against the superior articular facets of the lower vertebra, and this impaction will prevent further forward movement (see Fig. 3.5A).

Similarly, the medial orientation of the superior articular facets allows them to resist rotation. As the upper vertebra attempts to rotate, say, anticlockwise as viewed from above, its right inferior articular facet will impact against

the right superior articular facet of the vertebra below, and further rotation will be arrested (Fig. 3.5B).

Maximum resistance to forward displacement will be exerted by the superior articular facets that are orientated at 90° to the sagittal plane, for then the facets face fully backwards and the entire articular surface directly opposes the movement (Fig. 3.5C). Such facets, however, are less capable of resisting rotation, for during rotation the inferior articular facet impacts the superior articular facet at an angle and is able to glance off the superior articular facet (Fig. 3.5D).

Joints orientated parallel to the sagittal plane afford no resistance to forward displacement. The inferior articular facets are able simply to slide past the superior articular facets (Fig. 3.5E). However, such joints provide substantial resistance to rotation (Fig. 3.5F).

In essence, therefore, the closer a joint is orientated towards the sagittal plane, the less it is able to resist forward displacement. Resistance is greater the closer a joint is orientated to 90° to the sagittal plane.

In the case of joints with curved articular surfaces, the situation is modified to the extent that particular portions of the articular surface are involved in resisting different movements. In curved joints, the anteromedial end of the superior articular facet faces backwards, and it is this portion of the facet that will resist forward displacement. As the upper vertebra attempts to move forwards, its inferior articular facets will impact against the antero-medial portion of the superior articular facets of the

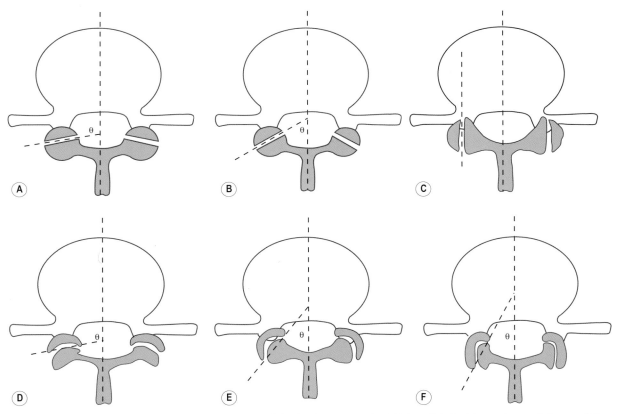

Figure 3.3 The varieties of orientation and curvature of the lumbar zygapophysial joints. (A) Flat joints orientated close to 90° to the sagittal plane. (B) Flat joints orientated at 60° to the sagittal plane. (C) Flat joints orientated parallel (0°) to the sagittal plane. (D) Slightly curved joints with an average orientation close to 90° to the sagittal plane. (E) C-shaped joints orientated at 45° to the sagittal plane. (F) J-shaped joints orientated at 30° to the sagittal plane.

vertebra below (Fig. 3.6A). The degree of resistance will be proportional to the surface area of the backward-facing, anteromedial portion of the superior articular facet. Thus, C-shaped facets (Fig 3.6A) have a larger surface area facing backwards and afford greater resistance than J-shaped facets (Fig. 3.6B), which have only a small portion of their articular surface facing backwards.

Rotation is well resisted by both C- and J-shaped facets, for virtually the entire articular surface is brought into contact by this movement (Fig. 3.6C,D).

The additional significance of variations in orientation of zygapophysial joints in relation to the biomechanical requirements of joints at different levels, the age changes they suffer and their liability to injury are explored in Chapters 5, 8, 13 and 15.

Articular cartilage

There are no particular or unique features of the cartilage of normal lumbar zygapophysial joints. However, it is appropriate to revise the histology of articular cartilage as it relates to the zygapophysial joints, to provide a foundation for later chapters on age-related changes in these joints.

Articular cartilage covers the facets of the superior and inferior articular processes, and as a whole assumes the same concave or convex curvature as the underlying facet. In a normal joint, the cartilage is thickest over the centre of each facet, rising to a height of about 2 mm.[4,5] Histologically, four zones may be recognised in the cartilage (Fig. 3.7).[5] The superficial, or tangential, zone consists of three to four layers of ovoid cells whose long axes are orientated parallel to the cartilage surface. Deep to this zone is a transitional zone in which cartilage cells are arranged in small clusters of three to four cells. Next deeper is a radial zone, which constitutes most of the cartilage thickness. It consists of clusters of six to eight large cells whose long axes lie perpendicular to the cartilage surface. The deepest zone is the calcified zone, which uniformly covers the subchondral bone plate and

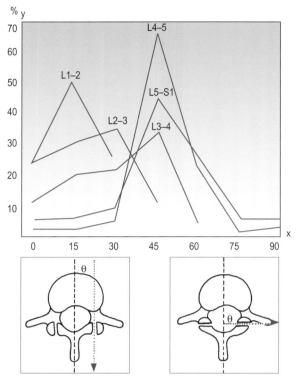

Figure 3.4 The orientation of lumbar zygapophysial joints with respect to the sagittal plane: incidence by level. (Based on Horwitz and Smith 1940.[3]) *x*-axis, orientation (degrees from sagittal plane); *y*-axis, proportion of specimens showing particular orientation.

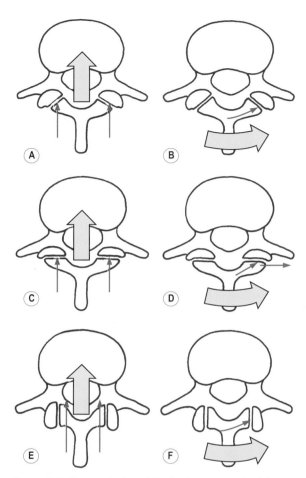

Figure 3.5 The mechanics of flat lumbar zygapophysial joints. A flat joint at 60° to the sagittal plane affords resistance to both forward displacement (A) and rotation (B). A flat joint at 90° to the sagittal plane strongly resists forward displacement (C) but during rotation (D) the inferior articular facet can glance off the superior articular facet. A flat joint parallel to the sagittal plane offers no resistance to forward displacement (E) but strongly resists rotation (F).

constitutes about one-sixth of the total cartilage thickness. Conspicuously, the radial zone of cartilage is identifiable only in the central regions of the cartilage. Towards the periphery, the calcified zone is covered only by the transitional and tangential zones. As is typical of all articular cartilage, the cartilage cells of the zygapophysial joints are embedded in a matrix of glycosaminoglycans and type II collagen; however, the most superficial layers of the tangential zone, forming the surface of the cartilage, lack glycosaminoglycans and consist only of collagen fibres running parallel to the cartilage surface. This thin strip is known as the lamina slendens.[6]

The articular cartilage rests on a thickened layer of bone known as the **subchondral bone** (see Fig. 3.7). In normal joints there are no particular features of the subchondral bone. However, the age changes and degenerative changes that affect the articular cartilage also affect the subchondral bone, and these changes are described in Chapter 13.

CAPSULE

Around its dorsal, superior and inferior margins, each lumbar zygapophysial joint is enclosed by a fibrous capsule, formed by collagen fibres passing more or less transversely from one articular process to the other (Figs 3.1, 3.8). Along the dorsal aspect of the joint, the outermost fibres of the capsule are attached about 2 mm from the edge of the articular cartilage but some of the deepest fibres attach into the margin of the articular cartilage

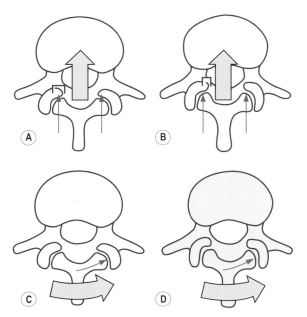

Figure 3.6 The mechanics of curved lumbar zygapophysial joints. (A) C-shaped joints have a wide anteromedial portion which faces backwards (indicated by the bracket), and this portion resists forward displacement. (B) J-shaped joints have a narrower anteromedial portion (bracket) that nonetheless resists forward displacement. (C,D) Both C- and J-shaped joints resist rotation as their entire articular surface impacts.

(Figs 3.8, 3.9).[7,8] At the superior and inferior poles of the joint, the capsule attaches further from the osteochondral junctions, creating subcapsular pockets over the superior and inferior edges of both the superior and inferior articular processes, which in the intact joint are filled with fat (see Fig. 3.8).[9] Anteriorly, the fibrous capsule of the joint is replaced entirely by the ligamentum flavum (see Ch. 4), which attaches close to the articular margin (Fig. 3.9).[9–11]

The capsule has been found to consist of two layers.[12] The outer layer consists of densely packed parallel collagen fibres. This layer is 13–17 mm long in the superior and middle regions of the joint, but 15–20 mm long over the inferior pole of the joint. The inner layer consists of irregularly orientated elastic fibres; it is 6–10 mm long over the superior and middle regions of the joint and 9–16 mm long over its inferior pole.

The joint capsule is thick dorsally and is reinforced by some of the deep fibres of the multifidus muscle (see Ch. 9).[5,7,12,13] At the superior and inferior poles of the joint, the capsule is abundant and loose.[9] Superiorly, it balloons upwards towards the base of the next transverse process. Inferiorly, it balloons over the back of the lamina (see Fig. 3.8). In both the superior and inferior parts of the capsule, there is a tiny hole, or foramen, that permits the passage of fat from within the capsule to the extracapsular space (see Fig. 3.10).[9]

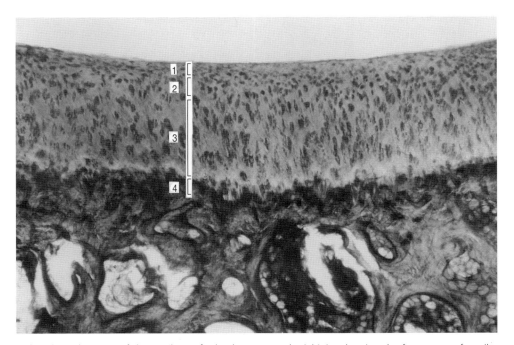

Figure 3.7 A histological section of the cartilage of a lumbar zygapophysial joint showing the four zones of cartilage: 1, superficial zone; 2, transitional zone; 3, radial zone; 4, calcified zone. *(Courtesy of Professor Lance Twomey.)*

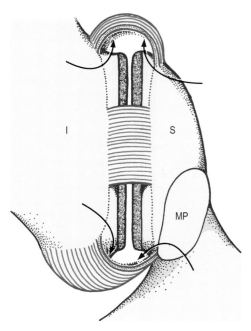

Figure 3.8 A posterior view of a right lumbar zygapophysial joint in which the posterior capsule has been partially removed to reveal the joint cavity and the subcapsular pockets (arrows). I, inferior articular process; MP, mamillary process; S, superior articular process.

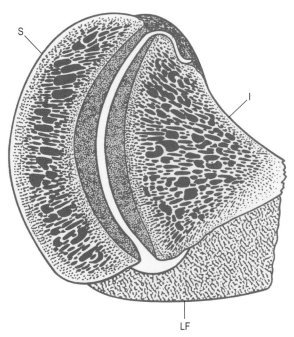

Figure 3.9 A transverse (horizontal) section through a lumbar zygapophysial joint. Note how the posterior capsule is fibrous and attaches to the inferior articular process (I) well beyond the articular margin, but at its other end it attaches to the superior articular process (S) and the margin of the articular cartilage. The anterior capsule is formed by the ligamentum flavum (LF).

SYNOVIUM

There are no particular features of the synovium of the lumbar zygapophysial joints that distinguish it from the synovium of any typical synovial joint. It attaches along the entire peripheral margin of the articular cartilage on one facet and extends across the joint to attach to the margin of the opposite articular cartilage. Basically, it lines the deep surface of the fibrous capsule and the ligamentum flavum but it is also reflected in parts to cover the various intra-articular structures of the lumbar zygapophysial joints.

INTRA-ARTICULAR STRUCTURES

There are two principal types of intra-articular structure in the lumbar zygapophysial joints. These are fat, and what may be referred to as 'meniscoid', structures. The fat basically fills any leftover space underneath the capsule. It is located principally in the subcapsular pockets at the superior and inferior poles of the joint (Fig. 3.10). Externally,

it is covered by the capsule, while internally it is covered by the synovium. It communicates with the fat outside the joint through the foramina in the superior and inferior capsules. Superiorly, this extracapsular fat lies lateral to the lamina and dorsal to the intervertebral foramen.[5,9] Inferiorly, it lies dorsal to the upper end of the lamina of the vertebra and separates the bone from the overlying multifidus muscle.

There have been many studies and differing interpretations of the meniscoid structures of the lumbar zygapophysial joints[3,9,14–28] but the most comprehensive study of these structures identifies three types.[29,30]

The simplest and smallest structure is the **connective tissue rim**. This is simply a wedge-shaped thickening of the internal surface of the capsule, which, along the dorsal and ventral margins of the joint, fills the space left by the curved margins of the articular cartilages (Fig. 3.11). The second type of structure is an **adipose tissue pad**. These are found principally at the superoventral and inferodorsal poles of the joint. Each consists of a fold of synovium enclosing some fat and blood vessels (see Fig. 3.11). At the base of the structure, the synovium is reflected onto the joint capsule to become continuous with the synovium of the rest of the joint, and the fat within the structure is continuous with other fat within the joint. These adipose tissue pads project into the joint cavity for a short distance (about 2 mm).

The largest of the meniscoid structures are the **fibro-adipose meniscoids**. These project from the inner surface of the superior and inferior capsules. They consist of a leaf-like fold of synovium which encloses fat, collagen and some blood vessels (see Fig. 3.11). The fat is located principally in the base of the structure, where it is continuous with the rest of the fat within the joint, and where

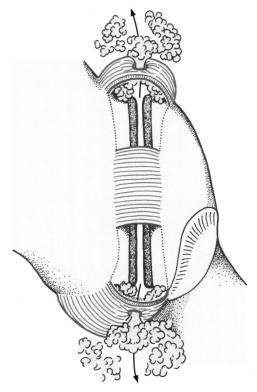

Figure 3.10 A right lumbar zygapophysial joint viewed from behind. Portions of the capsule have been removed to show how the fat in the subcapsular pockets communicates to the extracapsular fat through foramina in the superior and inferior capsules.

Figure 3.11 Intra-articular structures of the lumbar zygapophysial joints. (A) A coronal section of a left zygapophysial joint showing fibro-adipose meniscoids projecting into the joint cavity from the capsule over the superior and inferior poles of the joint. (B) A lateral view of a right zygapophysial joint, in which the superior articular process has been removed to show intra-articular structures projecting into the joint cavity across the surface of the inferior articular facet. The superior capsule is retracted to reveal the base of a fibro-adipose meniscoid (FM) and an adipose tissue pad (AP). Another fibro-adipose meniscoid at the lower pole of the joint is lifted from the surface of the articular cartilage. A connective tissue rim (CT) has been retracted along the posterior margin of the joint.

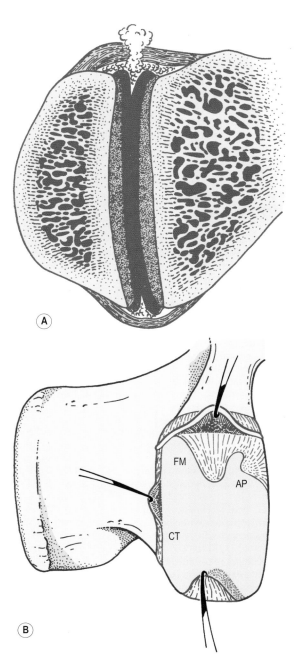

it communicates with the extracapsular fat through the superior and inferior capsular foramina. The collagen is densely packed and is located towards the apex of the structure. Fibro-adipose meniscoids are long and project up to 5 mm into the joint cavity.

Differing and conflicting interpretations have marked the literature on zygapophysial intra-articular structures, and there is no conventional, universal nomenclature that can be ascribed to them. However, it is clear from their histology that none is really a meniscus which resembles the menisci of the knee joint or the temporomandibular joint. They do, nonetheless, resemble the intra-articular structures found in the small joints of the hand.[31,32] The connective tissue rims described above are most easily interpreted as a thickening of the joint capsule that simply acts as a space filler, although it may be that they also serve to increase the surface area of contact when articular facets are impacted, and thereby transmit some load.[9,18]

The adipose tissue pads and the fibro-adipose meniscoids have been interpreted as serving a protective function.[29] During flexion of an intervertebral joint, the inferior articular facet slides upwards some 5–8 mm along the superior articular facet.[9,33] This movement results in cartilages of the upper portion of the inferior facet and the lower portion of the superior facet becoming exposed. The adipose tissue pads and the fibro-adipose meniscoids are suitably located to cover these exposed articular surfaces, and to afford them some degree of protection during this movement. By remaining in contact with the exposed articular cartilage, the synovium-covered pads and meniscoids can maintain a film of synovial fluid between themselves and the cartilage. This ensures that the cartilage is lubricated against friction as it moves back into its resting position against the surface of the apposing articular facet.

There is also another form of intra-articular structure derived from the articular cartilage but it is apparently formed artificially by traction on the cartilage. This structure is described in Chapter 13, and the clinical relevance of all intra-articular structures is considered in Chapter 15.

REFERENCES

1. Benini A. Das klein Gelenk der lenden Wirbelsaule. *Fortschr Med.* 1979;97:2103–2106.

2. Bogduk N, Engel R. The menisci of the lumbar zygapophysial joints. A review of their anatomy and clinical significance. *Spine.* 1984;9:454–460.

3. Horwitz T, Smith RM. An anatomical, pathological and roentgenological study of the intervertebral joints of the lumbar spine and of the sacroiliac joints. *Am J Roentgenol.* 1940;43:173–186.

4. Delmas A, Ndjaga-Mba M, Vannareth T. Le cartilage articulaire de L4-L5 et L5-S1. *Comptes Rendus de l'Association des Anatomistes.* 1970;147:230–234.

5. Dorr WM. Uber die Anatomie der Wirbelgelenke. *Arch Orthop Unfallchir.* 1958;50:222–234.

6. Dorr WM. Nochmals zu den Menisci in den Wirbelbo-gengelenken. *Z Orthop Ihre Grenzgeb.* 1962;96:457–461.

7. Emminger E. Les articulations interapophysaires et leurs structures meniscoides vues sous l'angle de la pathologie. *Ann Med Phys.* 1972;15:219–238.

8. Engel R, Bogduk N. The menisci of the lumbar zygapophysial joints. *J Anat.* 1982;135:795–809.

9. Giles LGF. Human lumbar zygapophyseal joint inferior recess synovial folds: a light microscope examination. *Anat Rec.* 1988;220:117–124.

10. Giles LGF. The surface lamina of the articular cartilage of human zygapophyseal joints. *Anat Rec.* 1992;233:350–356.

11. Giles LGF, Taylor JR. Inter-articular synovial protrusions. *Bull Hosp Joint Dis.* 1982;42:248–255.

12. Giles LGF, Taylor JR, Cookson A. Human zygapophyseal joint synovial folds. *Acta Anat.* 1986;126:110–114.

13. Guntz E. Die Erkrankungen der Zwischenwirbelgelenke. *Arch Orthop Unfallchir.* 1933–1934; 34:333–355.

14. Hadley LA. Anatomico-roentgenographic studies of the posterior spinal articulations. *Am J Roentgenol.* 1961;86:270–276.

15. Hadley LA. *Anatomico-roentgenographic Studies of the Spine.* Springfield: Thomas; 1964.

16. Hirsch C, Lewin T. Lumbosacral synovial joints in flexion-extension. *Acta Orthop Scand.* 1968;39: 303–311.

17. Kos J. Contribution a l'étude de l'anatomie et de la vascularisation des articulations intervertébrales. *Bull Ass Anat.* 1969;142:1088–1105.

18. Kos J, Wolf J. Les ménisques intervertébraux et leur rôle possible dans les blocages vertébraux. *Ann Med Phys.* 1972;15:203–218.

19. Kos J, Wolf J. Die 'Menisci' der Zwischenwirbelgelenke und ihre mogliche Rolle bei Wirbelblockierung. *Man Med.* 1972;10:105–114.

20. Lewin T. Osteoarthritis in lumbar synovial joints: a morphologic study. *Acta Orthop Scand.* 1964;176(Suppl. 73):1–112.

21. Lewin T, Moffet B, Viidik A. The morphology of the lumbar synovial intervertebral joints. *Acta Morphol Neerlando-Scand.* 1962;4:299–319.

22. Marchi GF. Le articolazioni intervertebrali. *La Clinica Ortopedica.* 1963;15:26–33.

23. Panjabi MM, Oxland T, Takata K, et al. Articular facets of the human spine: quantitative three-dimensional anatomy. *Spine.* 1993;18:1298–1310.

24. Ramsey RH. The anatomy of the ligamenta flava. *Clin Orthop.* 1966;44:129–140.

25. Santo E. Zur Entwicklung-dgeschichte und Histologie der Zwischenscheiben in den kleinen

Gelenken. *Z Anat Entwickl Gesch.* 1935;104:623–634.

26. Santo E. Die Zwischenscheiben in den kleinen Gelenken. *Anat Anz.* 1937;83:223–229.

27. Tager KH. Wirbelmeniskus oder synovial Forsatz. *Z Orthop Ihre Grenzgeb.* 1965;99:439–447.

28. Taylor JR, Twomey LT. Age changes in lumbar zygapophyseal joints. *Spine.* 1986;11:739–745.

29. Twomey LT, Taylor JR. Age changes in the lumbar articular triad. *Aust J Physio.* 1985;31:106–112.

30. Wolf J. The reversible deformation of the joint cartilage surface and its possible role in joint blockage. *Rehabilitacia.* 1975;8(Suppl. 10–11):30–36.

31. Yamashita T, Minaki Y, Ozaktay AC, et al. A morphological study of the fibrous capsule of the human lumbar facet joint. *Spine.* 1996;21:538–543.

32. Yong-Hing K, Reilly J, Kirkaldy-Willis WH. The ligamentum flavum. *Spine.* 1976;1:226–234.

33. Zaccheo D, Reale E. Contributo alla conoscenza delle articolazioni tra i processi articolari delle vertebre dell'uomo. *Archivio di Anatomia.* 1956;61:1–46.

The ligaments of the lumbar spine

Topographically, the ligaments of the lumbar spine may be classified into four groups:

1. Those ligaments that interconnect the vertebral bodies.
2. Those ligaments that interconnect the posterior elements.
3. The iliolumbar ligament.
4. False ligaments.

LIGAMENTS OF THE VERTEBRAL BODIES

The two named ligaments that interconnect the vertebral bodies are the **anterior** and **posterior longitudinal ligaments**. Intimately associated with these ligaments are the anuli fibrosi of the intervertebral discs, and it must be emphasised that although described as part of the intervertebral disc, each **anulus fibrosus** is both structurally and functionally like a ligament. In fact, on the basis of size and strength, the anuli fibrosi can be construed as the principal ligaments of the vertebral bodies, and for this reason their structure bears reiteration in the context of the ligaments of the lumbar spine.

Anuli fibrosi

As described in Chapter 2, each anulus fibrosus consists of collagen fibres running from one vertebral body to the next and arranged in concentric lamellae. Furthermore, the deeper lamellae of collagen are continuous with the collagen fibres in the fibrocartilaginous vertebral endplates (see Ch. 2). By surrounding the nucleus pulposus, these inner layers of the anulus fibrosus constitute a capsule or envelope around the nucleus, whereupon it could be inferred that their principal function is to retain the nucleus pulposus (Fig. 4.1).

In contrast, the outer fibres of the anulus fibrosus are attached to the ring apophysis (see Ch. 2). For various reasons it is these fibres that could be inferred to be the principal 'ligamentous' portion of the anulus fibrosus. Foremost, like other ligaments they are attached to separate bones, and like other ligaments they consist largely of type I collagen, which is designed to resist tension (see Ch. 2). Such tension arises during rocking or twisting movements of the vertebral bodies. During these movements the peripheral edges of the vertebral bodies undergo more separation than their more central parts, and the tensile stresses applied to the peripheral anulus are greater than those applied to the inner anulus. In resisting these

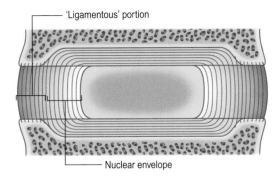

Figure 4.1 The anulus fibrosus as a ligament. The inner fibres of the anulus which attach to the vertebral endplate form an internal capsule that envelopes the nucleus pulposus. The outer fibres of the anulus which attach to the ring apophysis constitute the 'ligamentous' portion of the anulus fibrosus.

movements the peripheral fibres of the anulus fibrosus are subject to the same demands as conventional ligaments, and function accordingly.

As outlined in Chapter 2 and considered further in Chapter 8, the anulus fibrosus functions as a ligament in resisting distraction, bending, sliding and twisting movements of the intervertebral joint. Thus, the anulus fibrosus is called upon to function as a ligament whenever the lumbar spine moves. It is only during weight-bearing that it functions in concert with the nucleus pulposus.

Anterior longitudinal ligament

Conventional descriptions maintain that the anterior longitudinal ligament is a long band which covers the anterior aspects of the lumbar vertebral bodies and intervertebral discs (Fig. 4.2).[1] Although well developed in the lumbar region, this ligament is not restricted to that region. Inferiorly it extends into the sacrum, and superiorly it continues into the thoracic and cervical regions to cover the anterior surface of the entire vertebral column.

Structurally, the anterior longitudinal ligament is said to consist of several sets of collagen fibres.[1] There are short fibres that span each interbody joint, covering the intervertebral disc and attaching to the margins of the vertebral bodies (Figs 4.2, 4.3). These fibres are inserted into the bone of the anterior surface of the vertebral bodies or into the overlying periosteum.[2,3] Some early authors interpreted these fibres as being part of the anulus fibrosus,[4] and there is a tendency in some contemporary circles to interpret these fibres as constituting a 'disc capsule'. However, embryologically, their attachments are always associated with cortical bone, as are ligaments in general, whereas the anulus fibrosus proper is attached to the vertebral endplate.[2] Even those fibres of the adult anulus that attach to bone do so by being secondarily incorporated

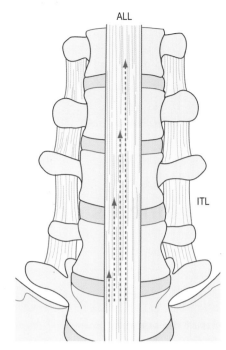

Figure 4.2 Classic descriptions of the anterior longitudinal ligament (ALL) and the intertransverse ligaments (ITL). The arrows indicate the span of various fibres in the anterior longitudinal ligament stemming from the L5 vertebra.

into the ring apophysis (Ch. 2), which is not cortical bone. Because of these developmental differences, the deep, short fibres of the anterior longitudinal ligament should not be considered to be part of the anulus fibrosus.

Covering the deep, unisegmental fibres of the anterior longitudinal ligament are several layers of increasingly longer fibres. There are fibres that span two, three and even four or five interbody joints. The attachments of these fibres, like those of the deep fibres, are into the upper and lower ends of the vertebral bodies.

Although the ligament is primarily attached to the anterior margins of the lumbar vertebral bodies, it is also secondarily attached to their concave anterior surfaces. The main body of the ligament bridges this concavity but some collagen fibres from its deep surface blend with the periosteum covering the concavity. Otherwise, the space between the ligament and bone is filled with loose areolar tissue, blood vessels and nerves. Over the intervertebral discs, the anterior longitudinal ligament is only loosely attached to the front of the anuli fibrosi by loose areolar tissue.

Because of its strictly longitudinal disposition, the anterior longitudinal ligament serves principally to resist vertical separation of the anterior ends of the vertebral bodies. In doing so, it functions during extension movements of

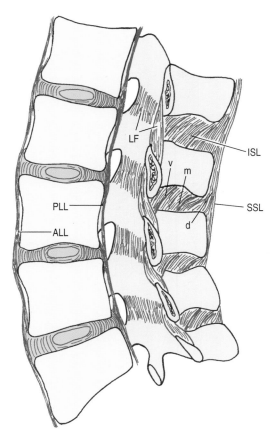

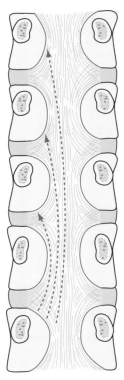

Figure 4.4 The posterior longitudinal ligament. The dotted lines indicate the span of some of the constituent fibres of the ligament arising from the L5 vertebra.

Figure 4.3 A median sagittal section of the lumbar spine to show its various ligaments. ALL, anterior longitudinal ligament; ISL, interspinous ligament: v, ventral part; m, middle part; d, dorsal part; PLL, posterior longitudinal ligament; SSL, supraspinous ligament. LF, ligamentum flavum, viewed from within the vertebral canal and in sagittal section at the midline.

the intervertebral joints and resists anterior bowing of the lumbar spine (see Ch. 5).

Comment

It is only in the thoracic spine that the anterior longitudinal ligament has an unambiguous structure, for there it stands in isolation from any prevertebral muscles. In the lumbar region the structure of the anterior longitudinal ligament is rendered ambiguous by the attachment of the crura of the diaphragm to the first three lumbar vertebrae. Although formal studies have not been completed, detailed examination of the crura and their attachments suggests that many of the tendinous fibres of the crura are prolonged caudally beyond the upper three lumbar vertebrae such that these tendons appear to constitute much of

what has otherwise been interpreted as the lumbar anterior longitudinal ligament. Thus, it may be that the lumbar anterior longitudinal ligament is, to a greater or lesser extent, not strictly a ligament but more a prolonged tendon attachment.

Posterior longitudinal ligament

Like the anterior longitudinal ligament, the posterior longitudinal ligament is represented throughout the vertebral column. In the lumbar region, it forms a narrow band over the backs of the vertebral bodies but expands laterally over the backs of the intervertebral discs to give it a serrated, or saw-toothed, appearance (Fig. 4.4). Its fibres mesh with those of the anuli fibrosi but penetrate through the anuli to attach to the posterior margins of the vertebral bodies.[3] The deepest and shortest fibres of the posterior longitudinal ligament span two intervertebral discs. Starting at the superior margin of one vertebra, they attach to the inferior margin of the vertebra two levels above, describing a curve concave laterally as they do so. Longer, more superficial fibres span three, four and even five vertebrae (see Figs 4.3 and 4.4).

41

The posterior longitudinal ligament serves to resist separation of the posterior ends of the vertebral bodies but because of its polysegmental disposition, its action is exerted over several interbody joints, not just one.

LIGAMENTS OF THE POSTERIOR ELEMENTS

The named ligaments of the posterior elements are the **ligamentum flavum**, the **interspinous** ligaments, and the **supraspinous** ligaments. In some respects, the capsules of the zygapophysial joints act like ligaments to prevent certain movements, and in a functional sense they can be considered to be one of the ligaments of the posterior elements. Indeed, their biomechanical role in this regard is quite substantial (see Ch. 8). However, their identity as capsules of the zygapophysial joints is so clear that they have been described formally in that context.

Ligamentum flavum

The ligamentum flavum is a short but thick ligament that joins the laminae of consecutive vertebrae. At each intersegmental level, the ligamentum flavum is a paired structure, being represented symmetrically on both left and right sides. On each side, the upper attachment of the ligament is to the lower half of the anterior surface of the lamina and the inferior aspect of the pedicle (Figs 4.3, 4.5). Its smooth surface blends perfectly with the smooth surface of the upper half of the lamina. Traced inferiorly, on each side the ligament divides into a medial and lateral portion.[5-7] The medial portion passes to the back of the next lower lamina and attaches to the rough area located on the upper quarter or so of the dorsal surface of that lamina (see Fig. 4.5). The lateral portion passes in front of the zygapophysial joint formed by the two vertebrae that the ligament connects. It attaches to the anterior aspects of the inferior and superior articular processes of that joint, and forms its anterior capsule. The most lateral fibres extend along the root of the superior articular process as far as the next lower pedicle to which they are attached.[7]

Histologically, the ligamentum flavum consists of 80% elastin and 20% collagen.[7,8] Elastic fibres proper are found throughout the ligament but at its terminal ends the ligament contains modified fibres consisting of elastin and microtubules, and known as elaunin.[8]

As an elastic ligament, the ligamentum flavum differs from all the other ligaments of the lumbar spine. This difference has prompted speculation as to its implied unique function. Its elastic nature has been said to aid in restoring the flexed lumbar spine to its extended position, while its lateral division is said to serve to prevent the anterior capsule of the zygapophysial joint being nipped

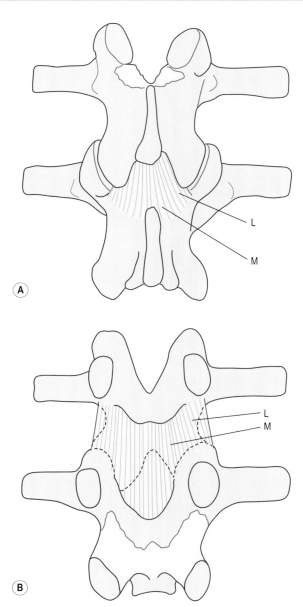

Figure 4.5 The ligamentum flavum at the L2–3 level. (A) Posterior view. (B) Anterior view (from within the vertebral canal). The medial (M) and lateral (L) divisions of the ligament are labelled. The shaded areas depict the sites of attachment of the ligamentum flavum at the levels above and below L2–3. In (B), the silhouettes of the laminae and inferior articular processes behind the ligament are indicated by the dotted lines.

within the joint cavity during movement. While all of these suggestions are consistent with the elastic nature of the ligament, the importance of these functions for the mechanics of the lumbar spine is unknown. It is questionable whether the ligamentum flavum contributes significantly to producing extension,[9] and no disabilities have been reported in patients in whom the ligamentum flavum has been excised, at single or even multiple levels. Biomechanical studies have revealed that the ligamentum flavum serves to pre-stress the intervertebral disc, exerting a disc pressure of about 0.70 kg cm^{-2},[10] but the biological significance of this effect remains obscure.

A plausible explanation for the unique nature of the ligamentum flavum relates more to its location than to its possible biomechanical functions. The ligamentum flavum lies immediately behind the vertebral canal, and therefore immediately adjacent to the nervous structures within the canal. As a ligament, it serves to resist excess separation of the vertebral laminae. A collagenous ligament in the same location would not function as well. A collagenous ligament could resist separation of the laminae, but when the laminae were approximated, a collagenous ligament would buckle. Were the ligament to buckle into the vertebral canal it would encroach upon the spinal cord or spinal nerve roots and possibly damage them. On the other hand, by replacing such a collagenous ligament with an elastic one, this buckling would be prevented. From a resting position, an elastic ligament stretches and thins. When relaxed again, the ligament simply assumes its original thickness. Buckling does not occur or is minimal. Therefore, by endowing the ligamentum flavum with elastic tissue, the risk of nerve root compromise is reduced.

Interspinous ligaments

The interspinous ligaments connect adjacent spinous processes. The collagen fibres of these ligaments are arranged in a particular manner, with three parts being identified (see Fig. 4.3).[11] The ventral part consists of fibres passing posterocranially from the dorsal aspect of the ligamentum flavum to the anterior half of the lower border of the spinous process above. The middle part forms the main component of the ligament, and consists of fibres that run from the anterior half of the upper border of one spinous process to the posterior half of the lower border of the spinous process above. The dorsal part consists of fibres from the posterior half of the upper border of the lower spinous process which pass behind the posterior border of the upper spinous process, to form the supraspinous ligament. Anteriorly, the interspinous ligament is a paired structure, the ligaments on each side being separated by a slit-like midline cavity filled with fat. This cavity is not present more posteriorly.

Histologically, the ligament consists essentially of collagen fibres, but elastic fibres occur with increasing density in the ventral part of the ligament, towards its junction with the ligamentum flavum.[8,12]

The fibres of the interspinous ligament are poorly disposed to resist separation of the spinous processes; they run almost perpendicularly to the direction of separation of the spinous processes. Indeed, X-ray diffraction studies have indicated a greater dispersal of fibre orientation than that indicated by dissection, with many fibres running roughly parallel to the spinous processes[13] instead of between them. Accordingly, contrary to traditional wisdom in this regard, the interspinous ligaments can offer little resistance to forward bending movements of the lumbar spine.[13]

Comment

Only the ventral and middle parts of the interspinous ligament constitute true ligaments, for only they exhibit connections to separate adjacent bones. The dorsal part of the ligament appears to pass from the upper border of one spinous process to the dorsal edge of the next above, but here the ligament does not assume a bony attachment: it blends with the supraspinous ligament whose actual identity as a ligament can be questioned (see below).

Supraspinous ligament

The supraspinous ligament lies in the midline. It runs posterior to the posterior edges of the lumbar spinous processes, to which it is attached, and bridges the interspinous spaces (see Fig. 4.3). The ligament is well developed only in the upper lumbar region; its lower limit varies. It terminates at the L3 spinous process in about 22% of individuals, and at L4 in 73%; it bridges the L4–5 interspace in only 5% of individuals, and is regularly lacking at L5–S1.[11,14]

Upon close inspection, the nature of the supraspinous ligament as a ligament can be questioned. It consists of three parts: a superficial; a middle; and a deep layer.[14] The superficial layer is subcutaneous and consists of longitudinally running collagen fibres that span three to four successive spinous processes. It varies considerably in size from a few extremely thin fibrous bundles to a robust band, 5–6 mm wide and 3–4 mm thick, with most individuals exhibiting intermediate forms.[14]

The middle layer is about 1 mm thick and consists of intertwining tendinous fibres of the dorsal layer of thoracolumbar fascia and the aponeurosis of longissimus thoracis (see Ch. 9).

The deep layer consists of very strong, tendinous fibres derived from the aponeurosis of longissimus thoracis. As these tendons pass to their insertions on the lumbar spinous processes, they are aggregated in a parallel fashion, creating a semblance of a supraspinous ligament, but they are clearly identifiable as tendons. The deepest of these tendons arch ventrally and caudally to reach the upper border of a spinous process, thereby constituting the dorsal part of the interspinous ligament at that level. The deep layer of the supraspinous ligament is reinforced by tendinous fibres of the multifidus muscle (see Ch. 9).

It is therefore evident that the supraspinous ligament consists largely of tendinous fibres derived from the back muscles and so is not truly a ligament. Only the superficial layer lacks any continuity with muscle, and this layer is not present at lower lumbar levels. Lying in the subcutaneous plane, dorsal to the other two layers and therefore displaced from the spinous processes, the superficial layer may be rejected as a true ligament and is more readily interpreted as a very variable condensation of the deep or membranous layer of superficial fascia that anchors the midline skin to the thoracolumbar fascia. It affords little resistance to separation of the spinous processes.[13]

At the L4 and L5 levels, where the superficial layer is lacking, there is no semblance of a longitudinally orientated midline supraspinous ligament, and the true nature of the 'ligament' is revealed. Here, the obliquely orientated tendinous fibres of the thoracolumbar fascia decussate dorsal to the spinous processes and are fused deeply with the fibres of the aponeurosis of longissimus thoracis that attach to the spinous processes.

ILIOLUMBAR LIGAMENT

The iliolumbar ligaments are present bilaterally, and on each side they connect the transverse process of the fifth lumbar vertebra to the ilium. In brief, each ligament extends from the tip of its transverse process to an area on the anteromedial surface of the ilium and the inner lip of the iliac crest. However, the morphology, and indeed the very existence of the iliolumbar ligament, has become a focus of controversy.

An early description, provided by professional anatomists with an eye for detail, accorded five parts to the ligament (Fig. 4.6).[15]

The **anterior iliolumbar ligament** is a well-developed ligamentous band whose fibres arise from the entire length of the anteroinferior border of the L5 transverse process, from as far medially as the body of the L5 vertebra to the tip of the transverse process. The fibres from the medial end of the transverse process cover those from the lateral end, and collectively they all pass posterolaterally, in line with the long axis of the transverse process, to attach to the ilium. Additional fibres of the anterior iliolumbar ligament arise from the very tip of the transverse process, so that beyond the tip of the transverse process the ligament forms a very thick bundle. The upper surface of this bundle forms the site of attachment for the fibres of the lower end of the quadratus lumborum muscle.

The **superior iliolumbar ligament** is formed by anterior and posterior thickenings of the fascia that surrounds the

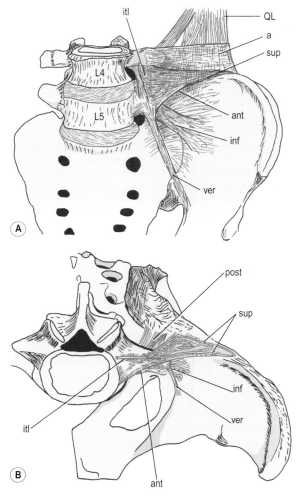

Figure 4.6 The left iliolumbar ligament. (Based on Shellshear and Macintosh 1949.[15]) (A) Front view. (B) Top view. a, anterior layer of thoracolumbar fascia; ant, anterior iliolumbar ligament; inf, inferior iliolumbar ligament; itl, intertransverse ligament; post, posterior iliolumbar ligament; QL, quadratus lumborum; sup, superior iliolumbar ligament; ver, vertical iliolumbar ligament.

base of the quadratus lumborum muscle. These thickenings are attached in common to the anterosuperior border of the L5 transverse process near its tip. Lateral to this, they separate to pass respectively in front of and behind the quadratus lumborum muscle to attach eventually to the ilium. Inferiorly, they blend with the anterior iliolumbar ligament to form a trough from which the quadratus lumborum arises.

The **posterior iliolumbar ligament** arises from the tip and posterior border of the L5 transverse process and inserts into the ligamentous area of the ilium behind the origin of the quadratus lumborum. The deepest fibres of the longissimus lumborum arise from the ligament in this area.

The **inferior iliolumbar ligament** arises from the lower border of the L5 transverse process and from the body of L5. Its fibres pass downwards and laterally across the surface of the anterior sacroiliac ligament to attach to the upper and posterior part of the iliac fossa. These fibres are distinguished from the anterior sacroiliac ligament by their oblique orientation.

The **vertical iliolumbar ligament** arises from the anteroinferior border of the L5 transverse process and descends almost vertically to attach to the posterior end of the iliopectineal line of the pelvis. Its significance lies in the fact that it forms the lateral margin of the channel through which the L5 ventral ramus enters the pelvis.

A modern study confirmed the presence of anterior and posterior parts of the iliolumbar ligament, but denied a superior part and did not comment on the inferior and vertical parts.[16] These differences can be resolved.

The recognition of the superior iliolumbar ligament is probably an overstatement. This tissue is clearly the anterior fascia of the quadratus lumborum and lacks the features of true ligament-orientated collagen fibres passing directly from one bone to another. The vertical and inferior iliolumbar ligaments are readily overlooked as part of the ventral sacroiliac ligament but their attachments are not sacral and iliac but lumbar and iliac. Therefore, they still deserve the name 'iliolumbar'.

Another study confirmed the incidence and attachments of the anterior, dorsal and inferior bands, but added a further part.[17] This was called the sacroiliac part. Its fibres passed between the sacrum and ilium, below the L5 transverse process, and blended superiorly with the lowest fibres of the anterior part.

Notwithstanding the details of its parts, the existence of the iliolumbar ligament has been questioned. One study has found it to be present only in adults. In neonates and children it was represented by a bundle of muscle.[18] The interpretation offered was that this muscle is gradually replaced by ligamentous tissue. Replacement starts near the transverse process and spreads towards the ilium. The structure is substantially ligamentous by the third decade, although some muscle fibres persist. From the fifth decade the ligament contains no muscle but exhibits hyaline degeneration. From the sixth decade the ligament exhibits fatty infiltration, hyalinisation, myxoid degeneration and calcification. The identity of the muscles that form the iliolumbar ligament is discussed in Chapter 9.

In contrast, another study unequivocally denied the absence of an iliolumbar ligament in fetuses.[19] It found the ligament to be present by 11.5 weeks of gestation. How this difference should be resolved is not clear. What may be critical are data from older fetuses and new data from infants. The embryological study was not able to examine fetuses older than 16.5 weeks, which leaves a gap between that age and infancy. The only reported data in that age range stipulate that the ligament was muscular.[18]

Regardless of what its structure may or may not be in children and adolescents, in the mature adult the iliolumbar ligament forms a strong bond between the L5 vertebra and the ilium, with different parts subserving different functions. As a whole, the ligament is disposed to prevent forward sliding of the L5 vertebra on the sacrum, and the relevance of this function is explored in Chapter 5. It also resists twisting, and forward, backward and lateral bending of the L5 vertebra.[20,21] Forward bending is resisted by the posterior band of the ligament, while lateral bending is resisted by its anterior band.[22]

FALSE LIGAMENTS

There are several structures in the lumbar spine that carry the name 'ligament' but for various reasons this is not a legitimate term. These structures are the intertransverse ligaments, the transforaminal ligaments and the mamillo-accessory ligament.

Intertransverse ligaments

The so-called intertransverse ligaments (see Fig. 4.2) have a complicated structure that can be interpreted in various ways. They consist of sheets of connective tissue extending from the upper border of one transverse process to the lower border of the transverse process above. Unlike other ligaments, they lack a distinct border medially or laterally, and their collagen fibres are not as densely packed, nor are they as regularly orientated as the fibres of true ligaments. Rather, their appearance is more like that of a membrane.[3] The medial and lateral continuations of these membranes suggest that rather than being true ligaments, these structures form part of a complex fascial system that serves to separate or demarcate certain paravertebral compartments. Indeed, the only 'true' ligament recognised in this area is the ligament of Bourgery which connects the base of a transverse process to the mamillary process below.[3]

In the intertransverse spaces, the intertransverse ligaments form a septum that divides the anterior musculature of the lumbar spine from the posterior musculature, and embryologically the ligaments arise from the tissue that separates the epaxial and hypaxial musculature (see Ch. 12). Laterally, the intertransverse ligaments can be interpreted as dividing into two layers: an anterior layer, otherwise known as the anterior layer of thoracolumbar fascia, which covers the front of the quadratus lumborum muscle and a posterior layer which blends with the aponeurosis of the transversus abdominis to form the middle layer of thoracolumbar fascia (see Ch. 9).

Towards the medial end of each intertransverse space, the intertransverse ligament splits into two leaves (Fig.

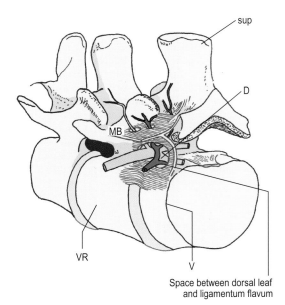

Space between dorsal leaf
and ligamentum flavum

Figure 4.7 The ventral and dorsal leaves of the intertransverse ligament. (Based on Lewin et al. 1962,[23] with permission.) D, dorsal leaf; MB, medial branch of dorsal ramus; V, ventral leaf; VR, ventral ramus of spinal nerve.

4.7).[23] The dorsal leaf continues medially to attach to the lateral margin of the lamina of the vertebra that lies opposite the intertransverse space. Inferiorly, it blends with the capsule of the adjacent zygapophysial joint. The ventral leaf curves forwards and extends forward over the lateral surface of the vertebral bodies until it eventually blends with the lateral margins of the anterior longitudinal ligament. In covering the lateral aspect of the vertebral column, it forms a membranous sheet that closes the outer end of the intervertebral foramen. This part of the leaf is marked by two perforations which transmit structures into and out of the intervertebral foramen. The superior opening transmits the nerve branches to the psoas muscle. The inferior opening transmits the ventral ramus of the spinal nerve and the spinal branches of the lumbar arteries and veins.

Enclosed between the ventral and dorsal leaves of the intertransverse ligament is a wedge-shaped space, called the superior articular recess. This recess serves to accommodate movements of the subadjacent zygapophysial joint. It is filled with fat that is continuous with the intra-articular fat in the joint below, through the foramen in its superior capsule. The superior articular process of this joint projects into the bottom end of the recess, and during extension movements of the joint, its inferior articular process moves inferiorly, pulling the superior articular recess, like a sleeve, over the medial end of the superior articular process. During this process the fat in the recess

acts as a displaceable space-filler. At rest, it maintains the space in the recess but is easily moved out to accommodate the superior articular process. A reciprocal mechanism operates at the inferior pole of the joint, where a pad of fat over the vertebral lamina maintains a space between the lamina and the multifidus muscle into which the inferior articular process can move.

Transforaminal ligaments

The transforaminal ligaments are narrow bands of collagen fibres that traverse the outer end of the intervertebral foramen. Five types of such bands have been described, according to their specific attachments (Fig. 4.8):[24]

- The superior corporotransverse ligaments connect the lower posterolateral corner of a vertebral body with the accessory process of the transverse process of the same vertebra.
- The inferior corporotransverse ligaments connect the lower posterolateral corner of a vertebral body with the transverse process below.
- The superior transforaminal ligaments bridge the inferior vertebral notches, and the inferior transforaminal ligaments bridge superior vertebral notches.
- The midtransforaminal ligaments run from the posterolateral corner of an anulus fibrosus to the zygapophysial joint capsule and ligamentum flavum behind.

Transforaminal ligaments are not always present. The overall incidence of all types is around 47%, with the superior corporotransverse being the most common type (27%).[24] For two reasons, they are not strictly ligaments. Firstly, their structure resembles bands of fascia more than ligaments proper. Secondly, except for the inferior corporotransverse ligament, they do not connect two separate bones, and the midtransforaminal variety is not connected to any bones. Accordingly, they are more correctly interpreted as bands of fascia, and in view of their location it is most likely that they represent thickenings in the ventral leaf of the intertransverse ligament.

Mamillo-accessory ligament

A tight bundle of collagen fibres of variable thickness bridges the tips of the ipsilateral mamillary and accessory processes of each lumbar vertebra (Fig. 4.9). This structure has been called the mamillo-accessory ligament[25] but it is not a true ligament because it connects two points on the same bone. Moreover, its cord-like structure resembles a tendon more than a ligament, and indeed it has been interpreted as representing a tendon of the semispinalis musculature in the lumbar region.[25] The ligament may be ossified, converting the mamillo-accessory notch into a bony foramen. The prevalence of this change was found

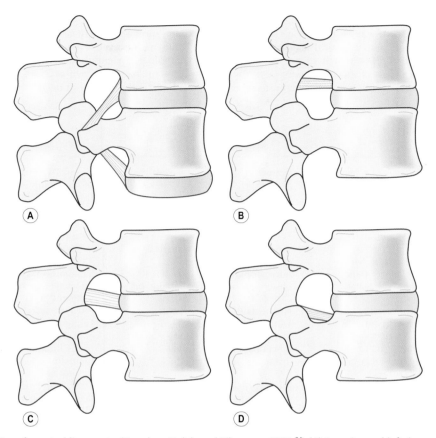

Figure 4.8 The transforaminal ligaments. (Based on Golub and Silverman 1969.[24]) (A) Superior and inferior corporotransverse ligaments. (B) Superior transforaminal ligament. (C) Middle transforaminal ligament. (D) Inferior transforaminal ligament.

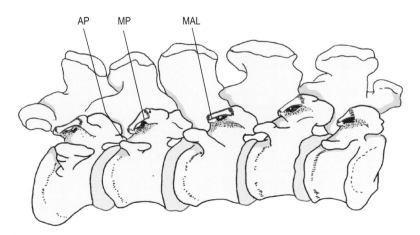

Figure 4.9 The mamillo-accessory ligaments (MAL). AP, accessory process; MP, mamillary process. Note the foramina under the ligaments, through which pass the medial branches of the lumbar dorsal rami.

in one study to be 10% at the L5 level,[25] while in another study it was 28% at L5, 10% at L4 and 3% at L3.[26]

The ligament has no biomechanical significance, but its significance lies in the fact that it covers the medial branch of the dorsal ramus of the spinal nerve as it runs through the mamillo-accessory notch. Furthermore, when the ligament is ossified, the foramen it forms can be an apparent anomaly evident on CT scans.[27] Ossification of the ligament, however, is a normal phenomenon without any pathological significance. It has been suggested that the ligament may be a site of entrapment of the nerve beneath it,[28] but this has not been verified clinically.

REFERENCES

1. Williams PL, ed. *Gray's Anatomy*, 38th ed. Edinburgh: Churchill Livingstone; 1995.

2. Francois RJ. Ligament insertions into the human lumbar vertebral body. *Acta Anat.* 1975;91:467–480.

3. Vallois HV. Arthologie. In: Nicolas A, ed. *Poirier and Charpy's Traité d'Anatomie Humaine*, Vol 1. Paris: Masson; 1926.

4. Coventry MB, Ghormley RK, Kernohan JW. The intervertebral disc: its microscopic anatomy and pathology. Part I. Anatomy, development and physiology. *J Bone Joint Surg.* 1945;27:105–112.

5. Naffziger HC, Inman V, Saunders JB, de CM. Lesions of the intervertebral disc and ligamenta flava. *Surg Gynecol Obstet.* 1938;66:288–299.

6. Ramsey RH. The anatomy of the ligamenta flava. *Clin Orthop.* 1966;44:129–140.

7. Yong-Hing K, Reilly J, Kirkaldy-Willis WH. The ligamentum flavum. *Spine.* 1976;1:226–234.

8. Yahia LH, Garzon S, Strykowski H, et al. Ultrastructure of the human interspinous ligament and ligamentum flavum: a preliminary study. *Spine.* 1990;15:262–268.

9. Twomey LT, Taylor JR. Sagittal movements of the human lumbar vertebral column: a quantitative study of the role of the posterior vertebral elements. *Arch Phys Med Rehab.* 1983;64:322–325.

10. Nachemson AL, Evans JH. Some mechanical properties of the third human lumbar interlaminar ligament (ligamentum flavum). *J Biomech.* 1968;1:211–220.

11. Heylings DJA. Supraspinous and interspinous ligaments of the human spine. *J Anat.* 1978;125:127–131.

12. Yahia LH, Drouin G, Maurais G, et al. Etude de la structure microscopique des ligaments postérieurs du rachis lombaire. *Int Orthop.* 1989;13:207–216.

13. Hukins DWL, Kirby MC, Sikoryn TA, et al. Comparison of structure, mechanical properties, and functions of lumbar spinal ligaments. *Spine.* 1990;15:787–795.

14. Rissanen PM. The surgical anatomy and pathology of the supraspinous and interspinous ligaments of the lumbar spine with special reference to ligament ruptures. *Acta Orthop Scand.* 1960;46(suppl.):1–100.

15. Shellshear JL, Macintosh NWG. The transverse process of the fifth lumbar vertebra. In: Shellshear JL, Macintosh NWG, eds. *Surveys of Anatomical Fields.* Sydney: Grahame; 1949:Ch. 3, 21–32.

16. Hanson P, Sonesson B. The anatomy of the iliolumbar ligament. *Arch Phys Med Rehab.* 1994;75:1245–1246.

17. Pool-Goudzwaard AL, Kleinrensink GJ, Snijders CJ, et al. The sacroiliac part of the iliolumbar ligament. *J Anat.* 2001;199:457–463.

18. Luk KDK, Ho HC, Leong JCY. The iliolumbar ligament. A study of its anatomy, development and clinical significance. *J Bone Joint Surg.* 1986;68B:197–200.

19. Uhtoff HK. Prenatal development of the iliolumbar ligament. *J Bone Joint Surg.* 1993;75B:93–95.

20. Chow DHK, Luk KDK, Leong JCY, et al. Torsional stability of the lumbosacral junction: significance of the iliolumbar ligament. *Spine.* 1989;14:611–615.

21. Yamamoto I, Panjabi MM, Oxland TR, et al. The role of the iliolumbar ligament in the lumbosacral junction. *Spine.* 1990;15:1138–1141.

22. Leong JCY, Luk KDK, Chow DHK, et al. The biomechanical functions of the iliolumbar ligament in maintaining stability of the lumbosacral junction. *Spine.* 1987;12:669–674.

23. Lewin T, Moffet B, Viidik A. The morphology of the lumbar synovial intervertebral joints. *Acta Morphol Neerlando-Scand.* 1962;4:299–319.

24. Golub BS, Silverman B. Transforaminal ligaments of the lumbar spine. *J Bone Joint Surg.* 1969;51A:947–956.

25. Bogduk N. The lumbar mamillo-accessory ligament. Its anatomical and neurosurgical significance. *Spine.* 1981;6:162–167.

26. Ninghsia Medical College. Anatomical observations on lumbar nerve posterior rami. *Chin Med J.* 1978;4:492–496.

27. Beers GJ, Carter AP, McNary WF. Vertical foramina in the lumbosacral region: CT appearance. *Am J Roentgenol.* 1984;143:1027–1029.

28. Bradley KC. The anatomy of backache. *Aust NZ J Surg.* 1974;44:227–232.

Chapter | 5 |

The lumbar lordosis and the vertebral canal

THE LUMBAR LORDOSIS

The intact lumbar spine is formed when the five lumbar vertebrae are articulated to one another (Fig. 5.1). Anteriorly the vertebral bodies are separated by the intervertebral discs and are held together by the anterior and posterior longitudinal ligaments. Posteriorly the articular processes form the zygapophysial joints, and consecutive vertebrae are held together by the supraspinous, interspinous and intertransverse ligaments and the ligamenta flava.

Although the lumbar vertebrae can be articulated to form a straight column of vertebrae, this is not the shape assumed by the intact lumbar spine in the upright posture. The reason for this is that the sacrum, on which the lumbar spine rests, is tilted forwards, so that its upper surface is inclined downwards and forwards. From radiographs taken in the supine position, the size of this angle with respect to the horizontal plane of the body has a mean value of about 42–45°,[1–3] and is said to increase by about 8° upon standing.[1]

If a straight lumbar spine articulated with the sacrum, it would consequently be inclined forwards. To restore an upward orientation and to compensate for the inclination of the sacrum, the intact lumbar spine must assume a curve (see Fig. 5.1). This curve is known as the lumbar **lordosis**.

The junction between the lumbar spine and the sacrum is achieved through joints like those between the lumbar vertebrae. Anteriorly, the body of the L5 vertebra forms an interbody joint with the first sacral vertebra, and the intervertebral disc of this joint is known as the lumbosacral disc. Posteriorly, the inferior articular processes of L5 and the superior articular processes of the sacrum form synovial joints, known either as the L5–S1 zygapophysial joints or as the lumbosacral zygapophysial joints. A ligamentum flavum is present between the laminae of L5 and the sacrum, and an interspinous ligament connects the L5 and S1 spinous processes. However, there is no supraspinous ligament at the L5–S1 level,[4] nor are there intertransverse ligaments, the latter having been replaced by the iliolumbar ligament.

The shape of the lumbar lordosis is achieved as a result of several factors. The first of these is the shape of the lumbosacral intervertebral disc. This disc is unlike any of the other lumbar intervertebral discs in that it is wedge shaped. Its posterior height is about 6–7 mm less than its anterior height.[5] Consequently, when the L5 vertebra is articulated to the sacrum, its lower surface does not lie parallel to the upper surface of the sacrum. It is still inclined forwards and downwards but less steeply than the top of the sacrum. The angle formed between the bottom of the L5 vertebra and the top of the sacrum varies from individual to individual over the range 6–29° and has an average size of about 16° (Fig. 5.2).[5]

The second factor that generates the lumbar lordosis is the shape of the L5 vertebra. Like the lumbosacral disc, the L5 vertebral body is also wedge shaped. The height of its posterior surface is some 3 mm less than the height of its

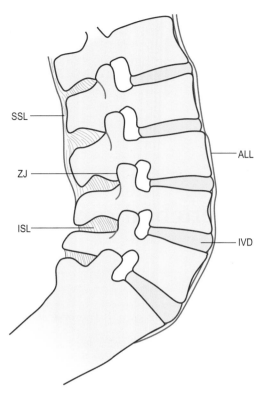

Figure 5.1 Lateral view of the intact, upright lumbar spine, showing its curved shape. ALL, anterior longitudinal ligament; IVD, intervertebral disc; ISL, interspinous ligament; SSL, supraspinous ligament; ZJ, zygapophysial joint.

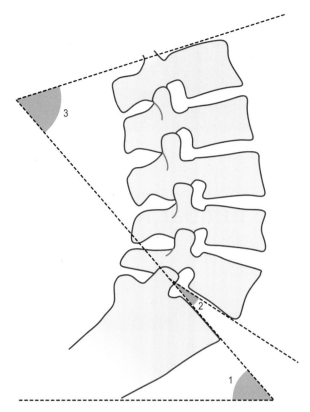

Figure 5.2 Some of the angles used to describe the lumbar spine. 1, angle formed by the top of the sacrum and the horizontal plane (mean value about 50°); 2, angle between the bottom of L5 and the top of the sacrum (mean value 16°); 3, angle between the top of L1 and the sacrum, used to measure the lumbar lordosis (mean value: about 70°).

anterior surface.[6] As a consequence of the wedge shape of both the L5 body and the lumbosacral disc, the upper surface of L5 lies much closer to a horizontal plane than does the upper surface of the sacrum.

The remainder of the lumbar lordosis is completed simply by inclination of the vertebrae above L5. Each vertebra is inclined slightly backwards in relation to the vertebra below. As a result of this inclination, the anterior parts of the anuli fibrosi and the anterior longitudinal ligament are stretched. Posteriorly, the intervertebral discs are compressed slightly, and the inferior articular processes slide downwards in relation to the superior articular processes of the vertebra below, and may impact either the superior articular process or the pedicle below. The latter phenomenon has particular bearing on the weight-bearing capacity of the zygapophysial joints and is described further in Chapter 8.

The form of the curve thus achieved is such that, in the upright posture, the L1 vertebra is brought to lie vertically above the sacrum. The exact shape of the lumbar lordosis at rest varies from individual to individual, and it is

difficult to define what might be called the 'normal' lumbar lordosis.

Magnitude

Various parameters have been used by different investigators to quantify the curvature of the lumbar lordosis, although they all involve measuring one or other of the angles formed by the lumbar vertebral bodies (see Fig. 5.2). Some have used the angle formed by the planes through the top surface of L1 and the top surface of the sacrum,[7,8] and this could be called the 'L1–S1 lordosis angle'. Fernand and Fox (1985)[9] measured the angles between the top of L2 and the top of the sacrum, and between the top of L2 and the bottom of L5, which they called, respectively, the 'lumbosacral lordotic angle' and the 'lumbolumbar lordotic angle'. Others have measured the angle between the top of L3 and the sacrum,[10] or the angle formed between planes that bisect the L1–L2 disc and the L5–S1 disc.[11,12] Consequently, the measures obtained in these various studies differ somewhat from one another. Nevertheless they all show substantial ranges of variation.

In radiographs taken in the supine position, the angle between the top of L1 and the top of the sacrum varies from 20° to more than 60° but has an average value of about 50°.[7] In the standing position, this same angle has been measured as 67° (±3° standard deviation, SD) in children, and 74° (±7° SD) in young males.[13] The angle between the top of L2 and the sacrum has a range of 16–80° and a mean value of 45°.[9] A value greater than 68° is considered to indicate a hyperlordotic curve.[9] However, despite a common belief that excessive lordosis is a risk factor for low back pain, comparison studies reveal that there is no correlation between the shape of the lumbar lordosis and the presence or absence of back pain symptoms.[7,10,12]

Stability

The foremost structural liability of the lumbar spine stems from the inclination of the sacrum. Because of the downward slope of the superior surface of the sacrum there is a constant tendency for the L5 vertebra, and hence the entire lumbar spine, to slide forwards down this slope under the influence of the weight of the trunk; more so whenever additional weights are borne by the lumbar spine. In turn there is a similar though lesser tendency for the L4 vertebra to slide down the upper surface of the L5 vertebra. However, the lumbar spine is adapted to offset these tendencies, and these adaptations are seen in the structure of the articular processes and ligaments of L5 and other lumbar vertebrae.

As described in Chapter 3, the lumbar zygapophysial joints provide a bony locking mechanism that resists forward displacement, and the degree to which a joint affords such resistance is determined by its orientation. The more a superior articular process faces backwards, the greater the resistance it offers to forward displacement.

To resist the tendency for the L5 vertebra to slip forwards, the superior articular processes of the sacrum face considerably backwards. The average orientation of the L5–S1 zygapophysial joints with respect to the sagittal plane is about 45° with most lumbosacral zygapophysial joints assuming this orientation (see Fig. 3.4). Only a minority of joints assume a greater or lesser angle. Joints with a greater angle, i.e. facing backwards to an even greater extent, provide greater resistance to forward displacement of L5, but they provide less resistance to axial rotation (twisting movements) of L5. Joints with an angle less than 45° provide greater protection against rotation but less against forward displacement. An angle of 45° is therefore a satisfactory compromise, allowing the lumbosacral zygapophysial joints to resist both rotation and forward displacement.

The L4–5 zygapophysial joints are also orientated at about 45° (see Fig. 3.4) and thereby resist forward displacement of the L4 vertebra. Above L4, the slopes of the upper surfaces of the vertebral bodies are horizontal or inclined backwards, and there is no tendency, at rest, for the upper lumbar vertebrae to slide forwards. Consequently, there is less need for the upper lumbar zygapophysial joints to face backwards, and their angle of orientation is progressively less than 45° (see Fig. 3.4). Such resistance as may be required to resist forward displacement of these joints during flexion of the lumbar spine is nevertheless afforded by the curved shape of their articular surfaces. Although their general orientation is closer to the sagittal plane, the anteromedial ends of the articular surfaces of the upper lumbar joints face backwards and can resist forward displacement, if required (see Ch. 3).

The second mechanism that stabilises the lumbar lordosis is provided by the ligaments of the lumbar spine. At all levels, any tendency for a vertebra to slide forwards will be resisted by the anulus fibrosus of the underlying intervertebral disc. However, the anuli fibrosi are spared undue strain in this regard by the bony locking mechanism of the zygapophysial joints. Bony impaction will occur before the intervertebral discs are strained. However, should the mechanism of the zygapophysial joints be compromised by unsuitable orientation, or by disease or injury, then the resistance of the anuli fibrosi will be invoked to a greater extent.

By connecting the L5 transverse processes to the ilium, the iliolumbar ligaments, through their sheer size, provide a strong additional mechanism that prevents the L5 vertebra from sliding forwards. The tension sustained through the iliolumbar ligament is evident in the size of the L5 transverse processes. These are unlike the transverse processes of any other lumbar vertebra. Instead of thin flat bars, they are thick and pyramidal. Moreover, instead of stemming just from the posterior end of the pedicle, they have an enlarged base that extends forwards along the pedicle as far as the vertebral body. This modification of structure can be interpreted as being due to the modelling of the bone in response to the massive forces transmitted through the L5 transverse processes and the iliolumbar ligaments.

The anterior longitudinal ligament, and in a similar way the anterior fibres of the anuli fibrosi, plays a further role in stabilising the lumbar lordosis. If the lumbar spine bows forwards, the anterior ends of the vertebral bodies will attempt to separate but this will be resisted by the anterior longitudinal ligament and the anterior fibres of the anuli fibrosi. Eventually an equilibrium will be established in which any force tending to separate the vertebral bodies will be balanced exactly by the tension in the anterior ligaments. Any increase in force will be met

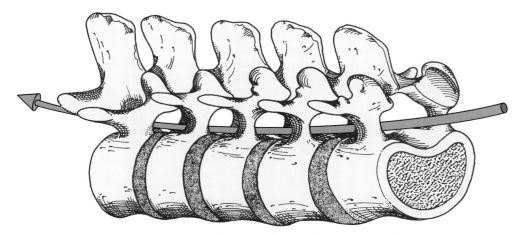

Figure 5.3 Lateral view of a prone lumbar spine with an arrow depicting the vertebral canal.

by increased tension in the ligaments. In this way, the anterior ligaments endow the curved lumbar spine with a resilience. This mechanism is analogous to the 'springiness' that can be felt in a long wooden rod or a plastic ruler that is stood on end and deformed into an arc.

One of the advantages of a curved lumbar spine lies in this resilience. By being curved, the lumbar spine is protected to an appreciable extent from compressive forces and shocks. In a straight lumbar spine, an axial compressive force would be transmitted through the vertebral bodies and intervertebral discs, and the only mechanism to protect the lumbar vertebrae would be the shock-absorbing capacity of the intervertebral discs (see Ch. 2). In contrast, in a curved lumbar spine, compressive forces are transmitted through the posterior ends of the intervertebral discs while the anterior ends of the vertebral bodies tend to separate. In other words, compression tends to accentuate the lumbar lordosis. This tendency will cause the anterior ligaments to become tense, which, in turn, will resist the accentuation. In this way, some of the energy of the compressive force is diverted into stretching the anterior ligaments instead of being transmitted directly into the next vertebral body.

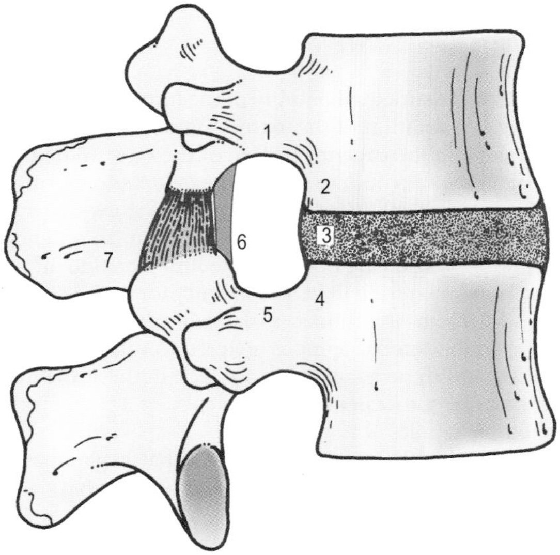

Figure 5.4 Lateral view of the boundaries of an intervertebral foramen. 1, pedicle; 2, back of vertebral body; 3, intervertebral disc; 4, back of vertebral body; 5, pedicle; 6, ligamentum flavum; 7, zygapophysial joint.

THE VERTEBRAL CANAL

In the intact lumbar spine, the vertebral foramina of the five lumbar vertebrae are aligned to form a continuous channel called the **vertebral canal** (Fig. 5.3). The anterior wall of this canal is formed by the posterior surfaces of the lumbar vertebrae, the intervening discs and the posterior longitudinal ligament. The posterior wall is formed by the laminae of the vertebrae and the intervening ligamenta flava. Because operations on the lumbar spine are most

frequently performed with the patient in the prone position, the anterior and posterior walls of the vertebral canal are, by convention, alternatively referred to as the **floor** and **roof** of the vertebral canal, respectively.

The floor of the vertebral canal is not absolutely flat because the posterior surfaces of the lumbar vertebral bodies exhibit slight curves, transversely and longitudinally. The posterior surfaces of the L1 to L3 vertebrae regularly exhibit a slight transverse concavity. In contrast L5 is slightly convex while L4 exhibits an intermediate curvature.[14] Along the sagittal plane, the lumbar vertebrae present a slightly concave posterior surface so that in profile the floor of the vertebral canal presents a scalloped appearance.[15] This scalloping is believed to be produced by the pulsatile, hydrostatic pressure of the cerebrospinal fluid in the dural sac, which occupies the vertebral canal.[15]

The lateral walls of the vertebral canal are formed by the pedicles of the lumbar vertebrae. Between the pedicles, the lateral wall is deficient where the superior and inferior vertebral notches appose one another to form the intervertebral foramina. Each intervertebral foramen is bounded anteriorly by an intervertebral disc, the adjacent lower third of the vertebral body above, and the uppermost portion of the vertebral body below (Fig. 5.4). Above

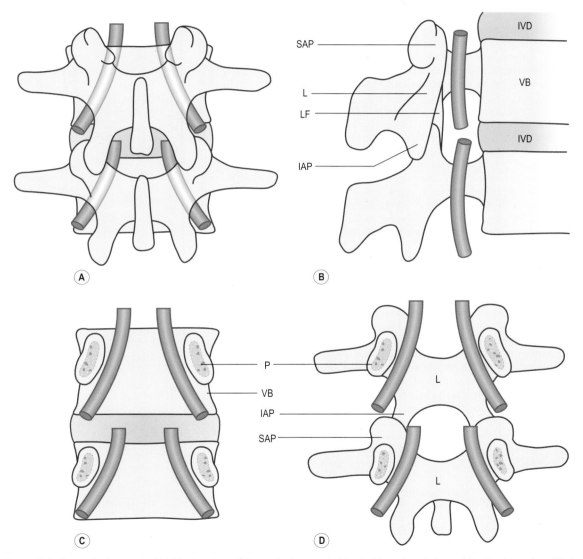

Figure 5.5 The radicular canals. (A) The location of the radicular canals (shaded) in a dorsal view of the lumbar spine. (B) A view of the radicular canals from within the vertebral canal, showing their lateral, anterior and posterior boundaries. (C) The anterior and lateral boundaries of the radicular canals, viewed from behind. (D) The posterior and lateral boundaries of the radicular canals, as seen from within the vertebral canal, looking at its roof. The ligamentum flavum has not been included (see also Fig. 4.5B). IAP, inferior articular process; IVD, intervertebral disc; L, lamina; LF, ligamentum flavum; P, pedicle; SAP, superior articular process; VB, vertebral body.

and below, each intervertebral foramen is bounded by a pedicle, while posteriorly it is bounded by a vertebral lamina and a zygapophysial joint. More accurately, the posterior boundary of each intervertebral foramen is the lateral portion of the ligamentum flavum that covers the anterior aspect of the lamina and zygapophysial joint (see Ch. 4).

Subdivisions of the vertebral canal, recognised by surgeons because of their relationship to the spinal nerve roots,[16–19] are the so-called **radicular canals**. These are not true canals because they do not have boundaries around all their aspects. More accurately, they are only subdivisions of the space of the vertebral canal and intervertebral foramina, through which the spinal nerve roots run (see Ch. 10), but in so far as they form a series of bony relations to the course of the nerve roots, they may be regarded as canals.

Each radicular canal is a curved channel running around the medial aspect of each pedicle in the lumbar spine, and each can be divided into three segments.[19] The uppermost, or retrodiscal segment, lies above the level of the pedicle. Its anterior wall is formed by the intervertebral disc in this region, while its posterior wall is formed by the uppermost end of a superior articular process (Fig. 5.5). This segment lacks a lateral wall because it lies opposite the level of an intervertebral foramen. Similarly, it has no medial wall for in this direction it is simply continuous with the rest of the vertebral canal.

The parapedicular segment lies immediately medial to the pedicle, which therefore forms its lateral wall. Anteriorly, this segment is related to the back of the vertebral body, while posteriorly it is covered by the vertebral lamina and the anteromedial edge of the superior articular process that projects from this lamina (see Fig. 5.5). Technically, this segment of the radicular canal is simply the lateral portion of the vertebral canal opposite the level of a pedicle, and for this reason this segment is also known as the **lateral recess** (of the vertebral canal). A lateral recess is therefore present on both sides of the vertebral canal opposite each of the lumbar pedicles.

The third segment of the radicular canal is formed by the upper part of the intervertebral foramen: that part behind the vertebral body and below the upper pedicle (see Fig. 5.5).

The anatomical relevance of the radicular canals is that the lumbar nerve roots run along them; the anatomy of these nerves is described in Chapter 10. The clinical relevance lies in the propensity for the nerve roots to be compressed by structural alterations in one or other of the structures that form boundaries to the canals.

Another concept of relevance to nerve root compression concerns narrowing of the vertebral canal. The shape and size of the lumbar vertebral canal govern the amount of space available for the nerves that the canal transmits, and if this space is in any way lessened by encroachment of the boundaries of the canal, the condition is referred to as **canal stenosis** or **spinal stenosis**.[20–26]

In transverse section, the lumbar vertebral canal varies in shape. It is oval at upper lumbar levels, becoming triangular more caudally, sometimes assuming a trefoil shape at lower lumbar levels (Fig. 5.6).[27]

The term 'trefoil' refers to a triangular shape in which the angles are stretched or accentuated.[28] The basal angles of the triangular or trefoil outline are formed by the lateral recesses of the vertebral canal.

The shape and size of the vertebral canal can be abnormally small as a result of aberrations in the development

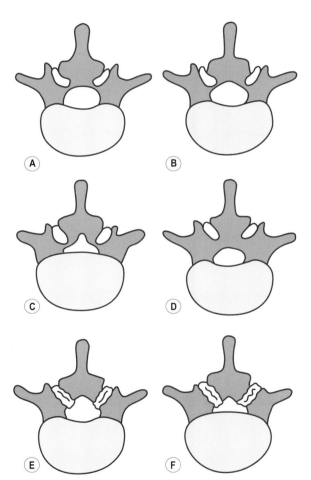

Figure 5.6 The shape of the vertebral canal in transverse section. (A) Oval outline of upper lumbar vertebrae. (B) Triangular shape of lower lumbar vertebrae. (C) Trefoil shape found at lower lumbar levels. (D) Congenital spinal stenosis. (E) Acquired spinal stenosis of a triangular vertebral canal due to arthrosis of the zygapophysial joints. (F) Acquired spinal stenosis of a trefoil vertebral canal due to arthrosis of the zygapophysial joints.

of the neural arch. In relation to the size of the vertebral canal, the pedicles may be too thick or the articular process may be too large. In effect, the space left in the vertebral canal becomes relatively too small for the volume of nerves that it has to transmit. This condition is called congenital or developmental spinal stenosis,[20] but by itself developmental stenosis does not cause compression of nerves. It only renders the patient more likely to compression in the face of the slightest aberration of the boundaries of the vertebral canal.[20,23]

Acquired spinal stenosis occurs whenever any of the structures surrounding the vertebral canal is affected by disease or degeneration that results in enlargement of the structure into the space of the vertebral canal. Examples of such processes include buckling of the ligamentum flavum, osteophytes from the zygapophysial joints or intervertebral discs, and intervertebral disc herniations or bulges.[17,20,23,25] Such changes may occur at single levels in the vertebral canal or at multiple levels, and symptoms may arise either from the disease process that caused the changes or as a result of compression of one or more nerves by the encroaching structure. The pathogenesis of symptoms in spinal stenosis is described further in Chapter 15.

REFERENCES

1. Arnoldi CC, Brodsky AE, Cauchoix J, et al. Lumbar spinal stenosis. *Clin Orthop*. 1976;115:4–5.

2. Bose K, Balasubramaniam P. Nerve root canals of the lumbar spine. *Spine*. 1984;9:16–18.

3. Crock HV. Normal and pathological anatomy of the lumbar spinal nerve root canals. *J Bone Joint Surg*. 1981;63B:487–490.

4. Dommisse GF. Morphological aspects of the lumbar spine and lumbosacral regions. *Orthop Clin North Am*. 1975;6:163–175.

5. Ehni G. Significance of the small lumbar spinal canal:cauda equina compression syndromes due to spondylosis. *J Neurosurg*. 1962;31:490–494.

6. Eisenstein S. The trefoil configuration of the lumbar vertebral canal. *J Bone Joint Surg*. 1980;62B:73–77.

7. Epstein JA, Epstein BS, Levine L. Nerve root compression associated with narrowing of the lumbar spinal canal. *J Neurol Neurosurg Psychiatry*. 1962;25:165–176.

8. Farfan HF, Huberdeau RM, Dubow HI. Lumbar intervertebral disc degeneration. The influence of geometrical features on the pattern of disc degeneration – a post-mortem study. *J Bone Joint Surg*. 1972;54A:492–510.

9. Fernand R, Fox DE. Evaluation of lumbar lordosis. A prospective and retrospective study. *Spine*. 1985;10:799–803.

10. Gilad I, Nissan M. Sagittal evaluation of elemental geometrical dimensions of human vertebrae. *J Anat*. 1985;143:115–120.

11. Hansson T, Bigos S, Beecher P, et al. The lumbar lordosis in acute and chronic low-back pain. *Spine*. 1985;10:154–155.

12. Hellems HK, Keates TE. Measurement of the normal lumbosacral angle. *Am J Roentgenol*. 1971;113:642–645.

13. Heylings DJA. Supraspinous and interspinous ligaments of the human spine. *J Anat*. 1978;125:127–131.

14. Kirkaldy-Willis WH, Wedge JH, Yong-Hing K, et al. Pathology and pathogenesis of lumbar spondylosis and stenosis. *Spine*. 1978;3:319–328.

15. Larsen JL. The posterior surface of the lumbar vertebral bodies. Part 1. *Spine*. 1985;10:50–58.

16. Larsen JL. The posterior surface of the lumbar vertebral bodies. Part 2. An anatomic investigation concerning the curvatures in the horizontal plane. *Spine*. 1985;10:901–906.

17. Parkin IG, Harrison GR. The topographical anatomy of the lumbar epidural space. *J Anat*. 1985;141:211–217.

18. Pearcy M, Portek I, Shepherd J. Three-dimensional X-ray analysis of normal movement in the lumbar spine. *Spine*. 1984;9:294–297.

19. Pelker RR, Gage JR. The correlation of idiopathic lumbar scoliosis and lumbar lordosis. *Clin Orthop*. 1982;163:199–201.

20. Pope MH, Bevins T, Wilder DG, et al. The relationship between anthropometric, postural, muscular, and mobility characteristics of males ages 18–55. *Spine*. 1985;10:644–648.

21. Schmorl G, Junghanns H. *The Human Spine in Health and Disease*, 2nd American ed. New York: Grune & Stratton; 1971:18.

22. Splithoff CA. Lumbosacral junction: roentgenographic comparisons of patients with and without backache. *JAMA*. 1953;152:199–201.

23. Torgerson WR, Dotter WE. Comparative roentgenographic study of the asymptomatic and symptomatic lumbar spine. *J Bone Joint Surg*. 1976;58A:850–853.

24. Verbiest H. A radicular syndrome from developmental narrowing of the lumbar vertebral canal. *J Bone Joint Surg*. 1954;36B:230–237.

25. Verbiest H. Pathomorphological aspects of developmental lumbar stenosis. *Orthop Clin North Am*. 1975;6:177–196.

26. Verbiest H. Fallacies of the present definition, nomenclature and classification of the stenoses of the lumbar vertebral canal. *Spine*. 1976;1:217–225.

27. Vital JM, Lavignolle B, Grenier N, et al. Anatomy of the lumbar radicular canal. *Anat Clin*. 1983;5:141–151.

28. Von Lackum HL. The lumbosacral region. An anatomic study and some clinical observations. *JAMA*. 1924;82:1109–1114.

Chapter | 6 |

The sacrum

The sacrum is a large block of bone located at the base of the vertebral column. It is designed to support the lumbar vertebral column and to transmit loads from the trunk to the pelvic girdle and into the lower limbs.

Its most obvious features are its triangular shape and its curvature. It has a broad, thick upper end but tapers to a blunt point inferiorly (Fig. 6.1). It has a relatively smooth anterior surface that is concave, and a rough posterior surface that is convex. Perforating its anterior surface is a series of paired holes, known as the **anterior sacral foramina**. Perforating its posterior surface is a corresponding series of holes, known as the **posterior sacral foramina**.

PARTICULAR FEATURES

Essentially, the sacrum consists of five fused vertebrae; the particular features of the sacrum can be discerned as the elements of these vertebrae or their vestiges.

In the midline anteriorly, the sacrum exhibits rectangular regions that resemble vertebral bodies embedded within the body of the sacrum (see Fig. 6.1). The top and bottom surfaces of each are marked by transverse ridges between which lie linear regions that resemble narrow intervertebral discs that have ossified. Laterally, bars of bone pass laterally from the vertebral bodies, above and below the anterior sacral foramina. Beyond the foramina, the bars expand, effectively into transverse processes.

Lateral to the foramina, consecutive transverse processes fuse with one another, and constitute the **lateral mass** of the sacrum.

Posteriorly, the posterior elements of the fused vertebrae are evident (Fig. 6.2). Along the midline, a series of prominences represent the spinous processes of the fused, sacral vertebrae. That of the first sacral vertebra (S1) is most prominent; at successively lower levels the spinous processes become less prominent. The line of spinous processes forms what is known as the **median sacral crest**. The laminae of the fifth sacral vertebrae fail to meet in the midline, and a fifth sacral spinous process is not formed. The defect in its place is known as the **sacral hiatus**. Lateral to the spinous processes, plates of bone extend laterally as far as the posterior sacral foramina. These represent the laminae of the sacral vertebrae, but consecutive laminae are fused with one another, there being no ligamentum flavum at sacral levels. Opposite the inferomedial corner of each posterior sacral foramen, the junction of consecutive laminae is marked by a tubercle that represents a fused sacral zygapophysial joint. The line of articular tubercles constitutes the intermediate crest of the sacrum. The tubercles of the S5 vertebra flank the sacral hiatus and form definitive right and left inferior articular process, called the sacral **cornua**, which articulate with the coccyx. The name is derived from the Latin *cornu*, meaning horn, because the cornua resemble little horns at the base of the sacrum.

Between and lateral to the posterior sacral foramina, the transverse processes from the front of the sacrum extend backwards and fuse with the lateral margins of the laminae, thereby enclosing the foramina around their superior, inferior and lateral aspects. Posteriorly, the lateral edge of the transverse processes is marked by a corrugated ridge, the summits of which mark the tips of the transverse

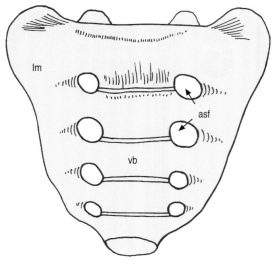

Figure 6.1 Anterior view of the sacrum. asf, anterior sacral foramina; lm, lateral mass; vb, vertebral bodies of the five sacral vertebrae.

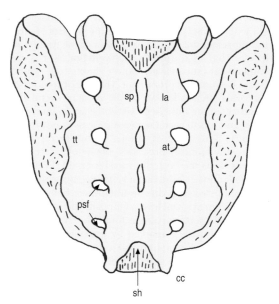

Figure 6.2 Posterior view of the sacrum. at, articular tubercles; cc, cornua; la, laminae; psf, posterior sacral foramina; sh, sacral hiatus; sp, spinous processes; tt, transverse tubercles.

processes and are called the **transverse tubercles**. The ridge forms the lateral crest of the sacrum.

The terminal end of the sacrum is the flattened bottom surface of the S5 vertebral body. It articulates with the coccyx through the sacrococcygeal intervertebral disc.

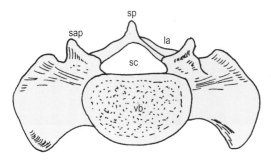

Figure 6.3 View of the upper end of the sacrum. la, lamina; sap, superior articular process; sc, sacral canal; sp, spinous process of S1; vb, vertebral body of S1.

The superior surface of the sacrum presents an appearance similar to that of the L5 vertebra (Fig. 6.3). An area representing the S1 vertebral body is clearly outlined. A broad transverse process extends from it laterally on each side and resembles a wing. For this reason, each is known as an **ala** of the sacrum, derived from the Latin *ala*, meaning wing. Posteriorly, the superior surface presents a pair of **superior articular processes**, which, with the inferior articular processes of the L5 vertebra, form the lumbosacral, or L5–S1, zygapophysial joint. Posterior to the S1 vertebral body, the elements of a neural arch are evident. Short pedicles support the superior articular processes and continue medially as the laminae of S1. The arch surrounds the upper opening of the **sacral canal**, which is the continuation of the vertebral canal from lumbar levels.

The sacral canal is patent throughout the entire length of the sacrum and is enclosed anteriorly by the sacral vertebral bodies, laterally by the transverse processes, and posteriorly by the laminae. Inferiorly, the canal opens through the sacral hiatus. Laterally, it communicates with the exterior of the sacrum through the anterior and posterior sacral foramina. A longitudinal section of the sacrum reveals the length of the sacral canal and the remains of the sacral intervertebral discs (Fig. 6.4).

A lateral view of the sacrum (Fig. 6.5) shows that the transverse processes of the lower two segments are quite narrow from front to back, but those of the first three segments are thick. It is this section of the sacrum that articulates with the ilium. It presents two distinct areas: a smooth surface that has the shape of an ear, for which reason it is called the **auricular surface**; and an irregular, rougher area behind that. The auricular surface is the articular surface for the sacroiliac joint. The rough area is a **ligamentous area** that receives the fibres of the interosseous sacroiliac ligament.

The auricular surface of the sacrum consists of two arms: a superior arm that extends across the lateral surface of the S1 segment and an inferior arm that extends across the S2

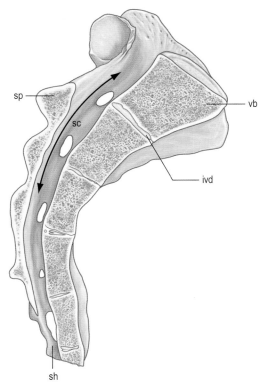

Figure 6.4 Longitudinal section through the sacrum. ivd, remnants of intervertebral disc; sc, sacral canal; sh, sacral hiatus; sp, spinous processes; vb, vertebral bodies.

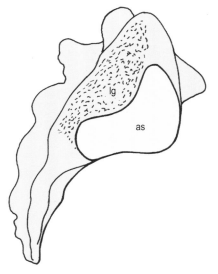

Figure 6.5 Lateral view of sacrum showing the auricular surface (as) and the ligamentous area (lg).

DESIGN FEATURES

segment and a variable distance across the S3 segment. The anterior edges of the superior and inferior arms co-incide with the anterior edge of the lateral surface of the sacrum. Consequently, the anterior edge of the sacroiliac joint coincides with the anterior surface of the sacrum.

The sacrum is massive but not because it bears the load of the vertebral column. After all, the L5 vertebra bears almost as much load as the sacrum but is considerably smaller. Rather, the sacrum is massive because it must be locked into the pelvis between the two ilia. The bulk of the sacrum lies in the bodies and transverse elements of its upper two segments and the upper part of the third segment. These segments are designed to allow the sacrum to be locked into the pelvic girdle and to transfer axial forces laterally into the lower limbs (and vice versa). Further aspects of this design are considered in the context of the sacroiliac joint (see Ch. 14).

Chapter | 7 |

Basic biomechanics

Because of its jargon and mathematical flavour, biomechanics is a subject that is often daunting and overwhelming to students of anatomy. However, certain biomechanical concepts are indispensable for the description and interpretation of the movements and age changes of the lumbar spine. It is therefore appropriate to review and summarise these concepts as a prelude to the chapters discussing these topics.

MOVEMENTS

There are two types of motion that a bone may undergo: **translation** and **rotation**. The essence of translation is that every point on the bone moves in the same direction and to the same extent (Fig. 7.1). Translation occurs whenever a single force or a net single force acts on a bone, and any force that tends to cause translation is called a **shear** force.

Rotation is characterised by all the points on a bone moving in parallel around a curved path centred on some fixed point. The points move in a similar direction but to different extents depending on their radial distance from the fixed point which is known as the centre of rotation (Fig. 7.2). Rotation occurs when two unaligned forces act in opposing directions on different parts of the bone, forming what is known as a force couple (see Fig. 7.2), and the net force tending to cause rotation is referred to as the **torque**. Depending on circumstances, torque may be the result of two opposed forces which may both be muscular actions, or they may be a muscular action and a ligamentous resistance, or they may be gravity opposed by either muscular action or ligamentous resistance.

When a rotating bone is considered in three dimensions it can be seen that all the points throughout the bone can be grouped into individual planes that lie parallel to the direction of motion (Fig. 7.3). In each plane, the points move about a centre located in that plane, and when all the centres of all the planes are lined up they depict a straight line that forms what is known as the **axis of rotation** of the bone.

There is nothing special about an axis of rotation in a biological sense. The points along an axis of rotation do not have any unique biological properties. An axis of rotation is only a mathematical phenomenon created by the net effect of forces acting on a bone. For any rotation, it can be shown that there is a region where all opposing forces cancel out and no net force acts, and this will be the axis of rotation. The axis remains stationary because no net force acts on it. Meanwhile, all the points surrounding the axis are subjected to a net force, and motion will occur around the stationary axis. Thus, a formal definition of an axis of rotation can be 'that region that does not move when two or more opposing, unaligned forces act on a bone'.

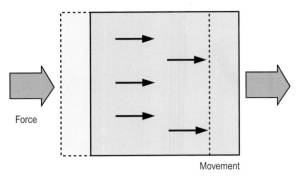

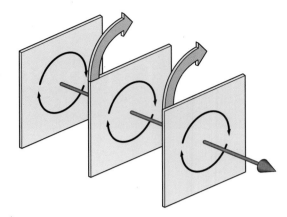

Figure 7.1 Translation. A single net force causes all points in a body to move in parallel, in the same direction and to the same extent.

Figure 7.3 During rotation, the points in any plane of a body move around a centre located in that plane. A line formed by these centres is the axis of rotation of the body.

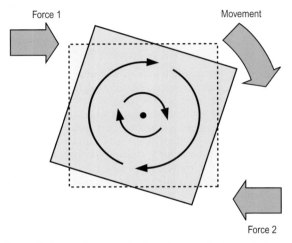

Figure 7.2 Rotation. Two unaligned, opposite forces (a force couple) cause the points in a body to move around a stationary centre.

The location of any axis of rotation is not an intrinsic property of the bone that moves around it. It is a property of the forces that may happen to act on the bone, and different forces will create a different axis of rotation. So-called 'normal' axes of rotation occur only when, during repetitions of a movement, the same forces are consistently applied. With each repetition, the axis of rotation occurs consistently in the same place. However, if at any time one of the applied forces is altered, a new axis will occur.

PLANES OF MOVEMENT

Both translation and rotation can occur in either of two opposite senses which can be variously defined according to circumstances or convention. For example, the motion

can be upwards or downwards, forwards or backwards, clockwise or anticlockwise, and in some conventions positive (+) or negative (−). Furthermore, in three-dimensional space, translation or rotation can occur in any of three fundamental planes. In anatomical terms, these planes are the sagittal, coronal and horizontal planes (Fig. 7.4). Backward or forward rotations are movements in the sagittal plane, as are translations in the backward or forward direction. Side-bending is rotation in the coronal plane, and twisting is rotation in the horizontal plane. A sideways gliding movement across the horizontal plane would be horizontal translation, while movements up or down are described as coronal translations.

Biomechanists prefer to define movements in relation to three imaginary axes drawn through the body, which are labelled X, Y and Z.[1,2] The X axis passes sideways through the body; the Y axis passes through it vertically; and the Z axis passes through it from back to front (Fig. 7.5). Movements can then be described as along or around any particular axis. Thus, sagittal translation is translation along the Z axis; sideways gliding movements are translations along the X axis; and up and down movements are along the Y axis. Forward bending is rotation around the X axis; side-bending is rotation about the Z axis; and twisting movements are rotations around the Y axis. The key to this nomenclature lies in the prepositions used. Translations are movements *along* one of the axes while rotations are movements *around* one of the axes.

The advantage of the biomechanists' convention is that the dimensions of movements are accurately and unambiguously defined. However, the terms 'X', 'Y' and 'Z' are unfamiliar and anonymous to all except to those who use them regularly. The terms 'sagittal', 'coronal' and 'horizontal' are somewhat more meaningful because of their use in other areas of anatomy, and these are the terms used in this text. In the anatomical system the movements are

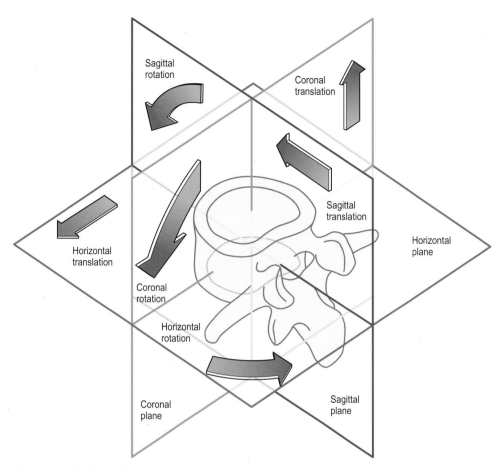

Figure 7.4 Planes and directions of motion: anatomical system.

perceived to occur *in* or *along* the plane in question, irrespective of whether the movement is a translation or a rotation. For reference, the equivalence of various terms derived from the anatomical system, the biomechanists' convention and colloquial vocabulary is shown in Table 7.1.

Because of difficulties in appreciating the distinctions between translations and rotations in the horizontal and coronal planes, the term 'axial' has been introduced in Table 7.1. Thus, the term 'axial rotation' replaces 'horizontal rotation' to refer to rotation in the horizontal plane, i.e. around the long axis of the body. The term 'axial translation' replaces 'coronal translation' to refer to movement up or down, or along the long axis of the body, and to distinguish this movement from sideways translations in the horizontal plane, which are described as horizontal or lateral translations.

To specify the direction of axial translations, the terms 'cephalad', meaning towards the head, and 'caudad', meaning towards the tail, are used in Table 7.1. Although

perhaps cumbersome and unfamiliar, these terms are accurate and applicable in all situations. The more familiar terms 'upward' and 'downward' are applicable for axial translations in the upright position but they are not strictly applicable in describing motions of vertebrae in patients who might be lying down. To overcome this difficulty, the more colloquial terms of 'distraction' and 'compression' are more usually used instead of 'cephalad' and 'caudad axial translation'. Similarly, the term 'lateral bending' is more convenient and is preferred to 'coronal rotation'.

In this text, the term 'sagittal' rotation is strictly used to refer to forward and backward rotatory movements. Although the terms 'flexion' and 'extension' are commonly used to describe this motion, these terms are insufficiently accurate when applied to movements of individual lumbar vertebrae. Flexion and extension are not pure movements of the lumbar vertebrae because, as will be shown in Chapter 8, these movements involve a combination of both sagittal translation and sagittal rotation. The terms 'flexion' and 'extension' may be used to describe forward

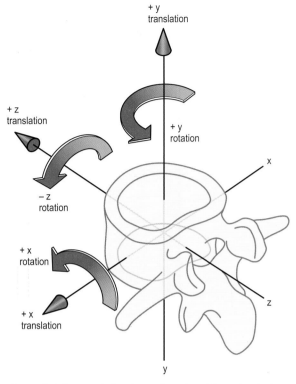

Figure 7.5 Axes and directions of motion: biomechanical system.

bending and backward bending of the lumbar spine in a general sense, but in relation to movements of individual vertebrae it should be understood that the terms refer to a combination of both sagittal rotation and sagittal translation.

The relevance of these explicit definitions of motion is extensive. In the first instance, the motion of individual vertebrae is often complex, and no single term can describe the motion. Nevertheless, it can always be described as some combination of the fundamental movements listed in Table 7.1. Furthermore, each component of motion of the lumbar spine is exerted and resisted by different mechanisms, and to appreciate how these mechanisms act, each needs to be analysed in relation to the particular component of motion that it controls. This type of analysis is undertaken in Chapter 8.

STRESS–STRAIN

To stretch a collagen fibre, a force must be applied to it. Once it starts to stretch, the fibre resists elongation by generating a resisting force due to the chemical bonds between collagen fibrils, between tropocollagen molecules, between collagen fibres, and between collagen fibres and proteoglycans (see Ch. 2). By convention, the applied or elongating force is known as the applied **stress** and the extent to which a fibre is elongated is known as the **strain**. Stress is measured in units of force (newtons) and strain is measured as the fractional or percentage increase in

Table 7.1 Descriptive terms of motion. By convention, the direction of any rotation is defined according to the direction of movement of the most anterior point on the bone

Anatomical system	Biomechanical system	Colloquial description
Anterior sagittal translation	+Z translation	Forward slide or glide
Posterior sagittal translation	–Z translation	Backward slide
Cephalad coronal translation	+Y translation	Longitudinal or axial distraction
Caudal coronal translation	–Y translation	Longitudinal or axial compression
Left horizontal translation	+X translation	Left lateral slide
Right horizontal translation	–X translation	Right lateral slide
Anterior sagittal rotation	+X rotation	Forward bend, 'flexion'
Posterior sagittal rotation	–X rotation	Backward bend, 'extension'
Left coronal rotation	–Z rotation	Left lateral bend
Right coronal rotation	+Z rotation	Right lateral bend
Left horizontal rotation	+Y rotation	Left axial rotation
Right horizontal rotation	–Y rotation	Right axial rotation

length relative to initial length. Thus a fibre of length L_0 when stretched to a new length L_1 undergoes a strain of L_1/L_0 or $L_1/L_0 \times 100\%$.

Particular terms are used to specify different types of stress and strain according to the direction in which a structure is deformed. When a structure is stretched longitudinally, the deforming force is known as **tension** and the structure undergoes tension strain. If a structure is squashed, the deforming stress is **compression** and it undergoes compression strain. The latter is measured as the fractional or percentage decrease in height of the structure. Forces that cause two vertebrae to slide with respect to one another are referred to as **shear** forces and the strain that occurs in the intervening intervertebral disc is referred to as shear strain. The distinction between shear and tension is that tension conventionally applies to forces exerted along the long axis of a structure, whereas shear forces are applied across this axis. When an object twists, it is said to undergo **torsion**. A force that causes torsion is a torque and the resultant strain is referred to as torsion strain.

At rest, single collagen fibres are usually buckled, and the wavy shape they assume is referred to as **crimp**.[3-6] When stress is applied to a collagen fibre, the first effect is to straighten this crimp. Little energy is required to do this as there are no major chemical bonds that maintain it. Thus, a crimped collagen fibre will elongate in response to little applied force. However, once crimp has been removed, the collagen fibre starts to resist strongly any further elongation. The stress attempts to break the bonds between the collagen fibrils and tropocollagen molecules. Energy is required to oppose strain and perhaps eventually to break these bonds. Consequently, more force is required to produce further elongation of the collagen fibre. If sufficient force is applied, the bonds may break, and when this occurs in a substantial number of bonds, the collagen fibre ceases to resist elongation and is said to 'fail'. Once the collagen fibre has failed, only small forces are required to tear apart its now unbonded component fibrils and molecules.

The mechanical behaviour of collagen fibres subject to stress can be depicted graphically,[7] as in Figure 7.6; such graphs are known as stress–strain curves. The curve exhibits three main regions. The first region, known as the 'toe' phase, reflects the phase when crimp is being removed from the collagen fibre. The second, or linear, region is the steep slope along the middle of the curve. Mathematical calculations reveal that the junction of the toe phase and the linear region represents the point where crimp has been maximally removed from the fibre and the stress starts to stretch the collagen fibre longitudinally.[6,7] The linear region represents the phase when bonds within and between collagen fibrils are being strained and some are being broken. The peak of the curve represents the phase of failure of the collagen fibre, when substantial numbers of bonds are irreversibly broken. As depicted by the last

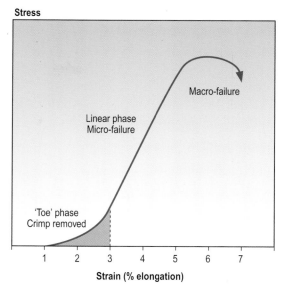

Figure 7.6 Stress–strain curve of collagen. *(Based on Abrahams 1967[7] and Shah et al.1977.[6])*

part of the curve, once failure has occurred, elongation can continue with ever decreasing amounts of stress being required.

A key feature of the mechanical properties of collagen is that bonds within and between collagen fibrils start to be strained and broken somewhere after 3% and 4% elongation of the fibre has occurred. Consequently, about 4% elongation is the maximum a fibre can sustain without risking microscopic damage.

Collagenous tissues, like ligaments and joint capsules, behave in a similar manner to isolated collagen fibres, and exhibit similar stress–strain curves[5,6,8,9] but certain additional mechanical events are involved (Fig. 7.7). In addition to the removal of crimp, the toe phase may represent the removal of any macroscopic slack in the ligament. During the second phase, collagen fibres are being rearranged in the stressed structure. Fibres that, at rest, are curved or run obliquely in the three-dimensional lattice of the ligament or capsule are straightened to line up with the applied force. Thus, when the three-dimensional lattice is stressed, any bonds between separate collagen fibres and between collagen fibres and their surrounding proteoglycan matrix are strained. Furthermore, to make way for the rearrangement of collagen fibres, water and proteoglycans may need to be displaced from between the collagen fibres.

All of these processes require energy: to strain the bonds to move the collagen fibres and proteoglycans; and to squeeze out water. Thus, to achieve continued elongation, more force must be applied and this creates the steep slope of the second phase (see Fig. 7.7). Eventually, after the

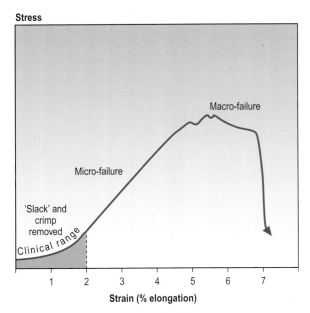

Figure 7.7 Stress–strain curve for a ligament. *(Based on Nordin and Frankel 1980[8] and Noyes 1977.[9])*

collagen fibres, proteoglycans and water have been rearranged, the bonds within individual collagen fibres are strained. In the face of increasing stress, these bonds and those between collagen fibres will fail and the entire structure fails.

The proportion of collagen fibres that needs to fail before macroscopic failure of a ligament or capsule occurs is not known, and it is not possible to predict the stress–strain curves for different structures on the basis of the number or nature of their constituent collagen fibres. Therefore the mechanical behaviour of different structures has to be derived empirically by subjecting several samples of the same structure to known stresses and obtaining average stress–strain curves representative of the particular structure.

The value of stress–strain curves is that they graphically depict the mechanical properties of collagenous (and other) structures, notably their strength and the way in which they resist elongation. In turn, the mechanical behaviour reflects the biochemical properties of the structure, for alterations in the proteoglycan content and the bonding within and between collagen fibres will affect the way a ligament or a capsule can resist applied forces.

To a certain extent, physical examination involves obtaining a stress–strain curve for a joint and its capsule or ligaments. When passive movement is induced, a stress is applied, and strain is reflected in terms of both the range of movement observed and the form of the palpated resistance to movement. It is important to realise, however, that clinical examination only studies the early part of the

stress–strain curve, no further than just beyond the toe phase.[8] The limit is well within the 4% elongation at which microscopic injury occurs. Physical examination rarely (and should not) enter into the second phase, for then it is actually inducing microfailure of the structure, and risks macrofailure. Physical examination therefore gains access to only a part of the total stress–strain curve possible. Nevertheless, it does detect some of the physical properties of the structure examined, which can be interpreted in the light of knowledge of the microstructure and biochemistry of the structure examined, and knowledge of its total mechanical behaviour as determined in cadaveric and post-mortem material.

STIFFNESS

The stiffness of a given structure is its resistance to deformation and can be measured by the force required to produce a unit elongation or deformation.[10] In mathematical terms, it is the slope of the stress–strain curve of a structure. Stiffer structures resist deformation and the slope of their stress–strain curves will be steeper. In biochemical terms, stiffness implies a greater degree of bonding between collagen fibres, or between collagen fibres and their surrounding matrix.

INITIAL RANGE OF MOVEMENT

If a joint is moved passively or actively by a constant force, a point is reached where no further movement appears possible. The resistance in the capsule and ligaments of the joint balances exactly the force attempting to move the joint. The distance moved by the joint up to this point is known as the **initial range of movement**. If a stress–strain curve were constructed for the joint, the initial range of movement would be found to occur somewhere early in the second phase of the curve, just after the toe phase when collagen bonding is starting to resist the movement.

Application of a greater force would strain the resisting structures further and a new, greater initial range of movement would be perceived. The amount of increased range would be dependent both on the increase in force and on the stiffness of the joint and its ligaments. However, to obtain a substantially greater initial range of movement, considerably larger forces would need to be applied to most joints and ligaments. Such larger forces are not usually possible during normal clinical examination.

With the forces used in clinical examination, the initial range of movement remains early in the second phase of the stress–strain curve, and even if the applied force varies somewhat with the strength of the examiner, the resistance of the joint is such that the differences in perceived range of movement are not great. Consequently, the initial range of movement as perceived from clinical examination falls in a narrow range and can be called the normal range of movement.

CREEP

Initial ranges of movement are usually measured on the basis of a brief application of force. The force is applied until the range of movement is maximal, and once the range is measured, the force is released. However, if a constant force is left applied to a collagenous structure for a more prolonged period, further movement is detectable. This movement is small in amplitude, occurs slowly, almost imperceptibly, and is consequently known as **creep**.

Graphically, creep is seen as continued displacement when a constant force is maintained at some point on a stress–strain curve (Fig. 7.8). The time over which creep can be measured is optional, and various studies have employed times varying from minutes to hours.[10–14]

The biochemical and structural basis of creep is not known for certain but it appears to be due to the gradual rearrangement of collagen fibres, proteoglycans and water in the ligament or capsule being stressed. Forces of short duration may not act long enough to squeeze water out of a ligament or to allow the rearrangement of collagen that could possibly occur. The force is removed before maximal displacement has had a chance to occur. In contrast,

sustained forces allow for these displacements to occur, whereupon the ligament or capsule can elongate slightly as a result of the internal readjustment of its constituents.

The academic relevance of creep is that it provides an indirect though readily obtainable measure of the interactions of collagen, proteoglycans and water in a ligament or capsule. By studying the creep of structures, one can determine how these interactions vary with age or in the face of disease processes or injury. However, creep is not just a laboratory phenomenon as it occurs regularly in activities of daily living.

Many occupational groups (e.g. stonemasons, bricklayers, roofing carpenters), regularly submit their lumbar spines to prolonged load-bearing in flexion. Once they achieve such a posture there is often little movement away from it, and their lumbar joints will creep. The possible significance of this phenomenon is discussed below.

HYSTERESIS

Most structures, and certainly all biological tissues, exhibit differences in mechanical behaviour during loading versus unloading. Loading produces a characteristic stress–strain curve but gradual release of the load produces a different stress–strain curve. Restoration of the initial length of a ligament occurs at a lesser rate and to a lesser extent than did the deformation (Fig. 7.9). This difference in behaviour is referred to as **hysteresis** and reflects the amount of energy lost when the structure was initially stressed.

When a structure is deformed, the energy applied to it goes into deforming the structure and into straining the bonds within it. For collagenous tissues, some of the energy goes into displacing proteoglycans and water, re-arranging the collagen fibres, and perhaps even into breaking some of the bonds between collagen fibres. Once used in this way, this energy is not immediately available to restore the structure to its original shape. Displaced water, for example, does not remain in the structure exerting some sort of back-pressure attempting to restore its original form. It is squeezed out of the structure, and the energy used to displace the water is no longer available to the system. If chemical bonds are broken they cannot act to restore the form of the structure.

Thus, with less energy available to restore the structure, the rate and extent of its restoration are reduced. When all applied forces are completely removed, the final length of the ligament or capsule may remain greater than its original length (or less in the case of compressed structures). This difference between initial and final length is referred to as a 'set'.

In general, hysteresis and a residual set do not occur if a structure is stressed only in the toe phase of its stress–strain curve, as bonds within and between the collagen

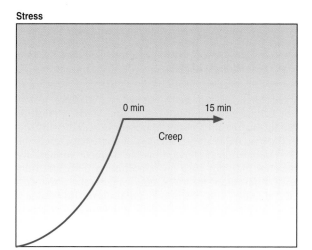

Figure 7.8 Stress–strain curve illustrating creep. Despite maintenance of a constant load, elongation occurs with the passage of time.

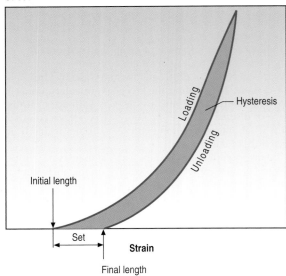

Figure 7.9 Stress–strain curve illustrating hysteresis. When unloaded, a structure regains shape at a rate different to that at which it deformed. Any difference between the initial and final shape is the 'set'.

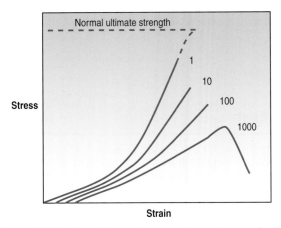

Figure 7.10 Fatigue failure. After a single application of an increasing force, a structure exhibits a typical stress–strain curve (1). However, after 10, 100 and 1000 repeated applications of a stress less than the initial ultimate tensile stress, the structure becomes less stiff and may fail at substantially less stress than its original ultimate tensile strain.

fibres are not broken. However, the further a structure is stressed beyond its toe phase, the more bonds are broken and the greater the hysteresis and set.[7]

In time, collagen fibres and proteoglycans in a structure may be rearranged into their usual configuration, and any displaced water is eventually reabsorbed, restoring the structure to its original form. Under these circumstances any set disappears, and the structure regains its original size.

A set often occurs after creep. When the applied force is released, the structure does not immediately spring back to its original shape, although it may do so in time. However, if bonds between or within collagen fibres have been broken, the set may not disappear until and unless the bonds are exactly reconstituted. If the original bonds are not reformed, or if new bonds are formed in the set position, the set may persist indefinitely.

This phenomenon has implications in the interpretation of trauma to ligaments or capsules. The energy lost in breaking the tissue may not be recoverable, and the original structure is not fully reformed. Healing may occur in a set position, and this may compromise the mechanical function of the structure. Healing in a set position effectively lengthens the ligament and it will therefore accommodate greater than normal initial ranges of movement, which may not be desirable.

The phenomena of creep and hysteresis are also of particular relevance to the interpretation of sustained insults to ligaments and capsules. A ligament may be subjected to forces well within its load-bearing capacity but if these forces are sustained for prolonged periods, the ligament will creep, and because of hysteresis, eventual release of the load does not result in the immediate restoration of the form and microstructure of the ligament. The ligament requires time to reform fully. In the meantime, the mechanical properties of the ligament have been altered. Its stress–strain capacity is different from normal, and until the structure is fully reformed it cannot be expected to sustain reapplied loads in the normal, or accustomed, way. Therefore, the structure may be liable to injury during this vulnerable period of restoration.

FATIGUE FAILURE

When forces are repeatedly applied to a material, it does not behave the same way each time. Each application produces a certain amount of hysteresis, and the structure of the material is altered slightly, albeit perhaps temporarily. However, if the repetitions are frequent enough, the material may not have an opportunity to recover fully. Each application, therefore, effectively weakens the material slightly. With one or two applications this weakness may not be apparent. However, following many repetitions, the small weaknesses accumulate, and weakness in the material becomes apparent. Indeed, after several frequent repetitions of a stress, the material may fail at a stress that is substantially less than that required to damage the material following a single application of a force.

This phenomenon is referred to as fatigue failure; its behaviour is illustrated graphically in Figure 7.10. An initial loading reveals the mechanical properties of the material. Its stiffness is evident, and the **ultimate tensile stress** is the force that would be required to disrupt the material completely upon one application of a force. However, if the material is repeatedly stressed, it exhibits an evolution of mechanical properties. Its stiffness decreases and, in particular, the stress at failure drops. As a result, by repeatedly stressing a material at forces less than those required to break it after one loading, the material can eventually be disrupted. A common analogy is the ability to break a wire or paper clip, not by pulling or bending it once but by repeatedly bending it.

Another way of plotting fatigue failure is to display the evolution of strain over time as a force of constant peak magnitude is applied (Fig. 7.11). The graph shows the repeated cycles of force being applied. Initially, the force applied results in a relatively constant strain but at some point the strain suddenly increases and the specimen operates at a new strain even though the stress has not changed. This behaviour indicates that something in the material has failed, allowing it to exhibit greater deformation for the same stress.

How rapidly a material undergoes fatigue failure is governed by the nature of the material itself and by the magnitude of the offending stress and its periodicity. Larger stresses are more likely to achieve failure sooner; smaller stresses will require more repetitions. Infrequent repetitions may allow biological materials to recover; frequent repetitions deny this recovery and may achieve failure sooner.

The clinical importance of fatigue failure is that damage to tissues may occur without a history of major or obvious trauma. Indeed, studies of human spinal tissues have shown that an anulus fibrosus typically fails after 3000 repetitions but can fail after as few as 20 repetitions of a force equal to 60% of the ultimate tensile stress.[15] Fractures of the vertebral endplate occur within 1000 repetitions but in some cases they occur after as few as 30–80 applications of a stress equal to 50–80% of ultimate compressive strength.[16] The forces involved are within the range of those encountered in activities of daily living, and these experimental studies warn that in the face of repetitive loading, elements of the lumbar spine can be injured by forces considerably less than those expected for an acute injury.

FORCES AND MOMENTS

When an object is free to move and is acted upon by a force, it will accelerate in the same direction as the applied force (Fig. 7.12). The force (F) is related to the acceleration (a) by the equation

$$F = ma$$

where 'm' is the mass of the object in kilograms. In the MKS system, the unit of force is a newton (N) and has the dimensions of kilogram metres per second squared (kg m s^{-2}).

For an object in the Earth's field of gravity, its weight is produced by the force of gravity trying to accelerate it towards the centre of the Earth (see Fig. 7.12). The mass of the object (m) is related to its weight by the acceleration produced by the Earth's gravitational field, i.e.

$$Weight = F = mg$$

where 'g' = 9.8 m s^{-2}. An object in the Earth's gravitational field therefore exerts a downward force whose magnitude in newtons is about 10 times its mass measured in kilograms.

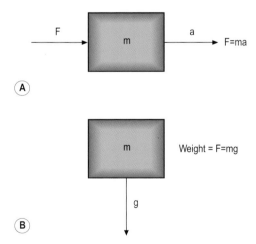

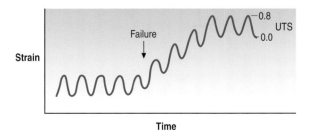

Figure 7.11 Fatigue failure. When a force of constant peak magnitude is applied cyclically, the material initially deforms repeatedly to the same extent, but at some point the strain increases even though the load has not changed. This point indicates the onset of fatigue failure. UTS, ultimate tensile stress.

Figure 7.12 The nature of forces. (A) A force (F) acting on a mass (m) imparts an acceleration (a) on the mass in the same direction as the force. (B) When gravity acts downwards on an object, the force it exerts is the weight of the object, which is proportional to its mass (m) and the gravitational acceleration of the Earth (g).

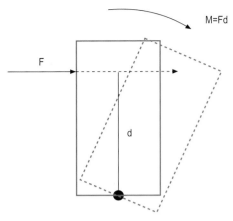

Figure 7.13 The nature of moments. When a force acts eccentrically on an object that is fixed at some point, the force tends to bend or rotate the object. This bending effect is a moment (M) whose magnitude is proportional to the magnitude of the force (F) and the perpendicular distance (d) between the fixed point and the direction of the force.

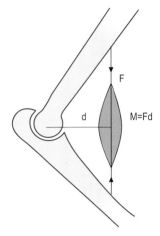

Figure 7.15 Muscles exert moments on joints that they move. The magnitude of the moment (M) is proportional to the force (F) exerted by the muscle and the perpendicular distance (d) between the line of action of the muscle and the axis of rotation of the joint.

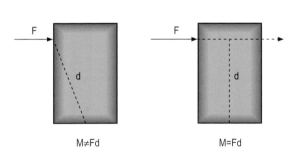

Figure 7.14 Moments (M) are calculated using not the distance (d) between the fixed point and the site of application of the force (F), but the perpendicular distance (d) between the fixed point and the direction of the force (F).

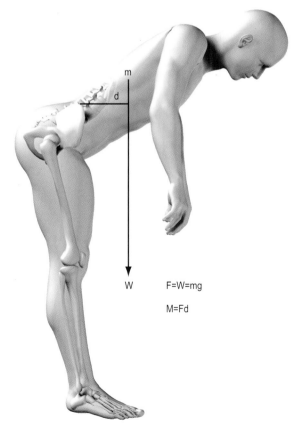

Figure 7.16 Flexion moments are exerted on the lumbar spine when the trunk leans forwards. The force (F) exerted is the weight (W) of the trunk above the lumbar spine. This force acts downwards from the centre of mass of the upper trunk (m). The moment arm (d) is the distance from the lumbar spine to the line of gravity (g) acting on the upper trunk. The magnitude of the flexion moment (M) is the product of the force and the moment arm.

If an object is acted upon by a force but is fixed at some point, the object is not free to move in the direction of the applied force. Instead, it will tend to bend or rotate about the fixed point (Fig. 7.13). A force that causes bending is known as a **moment**, and its magnitude is proportional to both the magnitude of the force applied and the perpendicular distance between the line of force and the fixed point, i.e.

$$Moment = Fd$$

The unit of measure of a moment is newton-metres, the dimensions of which are kg m^2 s^{-2}.

Intuitively, it should be obvious that the bending capacity of a moment will be greater either if the force applied is greater or if the distance from the fixed point is greater. (Compare the effort required to bend a short object versus a longer object of the same material.)

It is critical to appreciate that a moment is not calculated according to the distance between the fixed point and the point on the object at which the force is applied. It is calculated according to the perpendicular distance between the fixed point and the **direction** of the force (Fig. 7.14). This distance is referred to as the **moment arm**.

The concept of moments applies to all situations where joints bend, whether they are acted upon by muscles or gravity. The moment generated by a muscle is the product of the force exerted by the muscle and the perpendicular distance between the axis of rotation of the joint and the line of action of the muscle (Fig. 7.15). In the case of the vertebral column, movements such as flexion are frequently exerted by gravity. The force involved is the weight of the trunk leaning forwards of the lumbar spine and it is exerted vertically downwards on the centre of mass of the trunk (Fig. 7.16). The magnitude of the force acting on a given joint in the lumbar spine is calculated as the mass of the trunk above that joint multiplied by g. The moment arm is the perpendicular distance from the joint in question to the line of action of the force (see Fig. 7.16). Clearly, the further a subject leans forward, the longer this moment arm and the greater the resultant moment. Conversely, the more upright a subject stands, the shorter the moment arm and the smaller the flexion moment (Fig. 7.17).

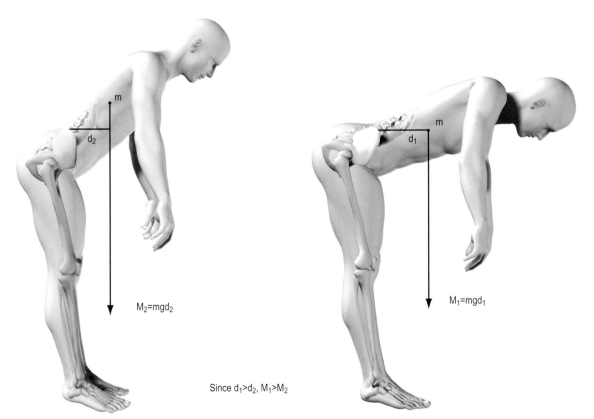

$M_2 = mgd_2$

$M_1 = mgd_1$

Since $d_1 > d_2$, $M_1 > M_2$

Figure 7.17 Different angles of flexion of the trunk result in moments (M) of different magnitude being applied to the lumbar spine. Even though the mass of the trunk (m) and the gravitational acceleration of the Earth (g) remains the same, different moments result from differences in the moment arms (d) that occur.

REFERENCES

1. White AA, Panjabi MM. *Clinical Biomechanics of the Spine*. Philadelphia: Lippincott; 1978.

2. White AA, Panjabi MM. The basic kinematics of the human spine. A review of past and current knowledge. *Spine*. 1978;3:12–20.

3. Diamant J, Keller A, Baer E, et al. Collagen ultrastructure and its relation to mechanical properties as a function of ageing. *Proc Roy Soc (series B)*. 1972;180:293–315.

4. Kirby MC, Sikoryn TA, Hukins DWL, et al. Structure and mechanical properties of the longitudinal ligaments and ligamentum flavum of the spine. *J Biomed Eng*. 1989;11:192–196.

5. Shah JS. Structure, morphology and mechanics of the lumbar spine. In: Jayson MIV, ed. *The Lumbar Spine and Backache*. 2nd ed. London: Pitman; 1980:Ch. 13, 359–405.

6. Shah JS, Jayson MIV, Hampson WGJ. Low tension studies of collagen fibres from ligaments of the human spine. *Ann Rheum Dis*. 1977;36:139–148.

7. Abrahams M. Mechanical behaviour of tendon in vitro. A preliminary report. *Med Biol Eng*. 1967;5:433–443.

8. Nordin M, Frankel VH. Biomechanics of collagenous tissues. In: Frankel VH, Nordin M, eds. *Basic Biomechanics of the Skeletal System*. Philadelphia: Lea & Febiger; 1980: Ch. 3, 87–110.

9. Noyes FR. Fundamental properties of knee ligaments and alterations induced by immobilization. *Clin Orthop*. 1977;123:210–242.

10. Twomey L, Taylor J. Flexion creep deformation and hysteresis in the lumbar vertebral column. *Spine*. 1982;7:116–122.

11. Kazarian LE. Dynamic response characteristics of the human lumbar vertebral column. *Acta Orthop Scand*. 1972;(Suppl)146:1–86.

12. Kazarian LE. Creep characteristics of the human spinal column. *Orthop Clin North Am*. 1975;6: 3–18.

13. Koreska J, Robertson D, Mills R H, et al. Biomechanics of the lumbar spine and its clinical significance. *Orthop Clin North Am*. 1977;8:121–123.

14. Markolf KL. Deformation of the thoracolumbar intervertebral joints in response to external loads. *J Bone Joint Surg*. 1972;54A:511–533.

15. Green TP, Adams MA, Dolan P. Tensile properties of the annulus fibrosus II. Ultimate tensile strength and fatigue life. *Eur Spine J*. 1993;2:209–214.

16. Hansson TH, Keller TS, Spengler DM. Mechanical behaviour of the human lumbar spine. II. Fatigue strength during dynamic compressive loading. *J Orthop Res*. 1987;5:479–487.

Chapter | 8 |

Movements of the lumbar spine

The principal movements exhibited by the lumbar spine and its individual joints are axial compression, axial distraction, flexion, extension, axial rotation and lateral flexion. Horizontal translation does not naturally occur as an isolated, pure movement, but is involved in axial rotation.

AXIAL COMPRESSION

Axial compression is the movement that occurs during weight-bearing in the upright posture, or as a result of contraction of the longitudinal back muscles (see Ch. 9). With respect to the interbody joints, the weight-bearing mechanisms of the intervertebral discs have already been described in Chapter 2, where it was explained how the nucleus pulposus and anulus fibrosus cooperate to transmit weight from one vertebra to the next. It is now appropriate to add further details.

During axial compression, both the anulus fibrosus and nucleus pulposus bear the load and transmit it to the vertebral endplates (see Ch. 2). In a normal disc, the outermost fibres of the anulus do not participate in bearing the load. Otherwise, the compression load is borne uniformly across the inner, anterior anulus and nucleus, but with a peak stress over the inner, posterior anulus (Fig. 8.1).[2–4] In older discs this posterior peak is larger.[3,4]

Compression squeezes water out of the disc.[5–7] Under a 100 kPa load, the nucleus loses some 8% of its water and the anulus loses 11%.[8–10] The loss of water results in a relative increase in the concentration of electrolytes remaining in the disc, and this increased concentration serves to re-imbibe water into the disc once compression is released.[9]

Under compression, the vertebral bodies around a disc approximate and the disc bulges radially.[6,8,11] The vertebral bodies approximate because the vertebral endplates bow away from the disc.[11–13] Indeed, the deflection of each endplate is almost equal to half the displacement of the vertebrae.[12] This amounts to a strain of approximately 3% in the endplate.[12] The disc bulges because, as the anulus loses height peripherally, the redundant length must somehow be accommodated, i.e. the lamellae of the anulus must buckle. Nuclear pressure normally prevents buckling inwards, leaving outward radial bulging as the only means of accommodating loss of disc height. The bulging is greater anteriorly than at the posterolateral corner of the disc, and induces a strain in the anulus fibrosus of about 2% per mm loss of disc height.[14] Removing part of the nucleus (as occurs in discectomy) increases both the loss of disc height and the radial bulge.[15]

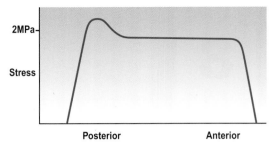

Figure 8.1 The stress profile of an intervertebral disc from the posterior to the anterior anulus during axial compression. *(Based on Adams et al. 1993.[1])*

The load on the endplate during compression is evenly distributed over its surface, there being no greater load over the nucleus pulposus than over the anulus fibrosus.[16] The endplate bows, however, because its periphery its strongly supported by the underlying cortical bone of the vertebra, whereas its central portion is supported by the slightly weaker trabecular bone of the vertebral body. This trabecular support is critical to the integrity of the endplate.

When excessive loads are applied to normal intervertebral discs, the trabeculae under the endplates fracture and the endplates themselves fracture, typically in their central region, i.e. over the nucleus pulposus, rather than over the anulus.[5,17–20] With the application of very great loads the entire endplate may fracture.[19–21]

In this context, it is noteworthy that the endplates are the weakest components of the intervertebral disc in the face of axial compression. Provided the anulus is healthy and intact, increasing the load causes one or other of the endplates to fail, by fracturing, sooner than the anulus fibrosus fails, by rupturing.[5,19,20] This phenomenon has particular ramifications in the pathology of compression injuries of the lumbar spine and disc degradation (see Ch. 15), and has its basis in the relative strengths of the anulus fibrosus and the bone of the vertebral body. Calculations have shown that the anulus fibrosus can withstand a pressure of 3.2×10^7 Nm^{-2} but cancellous bone yields at 3.4×10^6 Nm^{-2}.[8] Consequently, endplates would be expected to fail sooner than the anulus fibrosus when the disc is subjected to axial compression.

With respect to the vertebral bodies, in adults under the age of 40, between 25% and 55% of the weight applied to a vertebral body is borne by the trabecular bone;[11,22,23] the rest is borne by the cortical shell. In older individuals this proportion changes, for reasons explained in Chapter 13. Overall, the strength of a vertebral body is quite great but varies considerably between individuals. The ultimate compressive strength of a vertebral body ranges between 3 and 12 kN.[24,25] This strength is directly related to bone density[24,26,27] and can be predicted to within 1 kN on the basis of bone density and endplate area determined by CT

scanning.[28] It also seems to be inversely related to physical activity, in that active individuals have stronger vertebrae.[29]

Another factor that increases the load-bearing capacity of the vertebral body is the blood within its marrow spaces and intra-osseous veins (see Ch. 11). Compression of the vertebral body and bulging of the endplates causes blood to be extruded from the vertebra.[6] Because this process requires energy, it buffers the vertebral body, to some extent, from the compressive loads applied to it.[20]

During compression, intervertebral discs undergo an initial period of rapid creep, deforming about 1.5 mm in the first 2–10 min depending on the size of the applied load.[30–32] Subsequently, a much slower but definite creep continues at about 1 mm per hour.[32] Depending on age, a plateau is attained by about 90 min, beyond which no further creep occurs.[31]

Creep underlies the variation in height changes undergone by individuals during activities of daily living. Over a 16-hour day, the pressure sustained by intervertebral discs during walking and sitting causes loss of fluid from the discs, which results in a 10% loss in disc height[10] and a 16% loss of disc volume.[33] Given that intervertebral discs account for just under a quarter of the height of the vertebral column, the 10% fluid loss results in individuals being 1–2% shorter at the end of a day.[34–36] This height is restored during sleep or reclined rest, when the vertebral column is not axially compressed and the discs are rehydrated by the osmotic pressure of the disc proteoglycans.[10] Moreover, it has been demonstrated that rest in the supine position with the lower limbs flexed and raised brings about a more rapid return to full disc height than does rest in the extended supine position.[36]

The pressure within intervertebral discs can be measured using special needles,[37–39] and disc pressure measurement, or discometry, provides an index of the stresses applied to a disc in various postures and movements. Several studies have addressed this issue although for technical reasons virtually all have studied only the L3–4 disc.

In the upright standing posture, the load on the disc is about 70 kPa.[38] Holding a weight of 5 kg in this posture raises the disc pressure to about 700 kPa.[38,40] The changes in disc pressure during other movements and manoeuvres are described in Chapter 9.

Although the interbody joints are designed as the principal weight-bearing components of the lumbar spine (see Ch. 2), there has been much interest in the role that the zygapophysial joints play in weight-bearing. The earliest studies in this regard provided indirect estimates of the load borne by the zygapophysial joints based on measurements of intradiscal pressure, and it was reported that the zygapophysial joints carried approximately 20% of the vertical load applied to an intervertebral joint.[37] This conclusion, however, was later retracted.[41]

Subsequent studies have variously reported that the zygapophysial joints can bear 28%[42] or 40%[43] of a vertically applied load. To the contrary, others have reported that 'compression did not load the facet joints … very much',[44] and that 'provided the lumbar spine is slightly flattened … all the intervertebral compressive force is resisted by the disc'.[45]

Reasons for these differences in the conclusions relate to the experimental techniques used and to the differing appreciation of the anatomy of the zygapophysial joints and their behaviour in axial compression.

Although the articular surfaces of the lumbar zygapophysial joints are curved in the transverse plane (see Ch. 3), in the sagittal and coronal planes they run straight up and down (although see Ch. 11). Thus, zygapophysial joints, in a neutral position, cannot sustain vertically applied loads. Their articular surfaces run parallel to one another and parallel to the direction of the applied load. If an intervertebral joint is axially compressed, the articular surfaces of the zygapophysial joints will simply slide past one another. For the zygapophysial joints to participate in weight-bearing in erect standing, some aberration in their orientation must occur, and either of two mechanisms may operate singly or in combination to recruit the zygapophysial joints into weight-bearing.

If a vertebra is caused to rock backwards on its intervertebral disc without also being allowed to slide backwards, the tips of its inferior articular processes will be driven into the superior articular facets of the vertebra below (Fig. 8.2). Axial compression of the intervertebral joint will then result in some of the load being transmitted through the region of impaction of the zygapophysial joints. By rocking a pair of lumbar vertebrae, one can readily determine by inspection that the site of impaction in the zygapophysial joints falls on the inferior medial portion of the facets. Formal experiments have shown this to be the site where maximal pressure is detected in the zygapophysial joints of vertebrae loaded in extension.[46]

Another mechanism does not involve the zygapophysial joint surfaces but rather the tips of the inferior articular processes. With severe or sustained axial compression, intervertebral discs may be narrowed to the extent that the inferior articular processes of the upper vertebra are lowered until their tips impact the laminae of the vertebra below (Fig. 8.3).[47] Alternatively, this same impact may occur if an intervertebral joint is axially compressed while also tilted backwards, as is the case in a lordotic lumbar spine bearing weight.[46–49] Axial loads can then be transmitted through the inferior articular processes to the laminae.

It has been shown that under the conditions of erect sitting, the zygapophysial joints are not impacted and bear none of the vertical load on the intervertebral joint. However, in prolonged standing with a lordotic spine, the impacted joints at each segmental level bear an average of some 16% of the axial load.[45,48] In this regard, the lower joints (L3–4, L4–5, L5–S1) bear a relatively greater proportion (19%), while the upper joints (L1–2, L2–3) bear less (11%).[48] Other studies have shown that the actual load borne by impaction of inferior articular processes varies from 3–18% of the applied load, and critically depends on the tilt of the intervertebral joint.[49] It has also been estimated that pathological disc space narrowing can result in some 70% of the axial load being borne by the inferior articular processes and laminae.[45]

It is thus evident that weight-bearing occurs through the zygapophysial joints only if the inferior articular processes impact either the superior articular facets or the laminae of the vertebra below. Variations in the degree of such

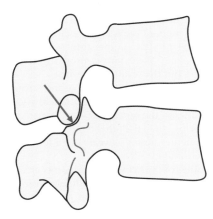

Figure 8.2 When a vertebra rocks backwards, its inferior articular processes impact the lower face of the superior articular processes of the vertebra below.

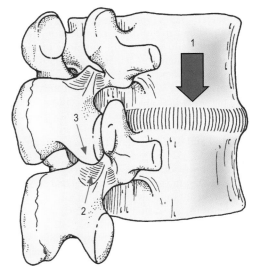

Figure 8.3 If an intervertebral joint is compressed (1), the inferior articular processes of the upper vertebra impact the laminae below (2), allowing weight to be transmitted through the inferior articular processes (3).

impactions account for the variations in the estimates of the axial load carried by the zygapophysial joints,[49] and explain why the highest estimates of the load borne are reported in studies in which the intervertebral joints have been loaded in the extended position.[42,43,50–52]

Although the preceding account of axial compression emphasises the role of the discs and zygapophysial joints in weight-bearing, other components of the lumbar spine also participate. The shape of the lordotic lumbar spine allows the anterior longitudinal ligament and the anterior portions of the anuli fibrosi to be involved in weight-bearing. Because of the curvature of the lordosis, the posterior parts of the intervertebral discs and the zygapophysial joints are compressed, but the anterior ligaments are stretched. Axial loading of a lordotic spine tends to accentuate the lordosis and, therefore, to increase the strain in the anterior ligaments. By increasing their tension, the anterior ligaments can resist this accentuation and share in the load-bearing.

In this way, the lordosis of the lumbar spine provides an axial load-bearing mechanism additional to those available in the intervertebral discs and the zygapophysial joints. Moreover, as described in Chapter 5, the tensile mechanism of the anterior ligaments imparts a resilience to the lumbar spine. The energy delivered to the ligaments is stored in them as tension and can be used to restore the curvature of the lumbar spine to its original form, once the axial load is removed.

Fatigue failure

Repetitive compression of a lumbar interbody joint results in fractures of the subchondral trabeculae and of one or other of the endplates. This damage occurs at loads substantially less than the ultimate compression strength of these structures, and well within the range of forces and repetitions encountered in activities of daily living, work and sporting activities.

Loads of between 37% and 80% of ultimate compression strength, applied at 0.5 Hz, can cause subchondral fractures after as few as 2000 or even 1000 cycles.[53] Loads between 50% and 80% of ultimate stress can cause subchondral and other vertebral fractures after fewer than 100 cycles.[26]

The probability of failure is a function of the load applied and the number of repetitions. Loads below 30% ultimate stress are unlikely to result in failure, even after 5000 repetitions; increasing the load increases the probability of failure after fewer repetitions.[24] At loads of 50–60% of ultimate stress, the probability of failure after 100 cycles is 39%; at loads of 60–70% ultimate strength, this probability rises to 63%.[24] The lesions induced range from subchondral trabecular fractures to impressions of an endplate, frank fractures of an endplate and fractures of the cortical bone of the vertebral body.[24] Repetitions of 100 and up to 1000 are within the calculated range for a variety

of occupational activities, as are loads of 60% ultimate stress of an average vertebral body.[24]

Endplate fractures result in a loss of disc height[17] and changes in the distribution of stress across the nucleus and anulus. The stress over the nucleus and anterior anulus decreases, while that over the posterior anulus rises.[1,11] This increase in stress causes the lamellae of the anulus to collapse inwards towards the nucleus, thereby disrupting the internal architecture of the disc.[11] Thus, even a small lesion can substantially compromise the normal biomechanics of a disc. The clinical significance of these phenomena is explored further in Chapter 15.

AXIAL DISTRACTION

Compared to axial compression and other movements of the lumbar spine, axial distraction has been studied far less. One study provided data on the stress–strain and stiffness characteristics of lumbar intervertebral discs as a whole, and revealed that the discs are not as stiff in distraction as in compression.[51] This is understandable, for the discs are designed principally for weight-bearing and would be expected to resist compression more than tension. In a biological sense, this correlates with the fact that humans spend far more time bearing compressive loads – in walking, standing and sitting – than sustaining tensile loads, as might occur in brachiating (tree-climbing) animals.

Other studies have focused on individual elements of the intervertebral joints to determine their tensile properties. When stretched along their length, isolated fibres of the anulus fibrosus exhibit a typical 'toe' region between 0% and 3% strain, a failure stress between 4 and 10 MPa, and a strain at failure between 9% and 15%; their stiffness against stretch ranges from 59 to 140 MPa.[54] If the anulus is tested while still attached to bone and distracted along the longitudinal axis of the vertebral column, as opposed to along the length of the fibres, the failure stress remains between 4 and 10 MPa but the stiffness drops to between 10 and 80 MPa.[55] These tensile properties seem to vary with location but the results between studies are conflicting. Isolated fibres seem to be stiffer and stronger in the anterior region than in the posterolateral region of the disc, and stiffer in the outer regions of the anulus than in the inner regions.[1] On the other hand, in intact specimens, the outer anterior anulus is weaker and less stiff than the outer posterior anulus.[55]

The capsules of the zygapophysial joints are remarkably strong when subjected to longitudinal tension. A single capsule can sustain 600 N before failing.[56] Figuratively, this means that a pair of capsules at a single level can bear twice the body weight if subjected to axial distraction.

However, the significance of these results lies not so much in the ability of elements of the lumbar spine to resist axial distraction but in their capacity to resist other movements that strain them. The anulus fibrosus will be strained by anterior sagittal rotation and axial rotation, and the zygapophysial joint capsules by anterior sagittal rotation. Those movements are considered below.

There has been one study[57] that has described the behaviour of the whole (cadaveric) lumbar spine during sustained axial distraction, to mimic the clinical procedure of traction. Application of a 9 kg weight to stretch the lumbar spine results in an initial mean lengthening of 7.5 mm. Lengthening is greater (9 mm) in lumbar spines of young subjects, and less in the middle-aged (5.5 mm) and the elderly (7.5 mm). Sustained traction over 30 min results in a creep of a further 1.5 mm. Removal of the load reveals an immediate 'set' of about 2.5 mm, which reduces to only 0.5 mm by 30 min after removal of the load. Younger spines demonstrate a more rapid creep and do not show a residual 'set'. The amount of distraction is greater in spines with healthy discs (11–12 mm) and substantially less (3–5 mm) in spines with degenerated discs.

Some 40% of the lengthening of the lumbar spine during traction occurs as a result of flattening of the lumbar lordosis, with 60% due to actual separation of the vertebral bodies. The major implication of this observation is that the extent of distraction achieved by traction (using a 9 kg load) is not great. It amounts to 60% of 7.5 mm of actual vertebral separation, which is equivalent to about 0.9 mm per intervertebral joint. This revelation seriously compromises those theories that maintain that lumbar traction exerts a beneficial effect by 'sucking back' disc herniations, and it is suggested that other mechanisms of the putative therapeutic effect of traction be considered.[57]

The other implication of this study relates to the fact that the residual 'set' after sustained traction is quite small (0.5 mm), amounting to about 0.1 mm per intervertebral joint. Moreover, this is the residual set in spines not subsequently reloaded by body weight. One would expect that, in living patients, a 0.1 mm set would naturally be obliterated the moment the patient rose and started to bear axial compression. Thus, any effect achieved by therapeutic traction must be phasic, i.e. occurring during the application of traction, and not due to some maintained lengthening of the lumbar spine.

FLEXION

During flexion, the entire lumbar spine leans forwards (Fig. 8.4). This is achieved basically by the 'unfolding' or straightening of the lumbar lordosis. At the full range of forward flexion, the lumbar spine assumes a straight alignment or is curved slightly forwards, tending to reverse the curvature of the original lordosis (see Fig. 8.3). The reversal occurs principally at upper lumbar levels. Reversal may occur at the L4–5 level but does not occur at the L5–S1 level.[58,59] Forward flexion is therefore achieved for the most part by each of the lumbar vertebrae rotating from their backward tilted position in the upright lordosis to a neutral position, in which the upper and lower surfaces of adjacent vertebral bodies are parallel to one another. This relieves the posterior compression of the intervertebral discs and zygapophysial joints, present in the upright lordotic lumbar spine. Some additional range of movement is achieved by the upper lumbar vertebrae rotating further forwards and compressing their intervertebral discs anteriorly.

It may appear that during flexion of the lumbar spine, the movement undergone by each vertebral body is simply anterior sagittal rotation. However, there is a concomitant component of forward translation as well.[59,60] If a vertebra rocks forwards over its intervertebral disc, its inferior articular processes are raised upwards and slightly backwards (Fig. 8.5A). This opens a small gap between each inferior articular facet and the superior articular facet in the zygapophysial joint. As the lumbar spine leans forwards, gravity or muscular action causes the vertebrae to slide forwards, and this motion closes the gap between the facets in the zygapophysial joints (Fig. 8.5B). Further forward translation will be arrested once impaction of the zygapophysial joints is re-established, but nonetheless a small forward translation will have occurred. At each intervertebral joint, therefore, flexion involves a combination of anterior sagittal rotation and a small amplitude anterior translation.

The zygapophysial joints play a major role in maintaining the stability of the spine in flexion, and much attention has been directed in recent years to the mechanisms involved. To appreciate these mechanisms, it is important to recognise that flexion involves both anterior sagittal rotation and anterior sagittal translation, for these two components are resisted and stabilised in different ways by the zygapophysial joints.

Anterior sagittal translation is resisted by the direct impaction of the inferior articular facets of a vertebra against the superior articular facets of the vertebra below, and this process has been fully described in Chapter 3. This mechanism becomes increasingly important the further the lumbar spine leans forward, for with a greater forward inclination of the lumbar spine, the upper surfaces of the lumbar vertebral bodies are inclined downwards (Fig. 8.6), and there will be a tendency for the vertebrae above to slide down this slope.

The cardinal ramification of the anatomy of the zygapophysial joints with respect to forward shear is that in joints with flat articular surfaces, the load will be borne evenly across the entire articular surface (see Ch. 3), but in joints with curved articular surfaces the load is concentrated on the anteromedial portions of the superior and inferior articular facets (see Ch. 3). Formal experiments have shown that during flexion, the highest pressures are

Flexion

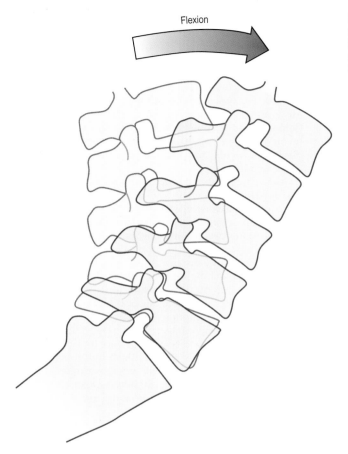

Figure 8.4 During flexion, the lumbar lordosis unfolds, and the lumbar spine straightens and leans forwards on the sacrum. The curvature of the lordosis may be reversed at upper lumbar levels but not at L5–S1.

recorded at the medial end of the lumbar zygapophysial joints,[46] and this has further bearing on the age changes seen in these joints (see Ch. 13).

The anterior sagittal rotation component of flexion is resisted by the zygapophysial joints in a different way. The mechanism involves tension in the joint capsule. Flexion involves an upward sliding movement of each inferior articular process, in relation to the superior articular process in each zygapophysial joint, and the amplitude of this movement is about 5–7 mm.[61] This movement will tense the joint capsule, and it is in this regard that the tensile strength of the capsule is recruited. Acting as a ligament, each capsule can resist as much as 600 N.[14,56] Indeed, the tension developed in the capsules during flexion is enough to bend the inferior articular processes downwards and forwards by some 5°.[62]

The other elements that resist the anterior sagittal rotation of flexion are the ligaments of the intervertebral joints. Anterior sagittal rotation results in the separation of the spinous processes and laminae. Consequently, the supraspinous and interspinous ligaments and the ligamenta flava will be tensed, and various types

of experiments have been performed to determine the relative contributions of these structures to the resistance of flexion. The experiments have involved either studying the range of motion in cadavers in which various ligaments have been sequentially severed,[60] or determining mathematically the stresses applied to different ligaments on the basis of the separation of their attachments during different phases of flexion.[3]

In young adult specimens, sectioning the supraspinous and interspinous ligaments and ligamenta flava results in an increase of about 5° in the range of flexion.[60] (Lesser increases occur in older specimens but this difference is discussed in Ch. 13.) Sectioning the zygapophysial joint capsules results in a further 4° of flexion. Transecting the pedicles, to remove the bony locking mechanism of the zygapophysial joints, results in a further 15° increase in range.

In a sense, these observations suggest the relative contributions of various structures to the resistance of flexion. The similar increases in range following the transection of ligaments and capsules suggest that the posterior ligaments and the zygapophysial joint capsules contribute

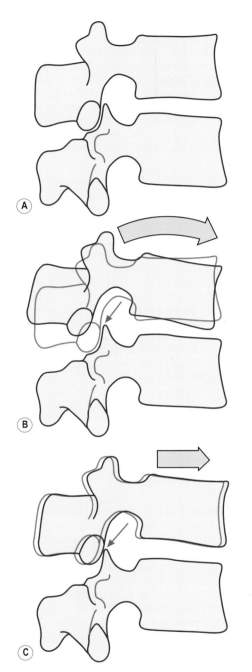

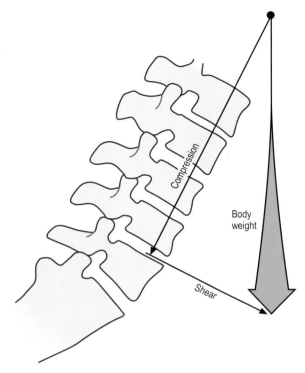

Figure 8.6 When the lumbar spine is flexed, the weight of the trunk exerts compressive and shearing forces on the intervertebral joints. The forces are proportional to the angle of inclination of the interbody joint.

Figure 8.5 The components of flexion of a lumbar intervertebral joint. (A) The lateral parts of the right superior articular process have been cut away to reveal the contact between the inferior and superior articular facets in the neutral position. (B) Sagittal rotation causes the inferior articular processes to lift upwards, leaving a gap between them and the superior articular facets. This gap allows for anterior sagittal translation. (C) Upon translation, the inferior articular facets once again impact the superior articular facets.

about equally, but their contribution is overshadowed by that of the bony locking mechanism, whose elimination results in a major increase in range of movement. However, such conclusions should be made with caution, for the experiments on which they are based involved sequential sectioning of structures. They do not reveal the simultaneous contributions of various structures, nor possible variations in the contribution by different structures at different phases of movement. Nevertheless, the role of the bony locking mechanism in the stability of the flexed lumbar spine is strikingly demonstrated.

To determine the simultaneous contribution by various structures to the resistance of flexion, mathematical analyses have been performed.[3] The results indicate that in a typical lumbar intervertebral joint, the intervertebral disc contributes about 29% of the resistance, the supraspinous and interspinous ligaments about 19%, the ligamentum flavum about 13%, and the capsules of the zygapophysial joints about 39%. It is emphasised that these figures relate only to the resistance of anterior sagittal rotation, which is the movement that tenses these ligaments. They do not relate to the role played by the bony locking mechanism in preventing anterior translation during flexion.

Within the disc, the posterior anulus is tensed during flexion and the anterior anulus is relaxed. The posterior anulus exhibits a strain of 0.6% per degree of rotation, and the anterior anulus exhibits a reciprocal strain of –0.6% per degree.[14] With respect to anterior translation, the anulus exhibits a strain of about 1% per mm of horizontal displacement.[14] An isolated disc can withstand a flexion moment of about 33 Nm, and can sustain flexion angles of about 18°,[63] but in an intact specimen it is protected by the posterior ligaments. In an intact intervertebral joint, the posterior ligaments protect the disc and resist 80% of the flexion moment and restrict the segment to 80% of the range of flexion that will damage the disc.[63]

Failure

If a lumbar spine is tested progressively to failure, it emerges that the first signs of injury (to the posterior ligaments) appear when the bending moment is about 60 Nm.[2] Gross damage is evident by 120 Nm and complete failure occurs at 140–185 Nm.[64,65] These data underscore the fact that ligaments alone are not enough to support the flexed lumbar spine and that they need support from the back muscles during heavy lifts that may involve moments in excess of 200 Nm (see Ch. 9). The disc fails by horizontal tears across the middle of the posterior anulus or by avulsion of the anulus from the ring apophysis.[63]

Speed of movement and sustained postures affect the resistance of the ligaments of the spine to flexion. Reducing the duration of movement from 10 s to 1 s increases resistance by 12%; holding a flexed posture for 5 min reduces resistance by 42%; holding for an hour reduces resistance by 67%.[2] These figures indicate that various work postures involving stooping can put the spine at risk by weakening its resistance to movement. Ostensibly, creep is the basis for this change in resistance.

Repetitive loading of the spine in flexion produces a variety of changes and lesions. Repeated pure bending has little effect on the intervertebral joints.[66] At most, it produces a 10% increase in the range of extension but no significant changes to other movements.[66] Repeated bending under compression, however, produces a variety of lesions in many specimens. Loading a lumbar joint in 9–12° of flexion, under 1500–6000 N, at 40 times per minute for up to 4 h causes endplate fractures in about one in four specimens, and a variety of internal disruptions of the anulus fibrosus, ranging from buckling of lamellae to overt radial fissures.[67] These lesions are similar to those observed under pure compression loading and should be ascribed not to bending but to the compression component of cyclic bending under compression.

The zygapophysial joints offer a resistance of up to 2000 N against the forward translation that occurs during flexion.[2] This resistance passes from the inferior articular processes, through the laminae and pedicles, into the vertebral body. As a result, a bending force is exerted on the pars interarticularis. Repetitive loading of the inferior articular facets results in failure of the pars interarticularis or the pedicles. Subject to a force of 380–760 N, 100 times per minute, many specimens can sustain several hundred thousand repetitions but others fail after as few as 1500, 300 and 139 repetitions.[68] These figures warn that, in addition to injuries to the disc, repeated flexion can induce fractures of the pars interarticularis.

EXTENSION

In principle, extension movements of the lumbar intervertebral joints are the converse of those that occur in flexion. Basically, the vertebral bodies undergo posterior sagittal rotation and a small posterior translation. However, certain differences are involved because of the structure of the lumbar vertebrae. During flexion, the inferior articular processes are free to move upwards until their movement is resisted by ligamentous and capsular tension. Extension, on the other hand, involves downward movement of the inferior articular processes and the spinous process, and this movement is limited not by ligamentous tension but by bony impaction.

Bony impaction usually occurs between the spinous processes.[69] As a vertebra extends, its spinous process approaches the next lower spinous process. The first limit to extension occurs as the interspinous ligament buckles and becomes trapped between the spinous processes. Further extension is met with further compression of this ligament until the spinous processes virtually come into contact (Fig. 8.7A).[69]

In individuals with wide interspinous spaces, extension may be limited before spinous processes come into contact.[69] Impaction occurs between the tip of one or other of the inferior articular processes of the moving vertebra and the subjacent lamina (Fig. 8.7B). This type of impaction is accentuated when the joint is subjected to the action of the back muscles,[47] for in addition to extending the lumbar spine, the back muscles also exert a substantial compression load on it (see Ch. 9). Consequently, during active extension, the inferior articular processes are drawn not only into posterior sagittal rotation but also downwards as the entire intervertebral joint is compressed. Under these circumstances, the zygapophysial joints become weight-bearing, as explained above (see 'Axial compression').

The posterior elements, however, are not critical for limiting extension. Resection of the zygapophysial joints has little impact on the capacity of a lumbar segment to bear an extension load.[70] The extension load, under these conditions, is adequately borne by the anterior anulus.[70]

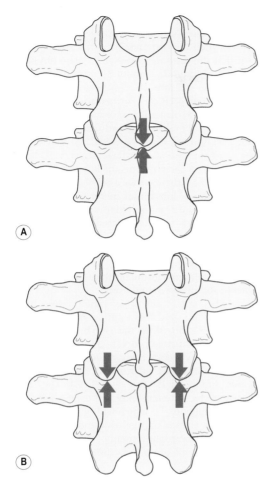

B

Figure 8.7 Factors limiting extension. Posterior sagittal rotation is usually limited by impaction of the spinous processes (A) but may be limited by impaction of the inferior articular processes of the laminae (B).

AXIAL ROTATION

Axial rotation of the lumbar spine involves twisting, or torsion, of the intervertebral discs and impaction of zygapophysial joints.

During axial rotation of an intervertebral joint, all the fibres of the anulus fibrosus that are inclined toward the direction of rotation will be strained. The other half will be relaxed (see Ch. 2). Based on the observation that elongation of collagen beyond about 4% of resting length leads to injury of the fibre (see Ch. 7), it can be calculated that the maximum range of rotation of an intervertebral disc without injury is about 3°.[8] Beyond this range the

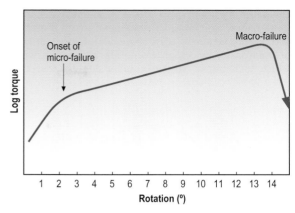

Figure 8.8 Stress–strain curve for torsion of the intervertebral disc. *(Based on Farfan et al. 1970.[71])*

collagen fibres will begin to undergo micro-injury. Moreover, observational studies have determined that the anulus fibrosus exhibits a strain of 1% per degree of axial rotation,[14] which also sets a limit of 3° before excessive strain is incurred.

Experiments on lumbar intervertebral discs have shown that they resist torsion more strongly than bending movements, and the stress–strain curves for torsion rise very steeply in the range 0–3° of rotation.[51] Very large forces have to be applied to strain the disc beyond 3°, and isolated discs (the posterior elements having being removed) fail macroscopically at about 12° of rotation.[71] This suggests that 12° is the ultimate range for rotation before disc failure occurs but this relates to total macroscopic failure. Analysis of the stress–strain curves for intervertebral discs under torsion (Fig. 8.8) reveals an inflection point just before 3° of rotation, which indicates the onset of microscopic failure in the anulus fibrosus.[71] The range between 3° and 12° represents continued microfailure until overt failure occurs.

In an intact intervertebral joint, the zygapophysial joints, and to a certain extent the posterior ligaments, protect the intervertebral disc from excessive torsion. Because the axis of rotation of a lumbar vertebra passes through the posterior part of the vertebral body,[72] all the posterior elements of the moving vertebra will swing around this axis during axial rotation. As the spinous process moves, the attachments of the supraspinous and interspinous ligaments will be separated, and these ligaments will be placed under slight tension. Furthermore, one of the inferior articular facets of the upper vertebra will be impacted against its apposing superior articular facet (Fig. 8.9). In the case of left axial rotation, it will be the right inferior articular facet that impacts (and vice versa). Once this impaction occurs, normal axial rotation is arrested.

Because the joint space of the zygapophysial joint is quite narrow, the range of movement before impaction occurs is quite small. Such movement as does occur is accommodated by compression of the articular cartilages, which are able to sustain compression because their

principal constituents are proteoglycans and water. Water is simply squeezed out of the cartilages, and is gradually reabsorbed when the compression is released.

Given that the distance between a zygapophysial joint and the axis of rotation is about 30 mm, it can be calculated that about 0.5 mm of compression must occur for every 1° of axial rotation. Furthermore, given that the articular cartilages of a lumbar zygapophysial joint are about 2 mm thick (see Ch. 3), and that articular cartilage is about 75% water,[73] it can be calculated that to accommodate 3° of rotation, the cartilages must be compressed to about 62% of their resting thickness and must lose more than half of their water. The zygapophysial joints therefore provide a substantial buffer during the first 3° of rotation, and the zygapophysial joint must be severely compressed before rotation exceeds the critical range of 3°, beyond which the anulus fibrosus risks torsional injury. Nevertheless, if sufficiently strong forces are applied, rotation can proceed beyond 3°, but then an 'impure' form of rotation occurs as the result of distortion of other elements in the intervertebral joint.

To rotate beyond 3°, the upper vertebra must pivot on the impacted joint, and this joint becomes the site of a new axis of rotation. Both the vertebral body and the opposite inferior articular process will then swing around this new axis. The vertebral body swings laterally and backwards, and the opposite inferior articular process swings backwards and medially (see Fig. 8.9C). The sideways movement of the vertebral body will exert a lateral shear on the underlying disc[71,72] which will be additional to any torsional stress already applied to the disc by the earlier rotation. The backward movement of the opposite inferior articular process will strain the capsule of its zygapophysial joint.

During this complex combination of forces and movements, the impacted zygapophysial joint is being strained by compression, the intervertebral disc is strained by torsion and lateral shear, and the capsule of the opposite zygapophysial joint is being stretched. Failure of any one of these elements can occur if the rotatory force is

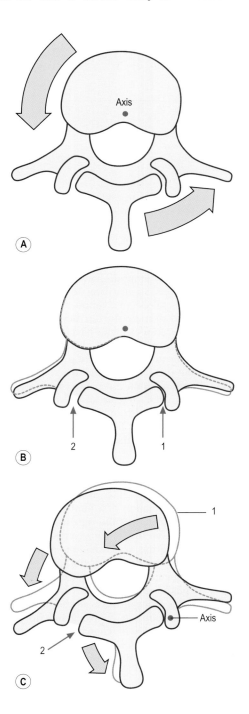

(A)

(B)

(C)

Figure 8.9 The mechanism of left axial rotation of a lumbar intervertebral joint. Two consecutive vertebrae, superimposed on one another, are viewed from above. The lower vertebra is depicted by a dotted line. (A) Initially, rotation occurs about an axis in the vertebral body. (B) As the posterior elements swing around, the right inferior articular process of the upper vertebra impacts the superior articular process of the lower vertebra (1). The opposite zygapophysial joint is gapped (2). (C) Rotation beyond 3° occurs about an axis located in the impacted zygapophysial joint. The intervertebral disc must undergo lateral shear (1), and the opposite zygapophysial joint is gapped and distracted posteriorly (2).

sufficiently strong, and this underlies the mechanism of torsional injury to the lumbar spine (see Ch. 15).

The relative contributions of various structures to the resistance of axial rotation have been determined experimentally, and it is evident that the roles played by the supraspinous and interspinous ligaments, and by the capsule of the tensed (the opposite) zygapophysial joint are not great.[74] The load is borne principally by the impacted zygapophysial joint and the intervertebral disc. Quantitative analysis[71] reveals that the disc contributes 35% of the resistance to torsion, the remaining 65% being exerted by the posterior elements: the tensed zygapophysial joint; the supraspinous and interspinous ligaments; and principally the impacted zygapophysial joint. Experimental studies, however, have established that the zygapophysial joints contribute only between 42% and 54% of the torsional stiffness of a segment, the rest stemming from the disc.[75]

Fatigue failure

Specimens vary in their susceptibility to repetitive axial rotation. If the segment does not rotate beyond 1.5°, it can sustain 10 000 repetitions without visible damage. Segments which exhibit a larger initial range of motion, however, exhibit failure after 2000 or 3000 repetitions but in some cases after as few as 200–500, or even 50, repetitions.[76] Failure occurs in the form of fractures of the facets, laminae or vertebral bodies, and tears in the anulus fibrosus and zygapophysial joint capsules.

LATERAL FLEXION

Lateral flexion of the lumbar spine does not involve simple movements of the lumbar intervertebral joints. It involves a complex and variable combination of lateral bending and rotatory movements of the interbody joints and diverse movements of the zygapophysial joints. Conspicuously, lateral flexion of the lumbar spine has not been subjected to detailed biomechanical analysis, probably because of its complexity and the greater clinical relevance of sagittal plane movements and axial rotation. However, some aspects of the mechanics of lateral flexion are evident when the range of this movement is considered below.

ROTATION IN FLEXION

There has been considerable interest in the movement of rotation in the flexed posture because this is a common movement associated with the onset of back pain. However, the studies offer conflicting results and opinions that stem from the complexities and subtleties of this movement, and differences in methods of study.

Using an external measuring device, Hindle and Pearcy[77] observed in 12 subjects that the range of axial rotation of the lumbar spine increased when these subjects sat in a flexed position. This, they argued, occurred because, upon flexion, the inferior articular facets are lifted out of the sockets formed by the apposed superior articular facets, and if the inferior facets are tapered towards one another, they gain an extra range of motion in the transverse direction. Subsequently, they demonstrated this phenomenon in cadavers.[78]

Gunzburg et al. (1991)[79] reported contrary data. They could not find increased rotation upon flexion either in cadavers or in living subjects in the standing position.

It has been argued that these differences can be explained by differences in compression loads.[80] If a cadaveric specimen is compressed when flexed, the zygapophysial joints will remain deeper in their sockets than when allowed simply to flex. In living subjects, stooping while standing imposes large external loads that must be resisted by the back muscles, whose contraction will compress the moving segments (see Ch. 9). Consequently, increased axial rotation may be prevented by axial compression. However, this compression is not as great during flexion in the sitting position, under which conditions the increased axial rotation becomes apparent.

The argument concludes that increased axial rotation during flexion will not be apparent if the back muscles are strongly contracted although it may be apparent during sitting or if sudden external loads are applied which exceed the force of the back muscles. Under these circumstances, the increased axial rotation renders the disc liable to injury. As long as the zygapophysial joints limit rotation to less than 3°, the anulus is protected from injury. However, if axial rotation is greater than this, the anulus must undergo a greater strain and, moreover, one that is superimposed on the strain already induced by flexion.[80]

RANGE OF MOVEMENT

The range of movement of the lumbar spine has been studied in a variety of ways. It has been measured in cadavers and in living subjects using either clinical measurements or measurements taken from radiographs. Studies of cadavers have the disadvantage that because of post-mortem changes and because cadavers are usually studied with the back musculature removed, the measurements obtained may not accurately reflect the mobility possible in living subjects. However, cadaveric studies have the advantage that motion can be directly and precisely measured and correlated with pathological changes determined by subsequent dissection or histological studies. Clinical studies have the advantage that they examine living subjects although they are limited by the accuracy of the instruments used and the reliability of identifying bony landmarks by palpation.

The availability and reliability of modern spondylometers, and the techniques for measuring the range of lumbar spinal motion are conveniently summarised in the AMA's *Guides to the Evaluation of Permanent Impairment*, which also provides modern normative data.[81] These, however, pertain to clinical measurements of spinal motion. They do not indicate exactly what happens in the lumbar spine and at each segment. That can be determined only by radiography.

Radiographic studies provide the most accurate measurements of living subjects but, although there have been many radiographic studies of segmental ranges of motion, these have now been superseded by the more accurate technique of biplanar radiography. Conventional radiography has the disadvantage that it cannot quantify movements that are not in the plane being studied. Thus, while lateral radiographs can be used to detect movement in the sagittal plane, they do not demonstrate the extent of any simultaneous movements in the horizontal and coronal planes. Such simultaneous movements can affect the radiographic image in the sagittal plane and lead to errors in the measurement of sagittal plane movements.[58,59,82]

The technique of biplanar radiography overcomes this problem by taking radiographs simultaneously through two X-ray tubes arranged at right angles to one another. Analysis of the two simultaneous radiographs allows movements in all three planes to be detected and quantified, allowing a more accurate appraisal of the movements that occur in any one plane.[58,59,82]

There have been two principal results stemming from the use of biplanar radiography. These are the accurate quantification of segmental motion in living subjects, and the demonstration and quantification of coupled movements.[58,59,83,84] The segmental ranges of motion in the sagittal plane (flexion and extension), horizontal plane (axial rotation) and coronal plane (lateral bending) are shown in Table 8.1. It is notable that, for the same age group and sex (25- to 36-year-old males), all lumbar joints have the same total range of motion in the sagittal plane, although the middle intervertebral joints have a relatively greater range of flexion, while the highest and lowest joints have a relatively greater range of extension.

As determined by biplanar radiography, the mean values of axial rotation are approximately equal at all levels (see Table 8.1), and even the greatest values fall within the limit of $3°$, which, from biomechanical evidence, is the range at which microtrauma to the intervertebral disc would occur. Conspicuously, the values obtained radiographically are noticeably smaller than those obtained both in cadavers and in living subjects using a spondylometer. The reasons for this discrepancy have not been investigated but may be due to the inability of clinical measurements to discriminate primary and coupled movements.

Coupled movements are movements that occur in an unintended or unexpected direction during the execution of a desired motion, and biplanar radiography reveals the patterns of such movements in the lumbar spine. Table 8.2 shows the ranges of movements coupled with flexion and extension of the lumbar spine and Table 8.3 shows the movements coupled with axial rotation and lateral flexion.

Flexion of lumbar intervertebral joints consistently involves a combination of $8–13°$ of anterior sagittal rotation and 1–3 mm of forward translation, and these movements are consistently accompanied by axial and coronal rotations of about $1°$ (see Table 8.2). Some vertical and lateral translations also occur but are of small amplitude. Conversely, extension involves posterior sagittal rotation and posterior translation, with some axial and coronal rotation, but little vertical or lateral translation (see Table 8.2).

Table 8.1 Ranges of segmental motion in males aged 25–36 years. (Based on Pearcy et al. 1984[59] and Pearcy and Tibrewal 1984.[84])

Level	Mean range (measured in degrees, with standard deviations)						
	Lateral flexion		Axial rotation		Flexion	Extension	Flexion and extension
	Left	Right	Left	Right			
L1–2	5	6	1	1	8 (5)	5 (2)	13 (5)
L2–3	5	6	1	1	10 (2)	3 (2)	13 (2)
L3–4	5	6	1	2	12 (1)	1 (1)	13 (2)
L4–5	3	5	1	2	13 (4)	2 (1)	16 (4)
L5–S1	0	2	1	0	9 (6)	5 (4)	14 (5)

Table 8.2 Movements coupled with flexion and extension of the lumbar spine. (Based on Pearcy et al. 1984.[59])

Primary movement and level	Coupled movements					
	Mean (SD) rotations (°)			Mean (SD) translations (mm)		
	Sagittal	Coronal	Axial	Sagittal	Coronal	Axial
Flexion						
L1	8 (5)	1 (1)	1 (1)	3 (1)	0 (1)	1 (1)
L2	10 (2)	1 (1)	1 (1)	2 (1)	1 (1)	1 (1)
L3	12 (1)	1 (1)	1 (1)	2 (1)	1 (1)	0 (1)
L4	13 (4)	2 (1)	1 (1)	2 (1)	0 (1)	0 (1)
L5	9 (6)	1 (1)	1 (1)	1 (1)	0 (1)	1 (1)
Extension						
L1	5 (1)	0 (1)	1 (1)	1 (1)	1 (1)	0 (1)
L2	3 (1)	0 (1)	1 (1)	1 (1)	0 (1)	0 (1)
L3	1 (1)	1 (1)	0 (1)	1 (1)	1 (1)	0 (1)
L4	2 (1)	1 (1)	1 (1)	1 (1)	0 (1)	1 (1)
L5	5 (1)	1 (1)	1 (1)	1 (1)	1 (1)	0 (1)

Axial rotation and lateral flexion are coupled with one another and with sagittal rotation (see Table 8.3). Axial rotation is variably coupled with flexion and extension. Either flexion or extension may occur during left or right rotation but neither occurs consistently. Consequently, the mean amount of flexion and extension coupled with axial rotation is zero (see Table 8.3). Similarly, lateral flexion may be accompanied by either flexion or extension of the same joint, but extension occurs more frequently and to a greater degree (see Table 8.3). Therefore, it might be concluded that lateral flexion is most usually accompanied by a small degree of extension.

The coupling between axial rotation and lateral flexion is somewhat more consistent and describes an average pattern. Axial rotation of the upper three lumbar joints is usually accompanied by lateral flexion to the other side, and lateral flexion is accompanied by contralateral axial rotation (see Table 8.3). In contrast, axial rotation of the L5–S1 joint is accompanied by lateral flexion to the same side, and lateral flexion of this joint is accompanied by ipsilateral axial rotation (see Table 8.2). The L4–5 joint exhibits no particular bias; in some subjects the coupling is ipsilateral while in others it is contralateral.[84]

While recognising these patterns, it is important to note that they represent average patterns. Not all individuals exhibit the same degree of coupling at any segment or necessarily in the same direction as the average; nor do all normal individuals necessarily exhibit the average direction of coupling at every segment. While exhibiting the average pattern of coupling at one level, a normal individual can exhibit contrary coupling at any or all other levels.[58] Consequently, no reliable rules can be formulated to determine whether an individual exhibits abnormal ranges or directions of coupling in the lumbar spine. All that might be construed is that an individual differs from the average pattern but this may not be abnormal.

The presence of coupling indicates that certain processes must operate during axial rotation to produce inadvertent lateral flexion, and vice versa. However, the details of these processes have not been determined. From first principles, they probably involve a combination of the way zygapophysial joints move and are impacted during axial rotation or lateral flexion, the way in which discs are subjected to torsional strain and lateral shear, the action of gravity, the line of action of the muscles that produce either axial rotation or lateral flexion, the shape of the lumbar lordosis and the location of the moving segment within the lordotic curve.

Clinical implications

Total ranges of motion are not of any diagnostic value, for aberrations of total movement indicate neither the nature of any disease nor its location. However, total ranges of motion do provide an index of spinal function that reflects the biomechanical and biochemical properties of the lumbar spine. Consequently, their principal value lies in comparing different groups to determine the influence of

Table 8.3 Coupled movements of the lumbar spine. (Based on Pearcy and Tibrewal 1984.[84])

Primary movement and level	Coupled movements					
	Axial rotation, degrees (+ve to left)		Flexion/extension, degrees (+ve flexion)		Lateral flexion, degrees (+ve to left)	
	Mean	Range	Mean	Range	Mean	Range
Right rotation						
L1	−1	(−2 to 1)	0	(−3 to 3)	3	(−1 to 5)
L2	−1	(−2 to 1)	0	(−2 to 2)	4	(1 to 9)
L3	−1	(−3 to 1)	0	(−2 to 2)	3	(1 to 6)
L4	−1	(−2 to 1)	0	(−9 to 5)	1	(−3 to 3)
L5	−1	(−2 to 1)	0	(−5 to 3)	−2	(−7 to 0)
Left rotation						
L1	1	(−1 to 1)	0	(−4 to 4)	−3	(−7 to −1)
L2	1	(−1 to 1)	0	(−4 to 4)	−3	(−5 to 0)
L3	2	(0 to 1)	0	(−3 to 2)	−3	(−6 to 0)
L4	2	(0 to 1)	0	(−7 to 2)	−2	(−5 to 1)
L5	0	(−2 to 1)	0	(−5 to 3)	1	(0 to 2)
Right lateral flexion						
L1	0	(−3 to 1)	−2	(−5 to 1)	−5	(−8 to −2)
L2	1	(−1 to 1)	−1	(−3 to 1)	−5	(−8 to −4)
L3	1	(−1 to 1)	−1	(−3 to 1)	−5	(−11 to 2)
L4	1	(0 to 1)	0	(−1 to 4)	−3	(−5 to 1)
L5	0	(−1 to 1)	2	(−3 to 8)	0	(−2 to 3)
Left lateral flexion						
L1	0	(−2 to 1)	−2	(−9 to 0)	6	(4 to 10)
L2	−1	(−3 to 1)	−3	(−4 to −1)	6	(2 to 10)
L3	−1	(−4 to 1)	−2	(−4 to 3)	5	(−3 to 8)
L4	−1	(−4 to 1)	−1	(−4 to 2)	3	(−3 to 6)
L5	−2	(−3 to 1)	0	(−5 to 5)	−3	(−6 to 1)

such factors as age and degeneration, and this is explored later in Chapter 13.

Of greater potential diagnostic significance is the determination of ranges of movement for individual lumbar intervertebral joints, for if focal disease is to affect movement it is more likely to be manifest to a greater degree at the diseased segment than in the total range of motion of the lumbar spine.

Armed with a detailed knowledge of the range of normal intersegmental motion and the patterns of coupled movements in the lumbar spine, investigators have explored the possibility that patients with back pain or specific spinal disorders might exhibit diagnostic abnormalities of range of motion or coupling. However, the results of such investigations have been disappointing. On biplanar radiography, patients with back pain, as a group, exhibit normal ranges of extension but a reduced mean range of flexion along with greater amplitudes of coupling; those patients with signs of nerve root tension exhibit reduced flexion but normal coupling.[85] However, patients with back pain exhibit such a range of movement that although their mean behaviour as a group differs from normal, biplanar radiography does not allow individual patients to be distinguished from normal with any worthwhile degree of sensitivity.[85] Patients with proven disc herniations exhibit reduced ranges of motion at all segments but the level of disc herniation exhibits no greater reduction.[86] Increased coupling occurs at the level above a herniation. However, these abnormalities are not sufficiently specific to differentiate between patients with disc herniations and those with low back pain of other origin.[86] Moreover, discectomy does not result in improvements in the range of motion nor does it restore normal coupling.[86]

Some investigators, however, have argued that abnormalities may not be evident if the spine is tested under active movements.[87] They argue that radiographs of passive motion may be more revealing of segmental hypermobility although appropriate studies to verify this conjecture have yet to be conducted.

AXES OF SAGITTAL ROTATION

The combination of sagittal rotation and sagittal translation of each lumbar vertebra which occurs during flexion and extension of the lumbar spine results in each vertebra exhibiting an arcuate motion in relation to the next lower vertebra (Fig. 8.10). This arcuate motion occurs about a centre that lies somewhere below the moving vertebra and can be located by applying elementary geometric techniques to flexion–extension radiographs of the moving vertebrae.[88]

For any arc of movement defined by a given starting position and a given end position of the moving vertebra, the centre of movement is known as the **instantaneous axis of rotation** or **IAR**. The exact location of the IAR is a function of the amount of sagittal rotation and the amount of simultaneous sagittal translation that occurs during the phase of motion defined by the starting and end positions selected. However, as a vertebra moves from full extension to full flexion, the amount of sagittal rotation versus sagittal translation is not regular. For different phases of motion the vertebra may exhibit relatively more rotation for the same change in translation, or vice versa. Consequently, the precise location of the IAR for each phase of motion differs slightly. In essence, the axis of movement of the joint is not constant but varies in location depending on the position of the joint.

The behaviour of the axis and the path it takes when it moves can be determined by studying the movement of the joint in small increments. If IARs are determined for each phase of motion and then plotted in sequence, they depict a locus known as the **centrode** of motion (Fig. 8.11). The centrode is, in effect, a map of the path taken

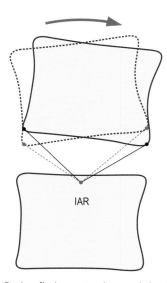

Figure 8.10 During flexion–extension, each lumbar vertebra exhibits an arcuate motion in relation to the vertebra below. The centre of this arc lies below the moving vertebra and is known as the instantaneous axis of rotation (IAR).

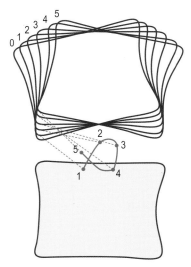

Figure 8.11 As a vertebra moves from extension to flexion, its motion can be reduced to small sequential increments. Five such phases are illustrated. Each phase of motion has a unique instantaneous axis of rotation (IAR). In moving from position 0 to position 1, the vertebra moved about IAR number 1. In moving from position 1 to position 2, it moved about IAR number 2, and so on. The dotted lines connect the vertebra in each of its five positions to the location of the IAR about which it moved. When the IARs are connected in sequence they describe a locus or a path known as the centrode.

by the moving axis during the full range of motion of the joint.

In normal cadaveric specimens the centrode is short and is located in a restricted area in the vicinity of the upper endplate of the next lower vertebra (Fig. 8.12A).[89,90] In specimens with injured or so-called degenerative intervertebral discs, the centrode differs from the norm in length, shape and average location (Fig. 8.12B).[89,90] These differences reflect the pathological changes in the stiffness properties of those elements of the intervertebral joint that govern sagittal rotation and translation. Changes in the resistance to movement cause differences in the IARs at different phases of motion and therefore in the size and shape of the centrode.

Increased stiffness or relative laxity in different structures such as the anulus fibrosus, the zygapophysial joints or the interspinous ligaments will affect sagittal rotation and translation to different extents. Therefore, different types of injury or disease should result in differences, if not characteristic aberrations, in the centrode pattern. Thus it could be possible to deduce the location and nature of a disease process or injury by examining the centrode pattern it produces. However, the techniques used to determine centrodes are subject to technical errors whenever small amplitudes of motion are studied.[88] Consequently, centrodes can be determined accurately only if metal markers can be implanted to allow exact registration of consecutive radiographic images. Without such markers, amplitudes of motion of less than 5° cannot be studied accurately in living subjects. Reliable observations in living subjects can only be made of the IAR for the movement of full flexion from full extension.[88] Such an IAR provides a convenient summary of the behaviour of the joint and

constitutes what can be taken as a reduction of the centrode of motion to a single point.

In normal volunteers, the IARs for each of the lumbar vertebrae fall in tightly clustered zones, centred in similar locations for each segment near the superior endplate of the next lower vertebra (Fig. 8.13).[88] Each segment operates around a very similar point, with little normal variation about the mean location. This indicates that the lumbar spine moves in a remarkably similar way in normal individuals: the forces governing flexion–extension must be similar from segment to segment, and are similar from individual to individual.

It has been shown[91] that the location of an IAR can be expressed mathematically as:

$$X_{IAR} = X_{CR} + T/2$$
$$Y_{IAR} = Y_{CR} + T/[2\tan(\theta/2)]$$

where (X_{IAR}, Y_{IAR}) are the coordinates of the IAR, (X_{CR}, Y_{CR}) are the coordinates of the centre of reaction, T is the translation exhibited by the moving vertebra and θ is the angular displacement of the vertebra (Fig. 8.14). These equations relate the location of the IAR to fundamental anatomical properties of the motion segment.

The centre of reaction is that point on the inferior endplate of the moving vertebra through which the compression forces are transmitted to the underlying intervertebral

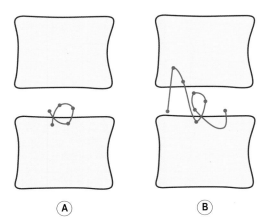

Figure 8.12 (A) The centrodes of normal cadaveric intervertebral joints are short and tightly clustered. (B) Degenerative specimens exhibit longer, displaced and seemingly erratic centrodes. *(Based on Gertzbein et al. 1985, 1986).*[89,90]

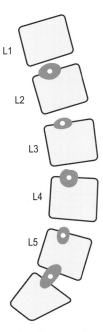

Figure 8.13 The mean location and distribution of instantaneous axes of rotation of the lumbar vertebrae. The central dot depicts the mean location, while the outer ellipse depicts the two SD range exhibited by 10 normal volunteers. *(Based on Pearcy and Bogduk 1988.*[88])

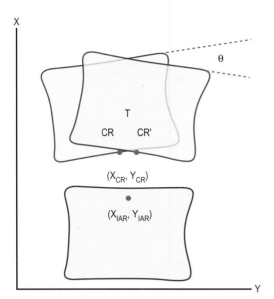

Figure 8.14 The location of an instantaneous axis of rotation (IAR) in relation to a coordinate system registered on the lower vertebral body, the location of the centre of reaction (CR) of the moving vertebra and the rotation and translation (T) which that vertebra exhibits.

disc; as a point it is the mathematical average of all the forces distributed across the endplate. A feature of the centre of reaction is that it is a point that undergoes no rotation: it exhibits only translation. Its motion therefore reflects the true translation of the moving vertebra. Other points that appear to exhibit translation exhibit a combination of true translation and a horizontal displacement due to sagittal rotation.

If the compression profile of the disc is altered, the centre of reaction will move. Consequently, the IAR will move. Similarly, if the amplitude of translation or rotation is altered, the IAR will move according to the equations.

These relationships allow the displacement of an IAR from normal to be interpreted in terms of those factors that can affect the centre of reaction, translation and angular rotation. For example, posterior muscle spasm will increase posterior compression loading and will reduce angular rotation. This will displace the IAR backwards and downwards.[92] Conversely, a joint whose IAR is located behind and below the normal location can be interpreted to be subject to excessive posterior muscle spasm.

In so far as IARs reflect the quality of movement of a segment, as opposed to its range of movement, determining the IARs in patients with spinal disorders could possibly provide a more sensitive way of detecting diagnostic movement abnormalities than simply measuring absolute ranges of movement. What remains to be seen is whether IARs in living subjects exhibit detectable aberrations analogous to the changes in centrode patterns seen in cadavers.

REFERENCES

1. Adams MA, McNally DS, Wagstaff J, et al. Abnormal stress concentrations in lumbar intervertebral discs following damage to the vertebral bodies: a cause of disc failure? *Eur Spine J.* 1993;1:214–221.

2. Adams MA. Spine update. Mechanical testing of the spine: an appraisal of methodology, results, and conclusions. *Spine.* 1995;20:2151–2156.

3. Adams MA, Hutton WC, Stott JRR. The resistance to flexion of the lumbar intervertebral joint. *Spine.* 1980;5:245–253.

4. McNally DS, Adams MA. Internal intervertebral disc mechanics as revealed by stress profilometry. *Spine.* 1992;17:66–73.

5. Brown T, Hansen RJ, Yorra AJ. Some mechanical tests on the lumbosacral spine with particular reference to the intervertebral discs. *J Bone Joint Surg.* 1957;39A: 1135–1164.

6. Roaf R. A study of the mechanics of spinal injuries. *J Bone Joint Surg.* 1960;42B:810–823.

7. Virgin WJ. Experimental investigations into the physical properties of the intervertebral disc. *J Bone Joint Surg.* 1951;33B:607–611.

8. Hickey DS, Hukins DWL. Relation between the structure of the annulus fibrosus and the function and failure of the intervertebral disc. *Spine.* 1980;5:100–116.

9. Kraemer J, Kolditz D, Gowin R. Water and electrolyte content of human intervertebral discs under variable load. *Spine.* 1985;10: 69–71.

10. Urban J, Maroudas A. The chemistry of the intervertebral disc in relation to its physiological function. *Clin Rheum Dis.* 1980;6:51–76.

11. Adams MA, Dolan P. Recent advances in lumbar spinal mechanics and their clinical significance. *Clin Biomech.* 1995;10:3–19.

12. Brinckmann P, Frobin W, Hierholzer E, et al. Deformation of the vertebral end-plate under axial loading of the spine. *Spine.* 1983;8:851–856.

13. Holmes AD, Hukins DWL, Freemont AJ. End-plate displacement during compression of lumbar vertebra-disc-vertebra segments and the mechanism of failure. *Spine.* 1993;18:128–135.

14. Stokes IAF. Surface strain on human intervertebral discs. *J Orthop Res.* 1987;5:348–355.

15. Brinckmann P, Grootenboer H. Change of disc height, radial disc

bulge, and intradiscal pressure from discectomy: an in vitro investigation on human lumbar discs. *Spine.* 1991;16:641–646.

16. Horst M, Brinckmann P. Measurement of the distribution of axial stress on the end-plate of the vertebral body. *Spine.* 1981;6:217–232.

17. Brinckmann P, Horst M. The influence of vertebral body fracture, intradiscal injection, and partial discectomy on the radial bulge and height of human lumbar discs. *Spine.* 1985;10:138–145.

18. Jayson MIV, Herbert CM, Barks JS. Intervertebral discs: nuclear morphology and bursting pressures. *Ann Rheum Dis.* 1973;32:308–315.

19. Perey O. Fracture of the vertebral end-plate in the lumbar spine. *Acta Orthop Scand.* 1957;25(suppl):1–101.

20. White AA, Panjabi MM. *Clinical Biomechanics of the Spine.* Philadelphia: Lippincott; 1978.

21. Twomey L, Taylor J, Furniss B. Age changes in the bone density and structure of the lumbar vertebral column. *J Anat.* 1983;136:15–25.

22. Rockoff SF, Sweet E, Bleustein J. The relative contribution of trabecular and cortical bone to the strength of human lumbar vertebrae. *Calcif Tissue Res.* 1969;3:163–175.

23. Yoganandan N, Myklebust JB, Wilson CR, et al. Functional biomechanics of the thoracolumbar vertebral cortex. *Clin Biomech.* 1988;3:11–18.

24. Brinckmann P, Biggemann M, Hilweg D. Fatigue fracture of human lumbar vertebrae. *Clin Biomech.* 1988;3(suppl 1):S1–S23.

25. Hutton WC, Adams MA. Can the lumbar spine be crushed in heavy lifting? *Spine.* 1982;7:586–590.

26. Hansson TH, Keller TS, Spengler DM. Mechanical behaviour of the human lumbar spine. II. Fatigue strength during dynamic compressive loading. *J Orthop Res.* 1987;5:479–487.

27. Hansson T, Roos B, Nachemson A. The bone mineral content and ultimate compressive strength of lumbar vertebrae. *Spine.* 1980;5:46–55.

28. Brinckmann P, Biggemann M, Hilweg D. Prediction of the compressive strength of human lumbar vertebrae. *Clin Biomech.* 1989;4(suppl 2):S1–S27.

29. Pope MH, Bevins T, Wilder DG, et al. The relationship between anthropometric, postural, muscular, and mobility characteristics of males ages 18–55. *Spine.* 1985;10:644–648.

30. Kazarian L. Dynamic response characteristics of the human lumbar vertebral column. *Acta Orthop Scand.* 1972;146(suppl):1–86.

31. Kazarian LE. Creep characteristics of the human spinal column. *Orthop Clin North Am.* 1975;6:3–18.

32. Markolf KL, Morris JM. The structural components of the intervertebral disc. *J Bone Joint Surg.* 1974;56A:675–687.

33. Bosford DJ, Esses SI, Ogilvie-Harris DJ. In vivo diurnal variation in intervertebral disc volume and morphology. *Spine.* 1994;19:935–940.

34. Krag MH, Cohen MC, Haugh LD, et al. Body height change during upright and recumbent posture. *Spine.* 1990;15:202–207.

35. Pukey P. The physiological oscillation of the length of the body. *Acta Orthop Scand.* 1935;6:338–347.

36. Tyrrell AJ, Reilly T, Troup JD. Circadian variation in stature and the effects of spinal loading. *Spine.* 1985;10:161–164.

37. Nachemson A. Lumbar intradiscal pressure. *Acta Orthop Scand.* 1960;43(suppl):1–104.

38. Nachemson A. Lumbar intradiscal pressure. In: Jayson MIV, ed. *The Lumbar Spine and Backache.* 2nd ed. London: Pitman; 1980:Ch 12, 341–358.

39. Nachemson AL. Disc pressure measurements. *Spine.* 1981;6:93–97.

40. Andersson GBJ, Ortengren R, Nachemson A. Quantitative studies of back loads in lifting. *Spine.* 1976;1:178–184.

41. Nachemson A. The influence of spinal movements on the lumbar intradiscal pressure and on the tensile stresses in the annulus fibrosus. *Acta Orthop Scand.* 1963;33:183–207.

42. Lorenz M, Patwardhan A, Vanderby R. Load-bearing characteristics of lumbar facets in normal and surgically altered spinal segments. *Spine.* 1983;8:122–130.

43. Hakim NS, King AI. Static and dynamic facet loads. Proceedings of the Twentieth Stapp Car Crash Conference. 1976, pp 607–639.

44. Miller JAA, Haderspeck KA, Schultz AB. Posterior element loads in lumbar motion segments. *Spine.* 1983;8:327–330.

45. Adams MA, Hutton WC. The mechanical function of the lumbar apophyseal joints. *Spine.* 1983;8:327–330.

46. Dunlop RB, Adams MA, Hutton WC. Disc space narrowing and the lumbar facet joints. *J Bone Joint Surg.* 1984;66B:706–710.

47. El-Bohy AA, Yang KH, King AI. Experimental verification of facet load transmission by direct measurement of facet lamina contact pressure. *J Biomech.* 1989;22:931–941.

48. Adams MA, Hutton WC. The effect of posture on the role of the apophyseal joints in resisting intervertebral compression force. *J Bone Joint Surg.* 1980;62B:358–362.

49. Yang KH, King AI. Mechanism of facet load transmission as a hypothesis for low-back pain. *Spine.* 1984;9:557–565.

50. Lin HS, Liu YK, Adams KH. Mechanical response of the lumbar intervertebral joint under physiological (complex) loading. *J Bone Joint Surg.* 1978;60A:41–54.

51. Markolf KL. Deformation of the thoracolumbar intervertebral joints in response to external loads. *J Bone Joint Surg.* 1972;54A:511–533.

52. Prasad P, King AI, Ewing CL. The role of articular facets during +Gz acceleration. *J Appl Mech.* 1974;41:321–326.

53. Liu YK, Njus G, Buckwalter J, et al. Fatigue response of lumbar intervertebral joints under axial cyclic loading. *Spine.* 1983;8:857–865.

54. Skaggs DL, Weidenbaum M, Iatridis JC, et al. Regional variation in tensile properties and biomechanical composition of the human lumbar anulus fibrosus. *Spine.* 1994;19:1310–1319.

55. Green TP, Adams MA, Dolan P. Tensile properties of the annulus

fibrosus II. Ultimate tensile strength and fatigue life. *Eur Spine J.* 1993;2:209–214.

56. Cyron BM, Hutton WC. The tensile strength of the capsular ligaments of the apophyseal joints. *J Anat.* 1981;132:145–150.

57. Twomey L. Sustained lumbar traction. An experimental study of long spine segments. *Spine.* 1985;10:146–149.

58. Pearcy MJ. Stereo-radiography of lumbar spine motion. *Acta Orthop Scand.* 1985;212(suppl):1–41.

59. Pearcy M, Portek I, Shepherd J. Three-dimensional X-ray analysis of normal movement in the lumbar spine. *Spine.* 1984;9:294–297.

60. Twomey LT, Taylor JR. Sagittal movements of the human lumbar vertebral column: a quantitative study of the role of the posterior vertebral elements. *Arch Phys Med Rehab.* 1983;64:322–325.

61. Lewin T, Moffet B, Viidik A. The morphology of the lumbar synovial intervertebral joints. *Acta Morphol Neerlando-Scand.* 1962;4:299–319.

62. Green TP, Allvey JC, Adams MA. Spondylolysis: bending of the inferior articular processes of lumbar vertebrae during simulated spinal movements. *Spine.* 1994;19:2683–2691.

63. Adams MA, Green TP, Dolan P. The strength in anterior bending of lumbar intervertebral discs. *Spine.* 1994;19:2197–2203.

64. Neumann P, Osvalder AL, Nordwall A, et al. The mechanism of initial flexion-distraction injury in the lumbar spine. *Spine.* 1992;17:1083–1090.

65. Osvalder AL, Neumann P, Lovsund P, et al. Ultimate strength of the lumbar spine in flexion – an in vitro study. *J Biomech.* 1990;23:453–460.

66. Goel VK, Voo LM, Weinstein JN, et al. Response of the ligamentous lumbar spine to cyclic bending loads. *Spine.* 1988;13:294–300.

67. Adams MA, Hutton WC. The effect of fatigue on the lumbar intervertebral disc. *J Bone Joint Surg.* 1983;65B:199–203.

68. Cyron BM, Hutton WC. The fatigue strength of the lumbar neural arch in spondylolysis. *J Bone Joint Surg.* 1978;60B:234–238.

69. Adams MA, Dolan P, Hutton WC. The lumbar spine in backward bending. *Spine.* 1988;13:1019–1026.

70. Haher TR, O'Brien M, Dryer JW, et al. The role of the lumbar facet joints in spinal stability: identification of alternative paths of loading. *Spine.* 1994;19:2667–2671.

71. Farfan HF, Cossette JW, Robertson GH, et al. The effects of torsion on the lumbar intervertebral joints: the role of torsion in the production of disc degeneration. *J Bone Joint Surg.* 1970;52A:468–497.

72. Cossette JW, Farfan HF, Robertson GH, et al. The instantaneous center of rotation of the third lumbar intervertebral joint. *J Biomech.* 1971;4:149–153.

73. Ham AW, Cormack DH. *Histology.* 8th ed. Philadelphia: Lippincott; 1979:373.

74. Adams MA, Hutton WC. The relevance of torsion to the mechanical derangement of the lumbar spine. *Spine.* 1981;6:241–248.

75. Asano S, Kaneda K, Umehara S, et al. The mechanical properties of the human L4–L5 functional spinal unit during cyclic loading: the structural effects of the posterior elements. *Spine.* 1992;17:1343–1352.

76. Liu YK, Goel VK, DeJong A, et al. Torsional fatigue of the lumbar intervertebral joints. *Spine.* 1985;10:894–900.

77. Hindle RJ, Pearcy MJ. Rotational mobility of the human back in forward flexion. *J Biomed Eng.* 1989;11:219–223.

78. Pearcy MJ, Hindle RJ. Axial rotation of lumbar intervertebral joints in forward flexion. *Proc Inst Mech Eng H.* 1991;205:205–209.

79. Gunzburg R, Hutton W, Fraser R. Axial rotation of the lumbar spine and the effect of flexion: an in vitro and in vivo biomechanical study. *Spine.* 1991;16:22–28.

80. Pearcy MJ. Twisting mobility of the human back in flexed postures. *Spine.* 1993;18:114–119.

81. American Medical Association. *1993 Guides to the Evaluation of Permanent Impairment.* 4th ed. Chicago: American Medical Association; 1993.

82. Benson DR, Schultz AB, Dewald RL. Roentgenographic evaluation of vertebral rotation. *J Bone Joint Surg.* 1976;58A:1125–1129.

83. Frymoyer JW, Frymoyer WW, Pope MH. The mechanical and kinematic analysis of the lumbar spine in normal living human subjects in vivo. *J Biomech.* 1979;12:165–172.

84. Pearcy MJ, Tibrewal SB. Axial rotation and lateral bending in the normal lumbar spine measured by three-dimensional radiography. *Spine.* 1984;9:582–587.

85. Pearcy MJ, Portek I, Shepherd J. The effect of low-back pain on lumbar spinal movements measured by three-dimensional X-ray analysis. *Spine.* 1985;10:150–153.

86. Tibrewal SB, Pearcy MJ, Portek I, et al. A prospective study of lumbar spinal movements before and after discectomy using biplanar radiography. *Spine.* 1985;10:455–460.

87. Dvořák J, Panjabi MM, Chang DG, et al. Functional radiographic diagnosis of the lumbar spine: flexion-extension and lateral bending. *Spine.* 1991;16:562–571.

88. Pearcy MJ, Bogduk N. Instantaneous axes of rotation of the lumbar intervertebral joints. *Spine.* 1988;13:1033–1041.

89. Gertzbein SD, Seligman J, Holtby R, et al. Tile M. Centrode characteristics of the lumbar spine as a function of segmental instability. *Clin Orthop.* 1986;208:48–51.

90. Gertzbein SD, Seligman J, Holtby R, et al. Centrode patterns and segmental instability in degenerative disc disease. *Spine.* 1985;10:257–261.

91. Bogduk N, Jull G. The theoretical pathology of acute locked back: a basis for manipulative therapy. *Man Med.* 1985;1:78–82.

92. Bogduk N, Amevo B, Pearcy M. A biological basis for instantaneous centres of rotation of the vertebral column. *Proc Inst Mech Eng H.* 1995;209:177–183.

The lumbar muscles and their fasciae

The lumbar spine is surrounded by muscles which, for descriptive purposes and on functional grounds, may be divided into three groups. These are:

1. Psoas major, which covers the anterolateral aspects of the lumbar spine.
2. Intertransversarii laterales and quadratus lumborum, which connect and cover the transverse processes anteriorly.
3. The lumbar back muscles, which lie behind and cover the posterior elements of the lumbar spine.

PSOAS MAJOR

The psoas major is a long muscle which arises from the anterolateral aspect of the lumbar spine and descends over the brim of the pelvis to insert into the lesser trochanter of the femur. It is essentially a muscle of the thigh whose principal action is flexion of the hip.

The psoas major has diverse but systematic attachments to the lumbar spine (Fig. 9.1). At each segmental level from T12–L1 to L4–5, it is attached to the medial three-quarters or so of the anterior surface of the transverse process, to the intervertebral disc, and to the margins of the vertebral bodies adjacent to the disc.[1] An additional fascicle arises from the L5 vertebral body. Classically, the muscle is also said to arise from a tendinous arch that covers the lateral aspect of the vertebral body.[2] Close dissection,[1] however, reveals that these arches constitute no more than the medial, deep fascia of the muscle, and that the fascia affords no particular additional origin; the most medial fibres of the muscle skirt the fascia and are anchored directly to the upper margin of the vertebral body. Nonetheless, the fascia forms an arcade deep to the psoas, over the lateral surface of the vertebral body, leaving a space between the arch and the bone that transmits the lumbar arteries and veins (see Ch. 11).

The muscle fibres from the L4–5 intervertebral disc, the L5 body and the L5 transverse process form the deepest and lowest bundle of fibres within the muscle. These fibres are systematically overlapped by fibres from the disc, vertebral margins and transverse process at successively

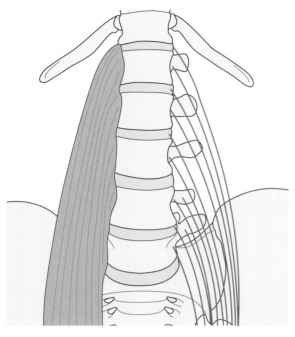

Figure 9.1 Psoas major. At each segmental level, the psoas major attaches to the transverse process, the intervertebral disc and adjacent vertebral margins.

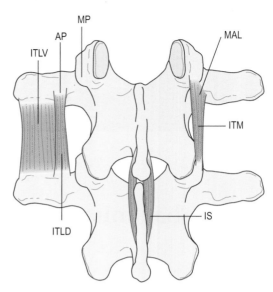

Figure 9.2 The short, intersegmental muscles. AP, accessory process; IS, interspinales; ITLD, intertransversarii laterales dorsales; ITLV, intertransversarii laterales ventrales; ITM, intertransversarii mediales; MAL, mamillo-accessory ligament; MP, mamillary process.

higher levels. As a result, the muscle in cross-section is layered circumferentially, with fibres from higher levels forming the outer surface of the muscle and those from lower levels buried sequentially, deeper within its substance. Within the muscle, bundles from individual lumbar segments have the same length, such that those from L1 become tendinous before those from successively lower levels. This isometric morphology indicates that the muscle is designed exclusively to act on the hip.[1]

Biomechanical analysis reveals that the psoas has only a feeble action on the lumbar spine with respect to flexion and extension. Its fibres are disposed so as to extend upper lumbar segments and to flex lower lumbar segments. However, the fibres act very close to the axes of rotation of the lumbar vertebrae and so can exert only very small moments, even under maximal contraction.[1] This denies the psoas any substantial action on the lumbar spine. Rather, it uses the lumbar spine as a base from which to act on the hip.

However, the psoas potentially exerts massive compression loads on the lower lumbar discs. The proximity of the lines of action of the muscle to the axes of rotation minimises its capacity as a flexor but maximises the axial compression that it exerts. Upon maximum contraction, in an activity such as sit-ups, the two psoas muscles can be expected to exert a compression load on the L5–S1 disc equal to about 100 kg of weight.[1]

INTERTRANSVERSARII LATERALES

The **intertransversarii laterales** consist of two parts: the intertransversarii laterales **ventrales** and the intertransversarii laterales **dorsales**. The ventral intertransversarii connect the margins of consecutive transverse processes, while the dorsal intertransversarii each connect an accessory process to the transverse process below (Fig. 9.2). Both the ventral and dorsal intertransversarii are innervated by the ventral rami of the lumbar spinal nerves,[3] and consequently cannot be classified among the back muscles which are all innervated by the dorsal rami (see Ch. 10). On the basis of their attachments and their nerve supply, the ventral and dorsal intertransversarii are considered to be homologous to the intercostal and levator costae muscles of the thoracic region.[3]

The function of the intertransversarii laterales has never been determined experimentally but it may be like that of the posterior, intersegmental muscles (see below).

QUADRATUS LUMBORUM

The quadratus lumborum is a wide, more or less rectangular, muscle that covers the lateral two-thirds or so of the anterior surfaces of the L1 to L4 transverse processes and extends laterally a few centimetres beyond the tips of the transverse processes. In detail, the muscle is a complex aggregation of various oblique and longitudinally running fibres that connect the lumbar transverse processes, the ilium and the 12th rib (Fig. 9.3).[4]

The muscle can be considered as consisting of four types of fascicle arranged in three layers.[5] Iliocostal fibres connect the ilium and the 12th rib. Iliolumbar lumbar fibres connect the ilium and the lumbar transverse processes. Lumbocostal fibres connect the lumbar transverse processes and the 12th rib. A fourth type of fascicle connects the ilium and the body of the 12th thoracic vertebra. Occasionally, fascicles may connect the lumbar transverse processes to the body of the 12th thoracic vertebra.

The posterior layer (see Fig. 9.3A) consists of iliolumbar fascicles inferiorly and medially, and iliocostal fascicles laterally.[5] The iliolumbar fibres arise from the iliac crest, and most consistently insert into the upper three lumbar transverse processes. Occasionally, some fascicles also insert into the L4 transverse process.

The middle layer (see Fig. 9.3B) typically arises by a common tendon from the anterior surface of the L3 transverse process. Its fascicles radiate to the inferior anterior aspect of the medial half or so of the 12th rib.[5] Occasionally these fascicles are joined by ones from the L2, L4 and L5 transverse processes.

The anterior layer (see Fig. 9.3C) consists of more or less parallel fibres stemming from the iliac crest and passing upwards. The more lateral fibres insert into the lower anterior aspect of the 12th rib. More medial fibres insert into a tubercle on the lateral aspect of the body of the 12th thoracic vertebra.[5] These latter fascicles may be joined at their insertion by fascicles from the lumbar transverse processes, most often from the L4 and L5 levels, when they occur.

Within each layer, different fascicles are interwoven, in a complex and irregular fashion. Also, the three layers blend in places, and may be difficult to distinguish, especially laterally where iliocostal fibres from the anterior and posterior layers wrap around the iliolumbar and lumbocostal fascicles of the middle and posterior layers.

The prevalence of fascicles with particular segmental attachments varies considerably from specimen to specimen. Not all are always represented. The most consistently represented fascicles are iliocostal fascicles from the outer end of the iliac origin of the muscle, iliolumbar fibres to the L3 transverse process, and lumbocostal fascicles from the L3 transverse process.

Fascicles also vary considerably in size, if and when present. The largest tend to be those from the ilium to the lumbar transverse processes, and those from the ilium to the 12th thoracic vertebra (when present).

The irregular and inconstant structure of the quadratus lumborum makes it difficult to discern exactly its function. Classically one of the functions of this muscle is said to be to fix the 12th rib during respiration.[2] This fits with many, although not most, of its fibres inserting into the 12th rib. The majority of fibres, and the largest, however, anchor the lumbar transverse processes and the 12th thoracic vertebra to the ilium. These attachments indicate that a major action of the muscle would be lateral flexion of the lumbar spine. However, the strength of the muscle is limited by the size of its fascicles and their moment arms. For lateral flexion, the quadratus lumborum can exert a maximum moment of about 35 Nm.[5]

Since the fascicles of the quadratus lumborum act behind the axes of sagittal rotation of the lumbar vertebrae, they are potentially extensors of the lumbar spine. However, in this role their capacity is limited to about 20 Nm,[5] which amounts to less than 10% of the moment exerted by the posterior back muscles.

These limitations in strength leave the actual function of the quadratus lumborum still an enigma.

THE LUMBAR BACK MUSCLES

The lumbar back muscles are those that lie behind the plane of the transverse processes and which exert an action on the lumbar spine. They include muscles that attach to the lumbar vertebrae and thereby act directly on the lumbar spine, and certain other muscles that, while not attaching to the lumbar vertebrae, nevertheless exert an action on the lumbar spine.

For descriptive purposes and on morphological grounds, the lumbar back muscles may be divided into three groups:

1. The short intersegmental muscles – the interspinales and the intertransversarii mediales.
2. The polysegmental muscles that attach to the lumbar vertebrae – the multifidus and the lumbar components of the longissimus and iliocostalis.
3. The long polysegmental muscles, represented by the thoracic components of the longissimus and iliocostalis lumborum, which in general do not attach to the lumbar vertebrae but cross the lumbar region from thoracic levels to find attachments on the ilium and sacrum.

The descriptions of the back muscles offered in this chapter, notably those of the multifidus and erector spinae, differ substantially from those given in standard textbooks. Traditionally, these muscles have been regarded as stemming from a common origin on the sacrum and ilium and passing upwards to assume diverse attachments to the lumbar and thoracic vertebrae and ribs. However, in the face of several studies of these muscles,[6–9] it is considered more appropriate to view them in the reverse direction – from above downwards. Not only is this more consistent with the pattern of their nerve supply[9,10] but it clarifies the identity of certain muscles and the identity of the erector spinae aponeurosis, and reveals the segmental biomechanical disposition of the muscles.

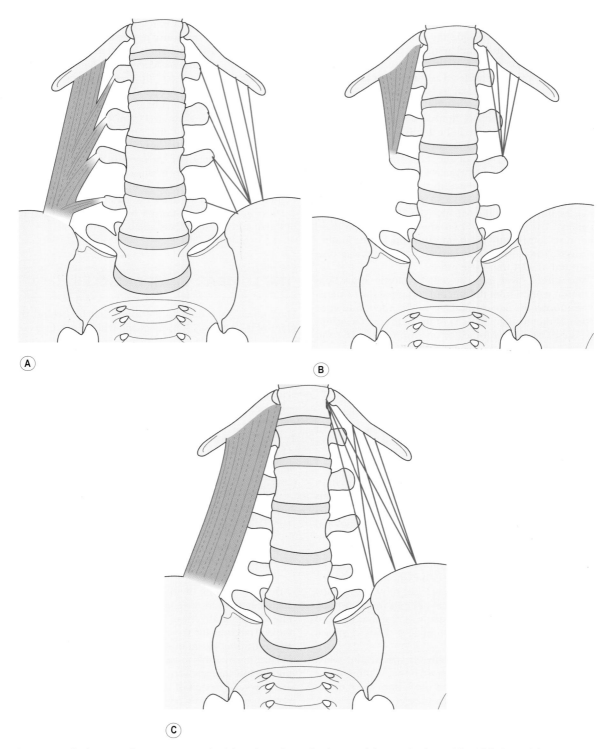

Figure 9.3 The layers and more common fascicles of quadratus lumborum. (A) Posterior layer. (B) Middle layer. (C) Anterior layer.

Interspinales

The lumbar interspinales are short paired muscles that lie on either side of the interspinous ligament and connect the spinous processes of adjacent lumbar vertebrae (see Fig. 9.2). There are four pairs in the lumbar region.

Although disposed to produce posterior sagittal rotation of the vertebra above, the interspinales are quite small and would not contribute appreciably to the force required to move a vertebra. This paradox is similar to that which applies for the intertransversarii mediales and is discussed further in that context.

Intertransversarii mediales

The intertransversarii mediales can be considered to be true back muscles for, unlike the intertransversarii laterales, they are innervated by the lumbar dorsal rami.[3,10] The intertransversarii mediales arise from an accessory process, the adjoining mamillary process and the mamillo-accessory ligament that connects these two processes.[11] They insert into the superior aspect of the mamillary process of the vertebra below (see Fig. 9.2).

The intertransversarii mediales lie lateral to the axis of lateral flexion and behind the axis of sagittal rotation. However, they lie very close to these axes and are very small muscles. Therefore, it is questionable whether they could contribute any appreciable force in either lateral flexion or posterior sagittal rotation. It might perhaps be argued that larger muscles provide the bulk of the power to move the vertebrae and the intertransversarii act to 'fine tune' the movement. However, this suggestion is highly speculative, if not fanciful, and does not account for their small size and considerable mechanical disadvantage.

A tantalising alternative suggestion is that the intertransversarii (and perhaps also the interspinales) act as large proprioceptive transducers; their value lies not in the force they can exert but in the muscle spindles they contain. Placed close to the lumbar vertebral column, the intertransversarii could monitor the movements of the column and provide feedback that influences the action of the surrounding muscles. Such a role has been suggested for the cervical intertransversarii, which have been found to contain a high density of muscle spindles.[12-14] Indeed, all unisegmental muscles of the vertebral column have between two and six times the density of muscles spindles found in the longer polysegmental muscles, and there is growing speculation that this underscores the proprioceptive function of all short, small muscles of the body.[15-17]

Multifidus

The multifidus is the largest and most medial of the lumbar back muscles. It consists of a repeating series of fascicles which stem from the laminae and spinous processes of the lumbar vertebrae and exhibit a constant pattern of attachments caudally.[9]

The shortest fascicles of the multifidus are the 'laminar fibres', which arise from the caudal end of the dorsal surface of each vertebral lamina and insert into the mamillary process of the vertebra two levels caudad (Fig. 9.4A). The L5 laminar fibres have no mamillary process into which they can insert, and insert instead into an area on the sacrum just above the first dorsal sacral foramen. Because of their attachments, the laminar fibres may be considered homologous to the thoracic rotatores.

The bulk of the lumbar multifidus consists of much larger fascicles that radiate from the lumbar spinous processes. These fascicles are arranged in five overlapping groups such that each lumbar vertebra gives rise to one of these groups. At each segmental level, a fascicle arises from the base and caudolateral edge of the spinous process, and several fascicles arise, by way of a common tendon, from the caudal tip of the spinous process. This tendon is referred to hereafter as 'the common tendon'. Although confluent with one another at their origin, the fascicles in each group diverge caudally to assume separate attachments to mamillary processes, the iliac crest and the sacrum.

The fascicle from the base of the L1 spinous process inserts into the L4 mamillary process, while those from the common tendon insert into the mamillary processes of L5, S1 and the posterior superior iliac spine (Fig. 9.4B).

The fascicle from the base of the spinous process of L2 inserts into the mamillary process of L5, while those from the common tendon insert into the S1 mamillary process, the posterior superior iliac spine, and an area on the iliac crest just caudoventral to the posterior superior iliac spine (Fig. 9.4C).

The fascicle from the base of the L3 spinous process inserts into the mamillary process of the sacrum, while those fascicles from the common tendon insert into a narrow area extending caudally from the caudal extent of the posterior superior iliac spine to the lateral edge of the third sacral segment (Fig. 9.4D). The L4 fascicles insert onto the sacrum in an area medial to the L3 area of insertion, but lateral to the dorsal sacral foramina (Fig. 9.4E), while those from the L5 vertebra insert onto an area medial to the dorsal sacral foramina (Fig. 9.4F).

It is noteworthy that while many of the fascicles of multifidus attach to mamillary processes, some of the deeper fibres of these fascicles attach to the capsules of the zygapophysial joints next to the mamillary processes (see Ch. 3).[18] This attachment allows the multifidus to protect the joint capsule from being caught inside the joint during the movements executed by the multifidus.

The key feature of the morphology of the lumbar multifidus is that its fascicles are arranged segmentally. Each lumbar vertebra is endowed with a group of fascicles that radiate from its spinous process, anchoring it below to

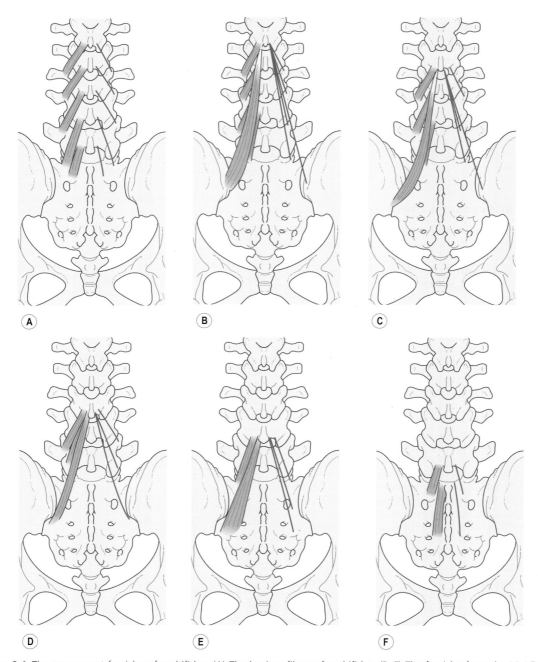

Figure 9.4 The component fascicles of multifidus. (A) The laminar fibres of multifidus. (B–F) The fascicles from the L1–L5 spinous processes, respectively.

mamillary processes, the iliac crest and the sacrum. This disposition suggests that the fibres of multifidus are arranged in such a way that their principal action is focused on individual lumbar spinous processes.[9] They are designed to act in concert on a single spinous process. This

contention is supported by the pattern of innervation of the muscle. All the fascicles arising from the spinous processes of a given vertebra are innervated by the medial branch of the dorsal ramus that issues from below that vertebra (see Ch. 10).[9,10] Thus, the muscles that directly act

98

on a particular vertebral segment are innervated by the nerve of that segment.

In a posterior view, the fascicles of multifidus are seen to have an oblique caudolateral orientation. Their line of action can therefore be resolved into two vectors: a large vertical vector and a considerably smaller horizontal vector (Fig. 9.5A).[7]

The small horizontal vector suggests that the multifidus could pull the spinous processes sideways, and therefore produce horizontal rotation. However, horizontal rotation of lumbar vertebrae is impeded by the impaction of the contralateral zygapophysial joints. Horizontal rotation occurs after impaction of the joints only if an appropriate shear force is applied to the intervertebral discs (see Ch. 7) but the horizontal vector of multifidus is so small that it is unlikely that the multifidus would be capable of exerting such a shear force on the disc by acting on the spinous process. Indeed, electromyographic studies reveal that the multifidus is inconsistently active in derotation and that, paradoxically, it is active in both ipsilateral and contralateral rotation.[19] Rotation, therefore, cannot be inferred to be a primary action of the multifidus. In this context, the multifidus has been said to act only as a 'stabiliser' in rotation,[18,19] but the aberrant movements, which it is supposed to stabilise, have not been defined (although see below).

The principal action of the multifidus is expressed by its vertical vector, and further insight is gained when this vector is viewed in a lateral projection (Fig. 9.5B). Each fascicle of multifidus, at every level, acts virtually at right angles to its spinous process of origin.[7] Thus, using the spinous process as a lever, every fascicle is ideally disposed to produce posterior sagittal rotation of its vertebra. The right-angle orientation, however, precludes any action as a posterior horizontal translator. Therefore, the multifidus can only exert the 'rocking' component of extension of the lumbar spine or control this component during flexion.

Having established that the multifidus is primarily a posterior sagittal rotator of the lumbar spine, it is possible to resolve the paradox about its activity during horizontal rotation of the trunk.[7] In the first instance, it should be realised that rotation of the lumbar spine is an indirect action. Active rotation of the lumbar spine occurs only if the thorax is first rotated, and is therefore secondary to thoracic rotation. Secondly, it must be realised that a muscle with two vectors of action cannot use these vectors independently. If the muscle contracts, then both vectors are exerted. Thus, the multifidus cannot exert axial rotation without simultaneously exerting a much larger posterior sagittal rotation.

The principal muscles that produce rotation of the thorax are the oblique abdominal muscles. The horizontal component of their orientation is able to turn the thoracic cage in the horizontal plane and thereby impart axial rotation to the lumbar spine. However, the oblique abdominal muscles also have a vertical component to their orientation. Therefore, if they contract to produce rotation they will also simultaneously cause flexion of the trunk, and therefore of the lumbar spine. To counteract this flexion, and maintain pure axial rotation, extensors of the lumbar

Figure 9.5 The force vectors of multifidus. (A) In a posteroanterior view, the oblique line of action of the multifidus at each level (bold arrows) can be resolved into a major vertical vector (V) and a smaller horizontal vector (H). (B) In a lateral view, the vertical vectors of the multifidus are seen to be aligned at right angles to the spinous processes.

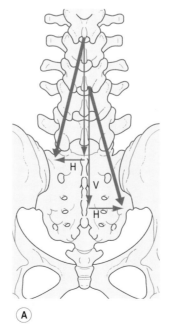

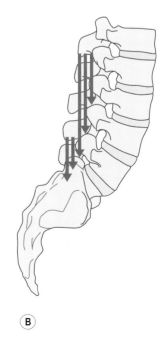

(A)

(B)

spine must be recruited, and this is how the multifidus becomes involved in rotation.

The role of the multifidus in rotation is not to produce rotation but to oppose the flexion effect of the abdominal muscles as they produce rotation. The aberrant motion 'stabilised' by the multifidus during rotation is, therefore, the unwanted flexion unavoidably produced by the abdominal muscles.[7]

Apart from its action on individual lumbar vertebrae, the multifidus, because of its polysegmental nature, can also exert indirect effects on any interposed vertebrae. Since the line of action of any long fascicle of multifidus lies behind the lordotic curve of the lumbar spine, such fascicles can act like bowstrings on those segments of the curve that intervene between the attachments of the fascicle. The bowstring effect would tend to accentuate the lumbar lordosis, resulting in compression of intervertebral discs posteriorly, and strain of the discs and longitudinal ligament anteriorly. Thus, a secondary effect of the action of the multifidus is to increase the lumbar lordosis and the compressive and tensile loads on any vertebrae and intervertebral discs interposed between its attachments.

Lumbar erector spinae

The lumbar erector spinae lies lateral to the multifidus and forms the prominent dorsolateral contour of the back muscles in the lumbar region. It consists of two muscles: the **longissimus thoracis** and the **iliocostalis lumborum**. Furthermore, each of these muscles has two components: a lumbar part, consisting of fascicles arising from lumbar vertebrae, and a thoracic part, consisting of fascicles arising from thoracic vertebrae or ribs.[6,8] These four parts may be referred to, respectively, as longissimus thoracis *pars lumborum*, iliocostalis lumborum *pars lumborum*, longissimus thoracis *pars thoracis* and iliocostalis lumborum *pars thoracis*.[8]

In the lumbar region, the longissimus and iliocostalis are separated from each other by the **lumbar intermuscular aponeurosis**, an anteroposterior continuation of the erector spinae aponeurosis.[6,8] It appears as a flat sheet of collagen fibres, which extend rostrally from the medial aspect of the posterior superior iliac spine for 6–8 cm. It is formed mainly by the caudal tendons of the rostral four fascicles of the lumbar component of longissimus (Fig. 9.6).

Longissimus thoracis pars lumborum

The longissimus thoracis pars lumborum is composed of five fascicles, each arising from the accessory process and the adjacent medial end of the dorsal surface of the transverse process of a lumbar vertebra (see Fig. 9.6).

The fascicle from the L5 vertebra is the deepest and shortest. Its fibres insert directly into the medial aspect of the posterior superior iliac spine. The fascicle from L4 also

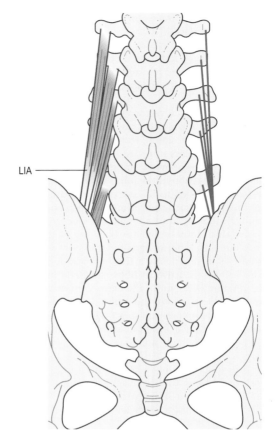

Figure 9.6 The lumbar fibres of longissimus (longissimus thoracis pars lumborum). On the left, the five fascicles of the intact muscle are drawn. The formation of the lumbar intermuscular aponeurosis (LIA) by the lumbar fascicles of longissimus is depicted. On the right, the lines indicate the attachments and span of the fascicles.

lies deeply, but lateral to that from L5. Succeeding fascicles lie progressively more dorsally, so that the L3 fascicle covers those from L4 and L5 but is itself covered by the L2 fascicle, while the L1 fascicle lies most superficially.

The L1–L4 fascicles all form tendons at their caudal ends. These converge to form the lumbar intermuscular aponeurosis, which eventually attaches to a narrow area on the ilium immediately lateral to the insertion of the L5 fascicle. The lumbar intermuscular aponeurosis thus represents a common tendon of insertion, or the aponeurosis, of the bulk of the lumbar fibres of longissimus.

Each fascicle of the lumbar longissimus has both a dorsoventral and a rostrocaudal orientation.[8] Therefore, the action of each fascicle can be resolved into a vertical vector and a horizontal vector, the relative sizes of which differ from L1 to L5 (Fig. 9.7A). Consequently, the relative

Figure 9.7 The force vectors of the longissimus thoracis pars lumborum. (A) In a lateral view, the oblique line of action of each fascicle of longissimus can be resolved into a vertical (V) and a horizontal (H) vector. The horizontal vectors of lower lumbar fascicles are larger. (B) In a posteroanterior view, the line of action of the fascicles can be resolved into a major vertical vector and a much smaller horizontal vector.

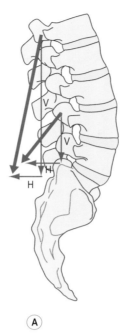

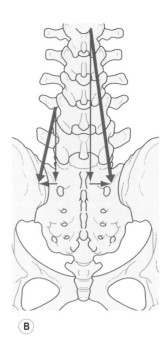

(A) (B)

actions of the longissimus differ at each segmental level. Furthermore, the action of the longissimus, as a whole, will differ according to whether the muscle contracts unilaterally or bilaterally.

The large vertical vector of each fascicle lies lateral to the axis of lateral flexion and behind the axis of sagittal rotation of each vertebra. Thus, contracting the longissimus unilaterally can laterally flex the vertebral column, but acting bilaterally the various fascicles can act, like the multifidus, to produce posterior sagittal rotation of their vertebra of origin. However, their attachments to the accessory and transverse processes lie close to the axes of sagittal rotation, and therefore their capacity to produce posterior sagittal rotation is less efficient than that of the multifidus, which acts through the long levers of the spinous processes.[8]

The horizontal vectors of the longissimus are directed backwards. Therefore, when contracting bilaterally the longissimus is capable of drawing the lumbar vertebrae backwards. This action of posterior translation can restore the anterior translation of the lumbar vertebrae that occurs during flexion of the lumbar column (see Ch. 7). The capacity for posterior translation is greatest at lower lumbar levels, where the fascicles of longissimus assume a greater dorsoventral orientation (Fig. 9.7B).

Reviewing the horizontal and vertical actions of longissimus together, it can be seen that longissimus expresses a continuum of combined actions along the length of the lumbar vertebral column. From below upwards, its capacity as a posterior sagittal rotator increases, while, conversely, from above downwards, the fascicles are better designed to resist or restore anterior translation. It is emphasised that the longissimus cannot exert its horizontal and vertical vectors independently. Thus, whatever horizontal translation it exerts must occur simultaneously with posterior sagittal rotation. The resolution into vectors simply reveals the relative amounts of simultaneous translation and sagittal rotation exerted at different segmental levels.

It might be deduced that because of the horizontal vector of longissimus, this muscle acting unilaterally could draw the accessory and transverse processes backwards and therefore produce axial rotation. However, in this regard, the fascicles of longissimus are orientated almost directly towards the axis of axial rotation and so are at a marked mechanical disadvantage to produce axial rotation.

Iliocostalis lumborum pars lumborum

The lumbar component of the iliocostalis lumborum consists of four overlying fascicles arising from the L1 through to the L4 vertebrae. Rostrally, each fascicle attaches to the tip of the transverse process and to an area extending 2–3 cm laterally onto the middle layer of the thoracolumbar fascia (Fig. 9.8).

The fascicle from L4 is the deepest, and caudally it is attached directly to the iliac crest just lateral to the posterior superior iliac spine. This fascicle is covered by the fascicle from L3 that has a similar but more dorsolaterally

101

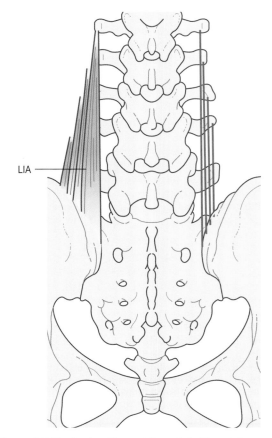

LIA

Figure 9.8 The lumbar fibres of iliocostalis (iliocostalis lumborum pars lumborum). On the left, the four lumbar fascicles of iliocostalis are shown. On the right, their span and attachments are indicated by the lines.

located attachment on the iliac crest. In sequence, L2 covers L3 and L1 covers L2, with insertions on the iliac crest becoming successively more dorsal and lateral. The most lateral fascicles attach to the iliac crest just medial to the attachment of the 'lateral raphe' of the thoracolumbar fascia (see below). The most medial fibres of iliocostalis contribute to the lumbar intermuscular aponeurosis but only to a minor extent.

Although an L5 fascicle of iliocostalis lumborum is not described in the literature, it is represented in the ilio-lumbar 'ligament'. In neonates and children this 'ligament' is said to be completely muscular in structure (see Ch. 4).[20] By the third decade of life, the muscle fibres are entirely replaced by collagen, giving rise to the familiar iliolumbar ligament.[20] On the basis of sites of attachment and relative orientation, the posterior band of the iliolumbar ligament would appear to be derived from the L5 fascicle of iliocostalis, while the anterior band of the ligament is a derivative of the quadratus lumborum.

The disposition of the lumbar fascicles of iliocostalis is similar to that of the lumbar longissimus, except that the fascicles are situated more laterally. Like that of the lumbar longissimus, their action can be resolved into horizontal and vertical vectors (Fig. 9.9A).

The vertical vector is still predominant, and therefore the lumbar fascicles of iliocostalis contracting bilaterally can act as posterior sagittal rotators (Fig. 9.9B), but because of the horizontal vector a posterior translation will be exerted simultaneously, principally at lower lumbar levels where the fascicles of iliocostalis have a greater forward orientation. Contracting unilaterally, the lumbar fascicles of iliocostalis can act as lateral flexors of the lumbar ver-tebrae, for which action the transverse processes provide very substantial levers.

Contracting unilaterally, the fibres of iliocostalis are better suited to exert axial rotation than the fascicles of lumbar longissimus, for their attachment to the tips of the transverse processes displaces them from the axis of hori-zontal rotation and provides them with substantial levers for this action. Because of this leverage, the lower fascicles of iliocostalis are the only intrinsic muscles of the lumbar spine reasonably disposed to produce horizontal rotation. Their effectiveness as rotators, however, is dwarfed by the oblique abdominal muscles that act on the ribs and produce lumbar rotation indirectly by rotating the tho-racic cage. However, because the iliocostalis cannot exert axial rotation without simultaneously exerting posterior sagittal rotation, the muscle is well suited to cooperate with the multifidus to oppose the flexion effect of the abdominal muscles when they act to rotate the trunk.

Longissimus thoracis pars thoracis

The thoracic fibres of longissimus thoracis typically consist of 11 or 12 pairs of small fascicles arising from the ribs and transverse processes of T1 or T2 down to T12 (Fig. 9.10). At each level, two tendons can usually be recog-nised, a medial one from the tip of the transverse process and a lateral one from the rib, although in the upper three or four levels, the latter may merge medially with the fascicle from the transverse process. Each rostral tendon extends 3–4 cm before forming a small muscle belly meas-uring 7–8 cm in length. The muscle bellies from the higher levels overlap those from lower levels. Each muscle belly eventually forms a caudal tendon that extends into the lumbar region. The tendons run in parallel, with those from higher levels being most medial. The fascicles from the T2 level attach to the L3 spinous process, while the fascicles from the remaining levels insert into spinous processes at progressively lower levels. For example, those from T5 attach to L5, and those from T7 to S2 or S3. Those from T8 to T12 diverge from the midline to find attach-ment to the sacrum along a line extending from the S3 spinous process to the caudal extent of the posterior supe-rior iliac spine.[8] The lateral edge of the caudal tendon of

Figure 9.9 The force vectors of the iliocostalis lumborum pars lumborum. (A) In a lateral view, the line of action of the fascicles can be resolved into vertical (V) and horizontal (H) vectors. The horizontal vectors are larger at lower lumbar levels. (B) In a posteroanterior view, the line of action is resolved into a vertical vector and a very small horizontal vector.

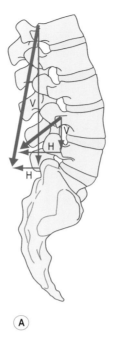

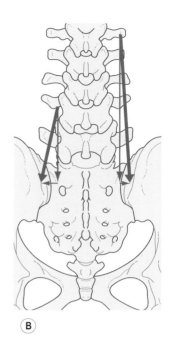

A

B

T12 lies alongside the dorsal edge of the lumbar intermuscular aponeurosis formed by the caudal tendon of the L1 longissimus bundle.

The side-to-side aggregation of the caudal tendons of longissimus thoracis pars thoracis forms much of what is termed the erector spinae aponeurosis, which covers the lumbar fibres of longissimus and iliocostalis but affords no attachment to them.

The longissimus thoracis pars thoracis is designed to act on thoracic vertebrae and ribs. Nonetheless, when contracting bilaterally it acts indirectly on the lumbar vertebral column and uses the erector spinae aponeurosis to produce an increase in the lumbar lordosis. However, not all of the fascicles of longissimus thoracis span the entire lumbar vertebral column. Those from the second rib and T2 reach only as far as L3, and only those fascicles arising between the T6 or T7 and the T12 levels actually span the entire lumbar region. Consequently, only a portion of the whole thoracic longissimus acts on all the lumbar vertebrae.

The oblique orientation of the longissimus thoracis pars thoracis also permits it to flex the thoracic vertebral column laterally and thereby to indirectly flex the lumbar vertebral column laterally.

Iliocostalis lumborum pars thoracis

The iliocostalis lumborum pars thoracis consists of fascicles from the lower seven or eight ribs that attach caudally to the ilium and sacrum (Fig. 9.11). These fascicles represent the thoracic component of iliocostalis lumborum and should not be confused with the iliocostalis thoracis, which is restricted to the thoracic region between the upper six and lower six ribs.

Each fascicle of the iliocostalis lumborum pars thoracis arises from the angle of the rib via a ribbon-like tendon 9–10 cm long. It then forms a muscle belly 8–10 cm long. Thereafter, each fascicle continues as a tendon, contributing to the erector spinae aponeurosis and ultimately attaching to the posterior superior iliac spine. The most medial tendons, from the more rostral fascicles, often attach more medially to the dorsal surface of the sacrum, caudal to the insertion of multifidus.

The thoracic fascicles of iliocostalis lumborum have no attachment to lumbar vertebrae. They attach to the iliac crest and thereby span the lumbar region. Consequently, by acting bilaterally, it is possible for them to exert an indirect 'bowstring' effect on the vertebral column, causing an increase in the lordosis of the lumbar spine. Acting unilaterally, the iliocostalis lumborum pars thoracis can use the leverage afforded by the ribs to laterally flex the thoracic cage and thereby laterally flex the lumbar vertebral column indirectly. The distance between the ribs and the ilium does not shorten greatly during rotation of the trunk, and therefore the iliocostalis lumborum pars thoracis can have little action as an axial rotator. However, contralateral rotation greatly increases this distance, and the iliocostalis lumborum pars thoracis can serve to de-rotate the thoracic cage and, therefore, the lumbar spine.

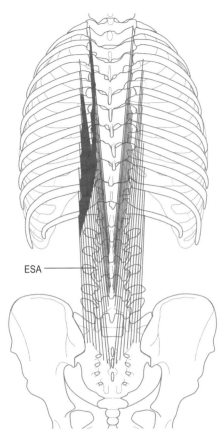

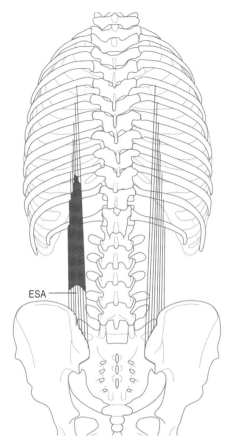

Figure 9.10 The thoracic fibres of longissimus (longissimus thoracis pars thoracis). The intact fascicles are shown on the left. The darkened areas represent the short muscle bellies of each fascicle. Note the short rostral tendons of each fascicle and the long caudal tendons, which collectively constitute most of the erector spinae aponeurosis (ESA). The span of the individual fascicles is indicated on the right.

Figure 9.11 The thoracic fibres of iliocostalis lumborum (iliocostalis lumborum pars thoracis). The intact fascicles are shown on the left, and their span is shown on the right. The caudal tendons of the fascicles collectively form the lateral parts of the erector spinae aponeurosis (ESA).

ERECTOR SPINAE APONEUROSIS

One of the cardinal revelations of studies of the lumbar erector spinae[6,8] is that this muscle consists of both lumbar and thoracic fibres. Modern textbook descriptions largely do not recognise the lumbar fibres, especially those of the iliocostalis.[6] Moreover, they do not note that the lumbar fibres (of both longissimus and iliocostalis) have attachments quite separate to those of the thoracic fibres. The lumbar fibres of longissimus and iliocostalis pass between the lumbar vertebrae and the ilium. Thus, through these muscles, the lumbar vertebrae are anchored directly to the ilium. They do not gain any attachment to the erector spinae aponeurosis, which is the implication of all modern textbook descriptions that deal with the erector spinae.

The erector spinae aponeurosis is described as a broad sheet of tendinous fibres that is attached to the ilium, the sacrum, and the lumbar and sacral spinous processes, and which forms a common origin for the lower part of erector spinae.[2] However, as described above, the erector spinae aponeurosis is formed virtually exclusively by the tendons of longissimus thoracis pars thoracis and iliocostalis pars thoracis.[6,8] The medial half or so of the aponeurosis is formed by the tendons of longissimus thoracis, and the lateral half is formed by the iliocostalis lumborum (Fig. 9.12). The only additional contribution comes from the most superficial fibres of multifidus from upper lumbar levels, which contribute a small number of fibres to the aponeurosis (see Figs 9.10, 9.11).[9] Nonetheless, the erector spinae aponeurosis is essentially formed only by the caudal attachments of muscles acting from thoracic levels.

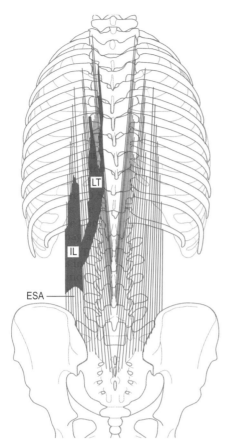

Figure 9.12 The erector spinae aponeurosis (ESA). This broad sheet is formed by the caudal tendons of the thoracic fibres of longissimus thoracis (LT) and iliocostalis lumborum (IL).

The lumbar fibres of erector spinae do not attach to the erector spinae aponeurosis. Indeed, the aponeurosis is free to move over the surface of the underlying lumbar fibres, and this suggests that the lumbar fibres, which form the bulk of the lumbar back musculature, can act independently from the rest of the erector spinae.

THORACOLUMBAR FASCIA

The thoracolumbar fascia consists of three layers of fascia that envelop the muscles of the lumbar spine, effectively separating them into three compartments. The **anterior layer** of thoracolumbar fascia is quite thin and is derived from the fascia of quadratus lumborum. It covers the anterior surface of quadratus lumborum and is attached medially to the anterior surfaces of the lumbar transverse

processes. In the intertransverse spaces, it blends with the intertransverse ligaments and may be viewed as one of the lateral extensions of the intertransverse ligaments (see Ch. 4). Lateral to the quadratus lumborum, the anterior layer blends with the other layers of the thoracolumbar fascia.

The **middle layer** of thoracolumbar fascia lies behind the quadratus lumborum. Medially, it is attached to the tips of the lumbar transverse processes and is directly continuous with the intertransverse ligaments. Laterally, it gives rise to the aponeurosis of the transversus abdominis. Its actual identity is debatable. It may represent a lateral continuation of the intertransverse ligaments, a medial continuation of the transversus aponeurosis, a thickening of the posterior fascia of the quadratus, or a combination of any or all of these.

The **posterior layer** of thoracolumbar fascia covers the back muscles. It arises from the lumbar spinous processes in the midline posteriorly and wraps around the back muscles to blend with the other layers of the thoracolumbar fascia along the lateral border of the iliocostalis lumborum. The union of the fasciae is quite dense at this site, and the middle and posterior layers, in particular, form a dense raphe which, for purposes of reference, has been called the **lateral raphe**.[21]

Traditionally, the thoracolumbar fascia has been ascribed no other function than to invest the back muscles and to provide an attachment for the transversus abdominis and the internal oblique muscles.[2] However, in recent years there has been considerable interest in its biomechanical role in the stability of the lumbar spine, particularly in the flexed posture and in lifting. This has resulted in anatomical and biomechanical studies of the anatomy and function of the thoracolumbar fascia, notably its posterior layer.[21–24]

The posterior layer of thoracolumbar fascia covers the back muscles from the lumbosacral region through to the thoracic region as far rostrally as the splenius muscle. In the lumbar region, it is attached to the tips of the spinous processes in the midline. Lateral to the erector spinae, between the 12th rib and the iliac crest, it unites with the middle layer of thoracolumbar fascia in the lateral raphe. At sacral levels, the posterior layer extends from the midline to the posterior superior iliac spine and the posterior segment of the iliac crest. Here it fuses with the underlying erector spinae aponeurosis and blends with fibres of the aponeurosis of the gluteus maximus.

On close inspection, the posterior layer exhibits a cross-hatched appearance, manifest because it consists of two laminae: a **superficial lamina** with fibres orientated caudomedially and a **deep lamina** with fibres oriented caudolaterally.[21,24]

The superficial lamina is formed by the aponeurosis of latissimus dorsi, but the disposition and attachments of its constituent fibres differ according to the portion of latissimus dorsi from which they are derived (Fig. 9.13).

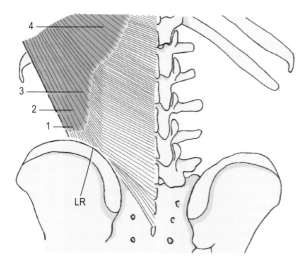

Figure 9.13 The superficial lamina of the posterior layer of thoracolumbar fascia. 1, aponeurotic fibres of the most lateral fascicles of latissimus dorsi insert directly into the iliac crest; 2, aponeurotic fibres of the next most lateral part of the latissimus dorsi glance past the iliac crest and reach the midline at sacral levels; 3, aponeurotic fibres from this portion of the muscle attach to the underlying lateral raphe (LR) and then deflect medially to reach the midline at the L3–L5 levels; 4, aponeurotic fibres from the upper portions of latissimus dorsi pass directly to the midline at thoracolumbar levels.

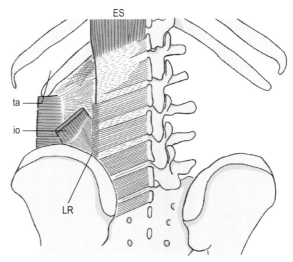

Figure 9.14 The deep lamina of the posterior layer of thoracolumbar fascia. Bands of collagen fibres pass from the midline to the posterior superior iliac spine and to the lateral raphe (LR). Those bands from the L4 and L5 spinous processes form alar-like ligaments that anchor these processes to the ilium. Attaching to the lateral raphe laterally are the aponeurosis of transversus abdominis (ta) and a variable number of the most posterior fibres of internal oblique (io). ES, erector spinae.

Those fibres derived from the most lateral 2–3 cm of the muscle are short and insert directly into the iliac crest without contributing to the thoracolumbar fascia. Fibres from the next most lateral 2 cm of the muscle approach the iliac crest near the lateral margin of the erector spinae, but then deflect medially, bypassing the crest to attach to the L5 and sacral spinous processes. These fibres form the sacral portion of the superficial lamina. A third series of fibres becomes aponeurotic just lateral to the lumbar erector spinae. At the lateral border of the erector spinae, they blend with the other layers of thoracolumbar fascia in the lateral raphe, but then they deflect medially, continuing over the back muscles to reach the midline at the levels of the L3, L4 and L5 spinous processes. These fibres form the lumbar portion of the superficial lamina of the posterior layer of thoracolumbar fascia.

The rostral portions of the latissimus dorsi cross the back muscles and do not become aponeurotic until some 5 cm lateral to the midline at the L3 and higher levels. These aponeurotic fibres form the thoracolumbar and thoracic portions of the thoracolumbar fascia.

Beneath the superficial lamina, the deep lamina of the posterior layer consists of bands of collagen fibres emanating from the midline, principally from the lumbar spinous processes (Fig. 9.14). The bands from the L4, L5 and S1

spinous processes pass caudolaterally to the posterior superior iliac spine. Those from the L3 spinous process and L3–4 interspinous ligament wrap around the lateral margin of the erector spinae to fuse with the middle layer of thoracolumbar fascia in the lateral raphe. Above L3 the deep lamina progressively becomes thinner, consisting of sparse bands of collagen that dissipate laterally over the erector spinae. A deep lamina is not formed at thoracic levels.

Collectively, the superficial and deep laminae of the posterior layer of thoracolumbar fascia form a retinaculum over the back muscles. Attached to the midline medially and the posterior superior iliac spine and lateral raphe laterally, the fascia covers or sheaths the back muscles, preventing their displacement dorsally.

Additionally, the deep lamina alone forms a series of distinct ligaments. When viewed bilaterally, the bands of fibres from the L4 and L5 spinous processes appear like alar ligaments anchoring these spinous processes to the ilia. The band from the L3 spinous process anchors this process indirectly to the ilium via the lateral raphe. Thirdly, the lateral raphe forms a site where the two laminae of the posterior layer fuse not only with the middle layer of thoracolumbar fascia but also with the transversus abdominis whose middle fibres arise from the lateral raphe (see Fig. 9.14). The posterior layer of thoracolumbar fascia thereby provides an indirect attachment for the transversus abdominis to the lumbar spinous processes. The mechanical significance of these three morphological features is explored in the following section.

FUNCTIONS OF THE BACK MUSCLES AND THEIR FASCIAE

Each of the lumbar back muscles is capable of several possible actions. No action is unique to a muscle and no muscle has a single action. Instead, the back muscles provide a pool of possible actions that may be recruited to suit the needs of the vertebral column. Therefore, the functions of the back muscles need to be considered in terms of the observed movements of the vertebral column. In this regard, three types of movement can be addressed: minor active movements of the vertebral column; postural movements; and major movements in forward bending and lifting. In this context, 'postural movements' refers to movements, usually subconscious, which occur to adjust and maintain a desired posture when this is disturbed, usually by gravity.

Minor active movements

In the upright position, the lumbar back muscles play a minor, or no active, role in executing movement, for gravity provides the necessary force. During extension, the back muscles contribute to the initial tilt, drawing the line of gravity backwards[25,26] but are unnecessary for further extension. Muscle activity is recruited when the movement is forced or resisted[27] but is restricted to muscles acting on the thorax. The lumbar multifidus, for example, shows little or no involvement.[28]

The lateral flexors can bend the lumbar spine sideways, but once the centre of gravity of the trunk is displaced lateral flexion can continue under the influence of gravity. However, the ipsilateral lateral flexors are used to direct the movement, and the contralateral muscles are required to balance the action of gravity and control the rate and extent of movement. Consequently, lateral flexion is accompanied by bilateral activity of the lumbar back muscles, but the contralateral muscles are relatively more active as they are the ones that must balance the load of the laterally flexing spine.[25,26,29–32] If a weight is held in the hand on the side to which the spine is laterally flexed, a greater load is applied to the spine, and the contralateral back muscles show greater activity to balance this load.[29,31]

Maintenance of posture

The upright vertebral column is well stabilised by its joints and ligaments but it is still liable to displacement by gravity or when subject to asymmetrical weight-bearing. The back muscles serve to correct such displacements and, depending on the direction of any displacement, the appropriate back muscles will be recruited.

During standing at ease, the back muscles may show slight continuous activity,[19,25–27,30,32–42] intermittent activity[25,27,32,42,43] or no activity,[36,39–42] and the amount of activity can be influenced by changing the position of the head or allowing the trunk to sway.[25]

The explanation for these differences probably lies in the location of the line of gravity in relation to the lumbar spine in different individuals.[27,36,41,42,44] In about 75% of individuals the line of gravity passes in front of the centre of the L4 vertebra, and therefore essentially in front of the lumbar spine.[36,41] Consequently, gravity will exert a constant tendency to pull the thorax and lumbar spine into flexion. To preserve an upright posture, a constant level of activity in the posterior sagittal rotators of the lumbar spine will be needed to oppose the tendency to flexion. Conversely, when the line of gravity passes behind the lumbar spine, gravity tends to extend it, and back muscle activity is not required. Instead, abdominal muscle activity is recruited to prevent the spine extending under gravity.[36,41]

Activities that displace the centre of gravity of the trunk sideways will tend to cause lateral flexion. To prevent undesired lateral flexion, the contralateral lateral flexors will contract. This occurs when weights are carried in one hand.[25,39] Carrying equal weights in both hands does not displace the line of gravity, and back muscle activity is not increased substantially on either side of the body.[25,39]

During sitting, the activity of the back muscles is similar to that during standing[34,35,45,46] but in supported sitting, as with the elbows resting on the knees, there is no activity in the lumbar back muscles,[25,32] and with arms resting on a desk, back muscle activity is substantially decreased.[34,35,45] In reclined sitting, the back rest supports the weight of the thorax, lessening the need for muscular support. Consequently, increasing the declination of the back rest of a seat decreases lumbar back muscle activity.[34,35,45,47,48]

Major active movements

Forward flexion and extension of the spine from the flexed position are movements during which the back muscles have their most important function. As the spine bends forwards, there is an increase in the activity of the back muscles;[19,25,26,28–30,32,33,43,49–52] this increase is proportional to the angle of flexion and the size of any load carried.[29,31,53,54] The movement of forward flexion is produced by gravity, but the extent and the rate at which it proceeds is controlled by the eccentric contraction of the back muscles. Movement of the thorax on the lumbar spine is controlled by the long thoracic fibres of longissimus and iliocostalis. The long tendons of insertion allow

107

these muscles to act around the convexity of the increasing thoracic kyphosis and anchor the thorax to the ilium and sacrum. In the lumbar region, the multifidus and the lumbar fascicles of longissimus and iliocostalis act to control the anterior sagittal rotation of the lumbar vertebrae. At the same time the lumbar fascicles of longissimus and iliocostalis also act to control the associated anterior translation of the lumbar vertebrae.

At a certain point during forward flexion, the activity in the back muscles ceases, and the vertebral column is braced by the locking of the zygapophysial joints and tension in its posterior ligaments (see Ch. 7). This phenomenon is known as 'critical point'.[26,43,44,55] However, critical point does not occur in all individuals or in all muscles.[19,25,32,42] When it does occur, it does so when the spine has reached about 90% maximum flexion, even though at this stage the hip flexion that occurs in forward bending is still only 60% complete.[44,55] Carrying weights during flexion causes the critical point to occur later in the range of vertebral flexion.[44,55]

The physiological basis for critical point is still obscure. It may be due to reflex inhibition initiated by proprioceptors in the lumbar joints and ligaments, or in muscle stretch and length receptors.[55] Whatever the mechanism, the significance of critical point is that it marks the transition of spinal load-bearing from muscles to the ligamentous system.

Extension of the trunk from the flexed position is characterised by high levels of back muscle activity.[19,25,26,43,52] In the thoracic region, the iliocostalis and longissimus, acting around the thoracic kyphosis, lift the thorax by rotating it backwards. The lumbar vertebrae are rotated backwards principally by the lumbar multifidus, causing their superior surfaces to be progressively tilted upwards to support the rising thorax.

COMPRESSIVE LOADS OF THE BACK MUSCLES

Because of the downward direction of their action, as the back muscles contract they exert a longitudinal compression of the lumbar vertebral column, and this compression raises the pressure in the lumbar intervertebral discs. Any activity that involves the back muscles, therefore, is associated with a rise in nuclear pressure. As measured in the L3–4 intervertebral disc, the nuclear pressure correlates with the degree of myoelectric activity in the back muscles.[29,31,48,56,57] As muscle activity increases, disc pressure rises.

Disc pressures and myoelectric activity of the back muscles have been used extensively to quantify the stresses applied to the lumbar spine in various postures and by various activities.[34,46–48,58–63] From the standing position, forward bending causes the greatest increase in disc pressure. Lifting a weight in this position raises disc pressure even further, and the pressure is greatly increased if a load is lifted with the lumbar spine both flexed and rotated. Throughout these various manoeuvres, back muscle activity increases in proportion to the disc pressure.

One of the prime revelations of combined discometric and electromyographic studies of the lumbar spine during lifting relates to the comparative stresses applied to the lumbar spine by different lifting tactics. In essence, it has been shown that, on the basis of changes in disc pressure and back muscle activity, there are no differences between using a 'stoop' lift or a 'leg' lift, i.e. lifting a weight with a bent back versus lifting with a straight back.[29,47,48,64] The critical factor is the distance of the load from the body. The further the load is from the chest the greater the stresses on the lumbar spine, and the greater the disc pressure and back muscle activity.[64] Performing a 'leg' lift with a straight back as opposed to maintaining a lordosis involves about 5% less electromyographic activity in the back muscles early in the lift but little difference thereafter.[65]

Strength of the back muscles

The strength of the back muscles has been determined in experiments on normal volunteers.[66] Two measures of strength are available: the absolute maximum force of contraction in the upright posture and the moment generated on the lumbar spine. The absolute maximum strength of the back muscles as a whole is about 4000 N. Acting on the short moment arms provided by the spinous processes and pedicles of the lumbar vertebrae, this force converts to an extensor moment of 200 Nm. These figures apply to average males under the age of 30; young females exhibit about 60% of this strength, while individuals over the age of 30 are about 10–30% weaker.[66]

Easy standing involves some 2–5% of maximum isometric strength; manual handling of heavy loads involves between 75% and 100%; sitting involves between 3% and 15% of maximum activity.[67]

Detailed dissection studies have allowed the strength of contraction to be apportioned to individual components of the back muscles.[68] Of the total extensor moment, the thoracic fibres of iliocostalis and longissimus account for some 50%. Thus, half of the extensor moment on the lumbar spine is exerted through the erector spinae aponeurosis. The other half is exerted by the muscles that act directly on the lumbar vertebrae, with the multifidus providing half of that 50% and the longissimus thoracis pars lumborum and iliocostalis lumborum pars lumborum providing the remainder. The compression loads exerted by the lumbar back muscles differ from segment to segment because of the different spans and attachments of the various muscles. However, at L5–S1 the thoracic fibres of the lumbar erector spinae exert about 42% of the total compression load, the lumbar fibres of this muscle contribute 36% and the multifidus contributes 22%.[68] At higher lumbar levels, relatively more of the total compression load on the segment is exerted by the thoracic fibres of the lumbar erector spinae.

With respect to shear forces, in the upright position the various lumbar back muscles exert forces that differ in magnitude and in direction at different levels.[68] This arises because of the different orientation of particular fascicles of the various muscles and because of the different orientation of particular vertebrae in the lumbar lordosis. As a result, the multifidus exerts mainly anterior shear forces at upper lumbar levels, but either anterior or posterior shear forces at lower levels; the lumbar fibres of erector spinae exert posterior shear forces on the vertebrae to which they are attached, but anterior shear forces on vertebrae below these; the thoracic fibres of lumbar erector spinae exert posterior shear forces on upper lumbar segments, but anterior shear forces on L4 and L5.[68] The net effect is that the back muscles exert posterior shear forces on upper lumbar segments in the upright spine but, paradoxically, they exert a net anterior shear force on L5.

Intriguingly, flexion of the lumbar spine does not compromise the strength of the back muscles.[69] The moment arms of some fascicles are reduced by flexion but those of others are increased, resulting in no significant change in the total capacity to generate moments. All fascicles, however, are elongated, but although this reduces their maximum force on active contraction, it increases the passive tension in the muscles, resulting in no reduction in total tension. Consequently, upon flexion, the total extensor moment of the back muscles and the compression load that they exert change little from those in the upright position. However, the shear forces change appreciably. The posterior shear forces on upper lumbar segments are reduced by flexion but the shear force on L5 reverses from an anterior shear force in the upright position to a posterior shear force in full flexion.[69]

With respect to axial rotation, although the back muscles have reasonable moment arms, they are compromised by their longitudinal orientation.[70] Only their horizontal vectors can exert axial rotation but these are very small components of the action of any of the muscles. As a result, the total maximal possible torque exerted by all the back muscles is next to trivial, and that exerted by any one muscle is negligible.[70] Consequently, the back muscles afford no stability to the lumbar spine in axial rotation. For that, the lumbar spine is reliant on the abdominal muscles.[70]

Histochemistry

As postural muscles, the back muscles are dominated by slow-twitch fibres. Furthermore, the density of slow-twitch and fast-twitch fibres differs from muscle to muscle.

Slow-twitch fibres constitute some 70% of the fibres of longissimus.[67] They constitute about 55% of the iliocostalis and multifidus. Conversely, fast-twitch type A fibres constitute 20% of the fibres of multifidus, iliocostalis and longissimus, and fast-twitch type B fibres constitute 25% of the fibres of multifidus and iliocostalis but only 11% of longissimus.[67]

These histochemical profiles seem to correlate with the fatigue resistance and endurance times of the back muscles, which are larger than most human muscles.[67] However, individuals exhibit a large variance in fatigue resistance.[67] The possibilities arise that endurance may be a direct function of the density of slow-twitch fibres in the back muscles, that lack of resistance to fatigue is a risk factor for back injury, and that conditioning can change the histochemical profile of an individual to overcome this risk. These possibilities, however, remain to be explored.

Some practitioners believe that muscle weakness, or muscle fatiguability, is the basis for back pain in some, if not many, patients. To them, data on muscle fibre types are attractive for they would seem to tally with the fact that patients with weak and fatiguable back muscles would show changes in fibre type towards type II fibres. This notion, however, has been dispelled.

A study has shown that there is no correlation between pain and either fatigue or fibre type.[71] Patients with back pain my exhibit less strength than asymptomatic individuals but not because of histochemical differences in their muscles.

Lifting

In biomechanical terms, the act of lifting constitutes a problem in balancing moments. When an individual bends forwards to execute a lift, flexion occurs at the hip joint and in the lumbar spine. Indeed, most of the forward movement seen during trunk flexion occurs at the hip joint.[55] The flexion forces are generated by gravity acting on the mass of the object to be lifted and on the mass of the trunk above the level of the hip joint and lumbar spine (Fig. 9.15). These forces exert flexion moments on both the hip joint and lumbar spine. In each case, the moment will be the product of the force and its perpendicular distance from the joint in question. The total flexion moment acting on each joint will be the sum of the moments exerted by the mass to be lifted and the mass of the trunk. For a lift to be executed, these flexion moments have to be overcome by a moment acting in the opposite direction. This could be exerted by longitudinal forces acting downwards behind the hip joint and vertebral column or by forces acting upwards in front of the joints, pushing the trunk upwards.

There are no doubts as to the capacity of the hip extensors to generate large moments and overcome the flexion moments exerted on the hip joint, even by the heaviest of loads that might be lifted.[72,73] However, the hip extensors

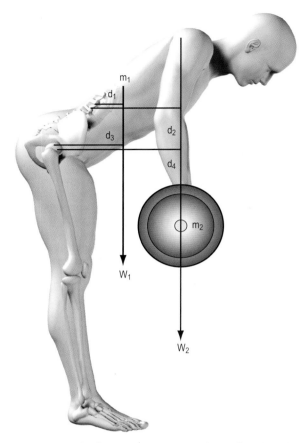

Figure 9.15 The flexion moments exerted on a flexed trunk. Forces generated by the weight of the trunk and the load to be lifted act vertically in front of the lumbar spine and hip joint. The moments they exert on each joint are proportional to the distance between the line of action of each force and the joint in question. The mass of the trunk (m_1) exerts a force (W_1) that acts at a measurable distance in front of the lumbar spine (d_1) and the hip joint (d_3). The mass to be lifted (m_2) exerts a force (W_2) that acts at a measurable distance from the lumbar spine (d_2) and the hip joint (d_4). The respective moments acting on the lumbar spine will be W_1d_1 and W_2d_2; those on the hip joint will be W_1d_3 and W_2d_4.

are only able to rotate the pelvis backwards on the femurs; they do not act on the lumbar spine. Thus, regardless of what happens at the hip joint, the lumbar spine still remains subject to a flexion moment that must be overcome in some other way. Without an appropriate mechanism, the lumbar spine would stay flexed as the hips extended; indeed, as the pelvis rotated backwards, flexion of the lumbar spine would be accentuated as its bottom end was pulled backwards with the pelvis while its top end remained stationary under the load of the flexion moment. A mechanism is required to allow the lumbar spine to

resist this deformation or to cause it to extend in unison with the hip joint.

Despite much investigation and debate, the exact nature of this mechanism remains unresolved. In various ways, the back muscles, intra-abdominal pressure, the thoracolumbar fascia and the posterior ligamentous system have been believed to participate.

For light lifts, the flexion moments generated are relatively small. In the case of a 70 kg man lifting a 10 kg mass in a fully stooped position, the upper trunk weighs about 40 kg and acts about 30 cm in front of the lumbar spine, while the arms holding the mass to be lifted lie about 45 cm in front of the lumbar spine. The respective flexion moments are, therefore, $40 \times 9.8 \times 0.30 = 117.6$ Nm, and $10 \times 9.8 \times 0.45 = 44.1$ Nm, a total of 161.7 Nm. This load is well within the capacity of the back muscles (200 Nm, see above). Thus, as the hips extend, the lumbar back muscles are capable of resisting further flexion of the lumbar spine, and indeed could even actively extend it, and the weight would be lifted.

Increasing the load to be lifted to over 30 kg increases the flexion moment to 132.2 Nm, which when added to the flexion moment of the upper trunk exceeds the capacity of the back muscles. To remain within the capacity of the back muscles such loads must be carried closer to the lumbar spine, i.e. they must be borne with a much shorter moment arm. Even so, decreasing the moment arm to about 15 cm limits the load to be carried to about 90 kg. The back muscles are simply not strong enough to raise greater loads. Such realisations have generated concepts of several additional mechanisms that serve to aid the back muscles in overcoming large flexion moments.

In 1957, Bartelink[74] raised the proposition that intra-abdominal pressure could aid the lumbar spine in resisting flexion by acting upwards on the diaphragm: the so-called intra-abdominal balloon mechanism. Bartelink himself was circumspect and reserved in raising this conjecture but the concept was rapidly popularised, particularly among physiotherapists. Even though it was never validated, the concept seemed to be treated as proven fact. It received early endorsement in orthopaedic circles,[28] and intra-abdominal pressure was adopted by ergonomists and others as a measure of spinal stress and safe-lifting standards.[75–82] In more contemporary studies, intra-abdominal pressure has been monitored during various spinal movements and lifting tasks.[29,64,83]

Reservations about the validity of the abdominal balloon mechanism have arisen from several quarters. Studies of lifting tasks reveal that, unlike myoelectric activity, intra-abdominal pressure does not correlate well with the size of the load being lifted or the applied stress on the vertebral column as measured by intradiscal pressure.[56,57,84] Indeed, deliberately increasing intra-abdominal pressure by a Valsalva manoeuvre does not relieve the load on the lumbar spine but actually increases it.[85] Clinical studies have shown that although abdominal muscles are weaker than normal in patients with back pain, intra-abdominal pressure is not different.[86] Furthermore, strengthening the abdominal muscles both in normal individuals[87] and in patients with back pain[88] does not influence intra-abdominal pressure during lifting.

The most strident criticism of the intra-abdominal balloon theory comes from bioengineers and others who maintain that:

1. To generate any significant anti-flexion moment the pressure required would exceed the maximum hoop tension of the abdominal muscles[89–91]

2. Such a pressure would be so high as to obstruct the abdominal aorta (a reservation raised by Bartelink himself[74,89])

3. Because the abdominal muscles lie in front of the lumbar spine and connect the thorax to the pelvis, whenever they contract to generate pressure they must also exert a flexion moment on the trunk, which would negate any anti-flexion value of the intra-abdominal pressure.[72,73,91,92]

These reservations inspired an alternative explanation of the role of the abdominal muscles during lifting. Farfan, Gracovetsky and colleagues[23,72,91,93] noted the criss-cross arrangement of the fibres in the posterior layer of thoracolumbar fascia and surmised that, if lateral tension was applied to this fascia, it would result in an extension moment being exerted on the lumbar spinous processes. Such tension could be exerted by the abdominal muscles that arise from the thoracolumbar fascia, and the trigonometry of the fibres in the thoracolumbar fascia was such that they could convert lateral tension into an appreciable extension moment: the so-called 'gain' of the thoracolumbar fascia.[91] The role of the abdominal muscles during lifting was thus to brace, if not actually extend, the lumbar spine by pulling on the thoracolumbar fascia. Any rises in intra-abdominal pressure were thereby only coincidental, occurring because of the contraction of the abdominal muscles acting on the thoracolumbar fascia.

Subsequent anatomic studies revealed several liabilities of this model.[21] First, the posterior layer of thoracolumbar fascia is well developed only in the lower lumbar region, but nevertheless its fibres are appropriately oriented to enable lateral tension exerted on the fascia to produce extension moments at least on the L2–L5 spinous processes (Fig. 9.16). However, dissection reveals that of the abdominal muscles the internal oblique offers only a few fibres that irregularly attach to the thoracolumbar fascia; the transversus abdominis is the only muscle that consistently attaches to the thoracolumbar fascia, but only its very middle fibres do this. The size of these fibres is such that, even upon maximum contraction, the force they exert is very small. Calculations revealed that the extensor moment they could exert on the lumbar spine amounted to less than 6 Nm.[94] Thus, the contribution that abdominal muscles might make to anti-flexion moments is trivial,

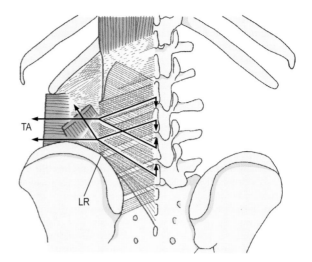

Figure 9.16 The mechanics of the thoracolumbar fascia. From any point in the lateral raphe (LR), lateral tension in the posterior layer of thoracolumbar fascia is transmitted upwards through the deep lamina of the posterior layer, and downwards through the superficial layer. Because of the obliquity of these lines of tension, a small downward vector is generated at the midline attachment of the deep lamina, and a small upward vector is generated at the midline attachment of the superficial lamina. These mutually opposite vectors tend to approximate or oppose the separation of the L2 and L4, and L3 and L5 spinous processes. Lateral tension on the fascia can be exerted by the transversus abdominis (TA) and to a lesser extent by the few fibres of the internal oblique when they attach to the lateral raphe.

a conclusion also borne out by subsequent independent modelling studies.[83]

A totally different model of lifting was elaborated by Farfan and Gracovetsky.[23,72,91] Noting the weakness of the back muscles, these authors proposed that extension of the lumbar spine was not required to lift heavy loads or loads with long moment arms. They proposed that the lumbar spine should remain fully flexed in order to engage, i.e. maximally stretch, what they referred to as the 'posterior ligamentous system', namely the capsules of the zygapophysial joints, the interspinous and supraspinous ligaments, and the posterior layer of thoracolumbar fascia, the latter acting passively to transmit tension between the lumbar spinous processes and the ilium.

Under such conditions the active energy for a lift was provided by the powerful hip extensor muscles. These rotated the pelvis backwards. Meanwhile, the external load acting on the upper trunk kept the lumbar spine flexed. Tension would develop in the posterior ligamentous system which bridged the thorax and pelvis. With the posterior ligamentous system so engaged, as the pelvis rotated backwards the lumbar spine would be passively raised while remaining in a fully flexed position. In essence, the posterior sagittal rotation of the pelvis would be transmitted through the posterior ligaments first to the L5 vertebra, then to L4 and so on, up through the lumbar spine into the thorax. All that was required was that the posterior ligamentous system be sufficiently strong to withstand the passive tension generated in it by the movement of the pelvis at one end and the weight of the trunk and external load at the other. The lumbar spine would thereby be raised like a long rigid arm rotating on the pelvis and raising the external load with it.

Contraction of the back muscles was not required if the ligaments could take the load. Indeed, muscle contraction was distinctly undesirable, for any active extension of the lumbar spine would disengage the posterior ligaments and preclude them from transmitting tension. The back muscles could be recruited only when the trunk had been raised sufficiently to shorten the moment arm of the external load, reducing its flexion moment to within the capacity of the back muscles.

The attraction of this model was that it overcame the problem of the relative weakness of the back muscles by dispensing with their need to act, which in turn was consistent with the myoelectric silence of the back muscles at full flexion of the trunk and the recruitment of muscle activity only once the trunk had been elevated and the flexion moment arm had been reduced. Support for the model also came from surgical studies which reported that if the midline ligaments and thoracolumbar fascia were conscientiously reconstructed after multilevel laminectomies, the postoperative recovery and rehabilitation of patients were enhanced.[95]

However, while attractive in a qualitative sense, the mechanism of the posterior ligamentous system was not validated quantitatively. The model requires that the ligaments be strong enough to sustain the loads applied. In this regard, data on the strength of the posterior ligaments are scant and irregular, but sufficient data are available to permit an initial appraisal of the feasibility of the posterior ligament model.

The strength of spinal ligaments varies considerably but average values can be calculated. Table 9.1 summarises some of the available data. It is evident that the strongest posterior 'ligaments' of the lumbar spine are the zygapophysial joint capsules and the thoracolumbar fascia forming the midline 'supraspinous ligament'. However, when the relatively short moment arms over which these ligaments act are considered, it transpires that the maximum moment they can sustain is relatively small. Even the sum total of all their moments is considerably less than that required for heavy lifting and is some four times less than the maximum strength of the back muscles. Of course, it is possible that the data quoted may not be representative of the true mean values of the strength of these ligaments but it does not seem likely that the literature quoted underestimated their strength by a factor of four or more. Under these conditions, it is evident that the posterior ligamentous system alone is not strong enough to perform the role required of it in heavy lifting. The posterior ligamentous system is not strong enough to replace the back muscles as a mechanism to prevent flexion of the lumbar spine during lifting. Some other mechanism must operate.

One such mechanism is that of the **hydraulic amplifier** effect.[93] It was originally proposed by Gracovetsky et al.[93] that because the thoracolumbar fascia surrounded the back muscles as a retinaculum it could serve to brace these muscles and enhance their power. The engineering basis for this effect is complicated, and the concept remained unexplored until very recently. A mathematical proof has been published which suggests that by investing the back muscles the thoracolumbar fascia enhances the strength of

Table 9.1 Strength of the posterior ligamentous system. The average force at failure has been calculated using raw data provided in the references cited. The moment arms are estimates based on inspection of a representative vertebra, measuring the perpendicular distance between the location of the axes of rotation of the lumbar spine and the sites of attachment of the various ligaments

Ligament	Ref.	Average force at failure (N)	Moment arm (m)	Maximum moment (Nm)
Posterior longitudinal	96	90	0.02	1.8
Ligamentum flavum	96	244	0.03	7.3
Zygapophysial joint capsule	96 97	680 672	0.04	27.2
Interspinous	96	107	0.05	5.4
Thoracolumbar fascia	96	500	0.06	30.0
Total				71.7

the back muscles by some 30%.[98] This is an appreciable increase and an attractive mechanism for enhancing the antiflexion capacity of the back muscles. However, the validity of this proof is still being questioned on the grounds that the principles used, while applicable to the behaviour of solids, may not be applicable to muscles; and the concept of the hydraulic amplifier mechanism still remains under scrutiny.

Quite a contrasting model has been proposed to explain the mechanics of the lumbar spine in lifting. It is based on arch theory and maintains that the behaviour, stability and strength of the lumbar spine during lifting can be explained by viewing the lumbar spine as an arch braced by intra-abdominal pressure.[99,100] This intriguing concept, however, has not met with any degree of acceptance and indeed, has been challenged from some quarters.[101]

In summary, despite much effort over recent years, the exact mechanism of heavy lifting still remains un-explained. The back muscles are too weak to extend the lumbar spine against large flexion moments, the intra-abdominal balloon has been refuted, the abdominal mechanism and thoracolumbar fascia have been refuted, and the posterior ligamentous system appears too weak to replace the back muscles. Engineering models of the hydraulic amplifier effect and arch model are still subject to debate.

What remains to be explained is what provides the missing force to sustain heavy loads, and why intra-abdominal pressure is so consistently generated during lifts if it is neither to brace the thoracolumbar fascia nor to provide an intra-abdominal balloon. At present these questions can only be addressed by conjecture but certain concepts appear worthy of consideration.

With regard to intra-abdominal pressure, one concept that has been overlooked in studies of lifting is the role of the abdominal muscles in controlling axial rotation of the trunk. Investigators have focused their attention on movements in the sagittal plane during lifting and have ignored the fact that when bent forward to address an object to be lifted, the trunk is liable to axial rotation. Unless the external load is perfectly balanced and lies exactly in the midline, it will cause the trunk to twist to one side. Thus, to keep the weight in the midline and in the sagittal plane, the lifter must control any twisting effect. The oblique abdominal muscles are the principal rotators of the trunk and would be responsible for this bracing. In contracting to control axial rotation, the abdominal muscles would secondarily raise intra-abdominal pressure. This pressure rise is therefore an epi-phenomenon and would reflect not the size of any external load but its tendency to twist the flexed trunk.

With regard to loads in the sagittal plane, the passive strength of the back muscles has been neglected in discussions of lifting. From the behaviour of isolate muscle fibres, it is known that as a muscle elongates, its maximum contractile force diminishes but its passive elastic tension rises, so much so that in an elongated muscle the total passive and active tension generated is at least equal to the maximum contractile capacity of the muscle at resting length. Thus, although they become electrically silent at full flexion, the back muscles are still capable of providing passive tension equal to their maximum contractile strength. This would allow the silent muscles to supplement the engaged posterior ligamentous system. With the back muscles providing some 200 Nm and the ligaments some 50 Nm or more, the total antiflexion capacity of the lumbar spine rises to about 250 Nm which would allow some 30 kg to be safely lifted at 90° trunk flexion. Larger loads could be sustained by proportionally shortening the moment arm. Consequently, the mechanism of lifting may well be essentially as proposed by Farfan and Gracovetsky[22,72,93] except that the passive tension in the back muscles constitutes the major component of the 'posterior ligamentous system'.

REFERENCES

1. Bogduk N, Pearcy M, Hadfield G. Anatomy and biomechanics of psoas major. *Clin Biomech.* 1992;7:109–119.

2. Williams PL, ed. *Gray's Anatomy.* 38th ed. Edinburgh: Churchill Livingstone; 1995.

3. Cave AJE. The innervation and morphology of the cervical intertransverse muscles. *J Anat.* 1937;71:497–515.

4. Poirier P. Myologie. In: Poirier P, Charpy A, eds. *Traité d'Anatomie Humaine.* 3rd ed. vol. 2, Fasc.

1. Paris: Masson; 1912:139–140.

5. Phillips S, Mercer S, Bogduk N. Anatomy and Biomechanics of Quadratus Lumborum. *J Engineering in Medicine.* 2008;222:151–159.

6. Bogduk N. A reappraisal of the anatomy of the human lumbar erector spinae. *J Anat.* 1980;131:525–540.

7. Macintosh JE, Bogduk N. The biomechanics of the lumbar multifidus. *Clin Biomech.* 1986;1:205–213.

8. Macintosh JE, Bogduk N. The morphology of the lumbar erector spinae. *Spine.* 1986;12:658–668.

9. Macintosh JE, Valencia F, Bogduk N, et al. The morphology of the lumbar multifidus muscles. *Clin Biomech.* 1986;1:196–204.

10. Bogduk N, Wilson AS, Tynan W. The human lumbar dorsal rami. *J Anat.* 1982;134:383–397.

11. Bogduk N. The lumbar mamillo-accessory ligament. Its anatomical and neurosurgical significance. *Spine.* 1981;6:162–167.

12. Abrahams VC. The physiology of neck muscles; their role in head movement and maintenance of posture. *Can J Physiol Pharmacol.* 1977;55:332–338.

13. Abrahams VC. Sensory and motor specialization in some muscles of the neck. *TINS.* 1981;4:24–27.

14. Cooper S, Danial PM. Muscle spindles in man, their morphology in the lumbricals and the deep muscles of the neck. *Brain.* 1963;86:563–594.

15. Bastide G, Zadeh J, Lefebvre D. Are the 'little muscles' what we think they are? *Surg Radiol Anat.* 1989;11:255–256.

16. Nitz AJ, Peck D. Comparison of muscle spindle concentrations in large and small human epaxial muscles acting in parallel combinations. *Am Surg.* 1986;52:273–277.

17. Peck D, Buxton DF, Nitz A. A comparison of spindle concentrations in large and small muscles acting in parallel combinations. *J Morphol.* 1984;180:243–252.

18. Lewin T, Moffet B, Viidik A. The morphology of the lumbar synovial intervertebral joints. *Acta Morphol Neerlando-Scand.* 1962;4:299–319.

19. Donisch EW, Basmajian JV. Electromyography of deep back muscles in man. *Am J Anat.* 1972;133:25–36.

20. Luk KDK, Ho HC, Leong JCY. The iliolumbar ligament. A study of its anatomy, development and clinical significance. *J Bone Joint Surg.* 1986;68B:197–200.

21. Bogduk N, Macintosh J. The applied anatomy of the thoracolumbar fascia. *Spine.* 1984;9:164–170.

22. Fairbank JCT, O'Brien JP. *The abdominal cavity and thoracolumbar fascia as stabilisers of the lumbar spine in patients with low back pain. Vol 2. Engineering Aspects of the Spine.* London: Mechanical Engineering Publications; 1980:83–88.

23. Gracovetsky S, Farfan HF, Lamy C. The mechanism of the lumbar spine. *Spine.* 1981;6:249–262.

24. Vleeming A, Pool-Goudzwaard AL, Stoeckart R, et al. The posterior layer of the thoracolumbar fascia: its function in load transfer from spine to legs. *Spine.* 1995;20:753–758.

25. Floyd WF, Silver PHS. The function of the erectores spinae muscles in certain movements and postures in man. *J Physiol.* 1955;129:184–203.

26. Morris JM, Benner G, Lucas DB. An electromyographic study of the intrinsic muscles of the back in man. *J Anat.* 1962;96:509–520.

27. Ortengren R, Andersson GBJ. Electromyographic studies of trunk muscles with special reference to the functional anatomy of the lumbar spine. *Spine.* 1977;2:44–52.

28. Morris JM, Lucas DB, Bresler B. Role of the trunk in stability of the spine. *J Bone Joint Surg.* 1961;43A:327–351.

29. Andersson GBJ, Ortengren R, Nachemson A. Intradiscal pressure, intra-abdominal pressure and myoelectric back muscle activity related to posture and loading. *Clin Orthop.* 1977;129:156–164.

30. Carlsoo S. The static muscle load in different work positions: an electromyographic study. *Ergonomics.* 1961;4:193–211.

31. Ortengren R, Andersson G, Nachemson A. Lumbar loads in fixed working postures during flexion and rotation. In: Asmussen E, Jorgensen K, eds. *Biomechanics VI-B, International Series on Biomechanics.* Vol 2B. Baltimore: University Park Press; 1978:159–166.

32. Portnoy H, Morin F. Electromyographic study of the postural muscles in various positions and movements. *Am J Physiol.* 1956;186:122–126.

33. Allen CEL. Muscle action potentials used in the study of dynamic anatomy. *Br J Phys Med.* 1948;11:66–73.

34. Andersson BJ, Ortengren R. Myoelectric back muscle activity during sitting. *Scand J Rehabil Med Suppl.* 1974;3:73–90.

35. Andersson BJ, Jonsson B, Ortengren R. Myoelectric activity in individual lumbar erector spinae muscles in sitting. A study with surface and wire electrodes. *Scand J Rehabil Med Suppl.* 1974;3:91–108.

36. Asmussen E, Klausen K. Form and function of the erect human spine. *Clin Orthop.* 1962;25:55–63.

37. Carlsoo S. Influence of frontal and dorsal loads on muscle activity and on the weight distribution in the feet. *Acta Orthop Scand.* 1964;34:299–309.

38. De Vries HA. Muscle tonus in postural muscles. *Am J Phys Med.* 1965;44:275–291.

39. Jonsson B. The functions of the individual muscles in the lumbar part of the spinae muscle. *Electromyography.* 1970;10:5–21.

40. Joseph J, McColl I. Electromyography of muscles of posture: posterior vertebral muscles in males. *J Physiol.* 1961;157:33–37.

41. Klausen K. The form and function of the loaded human spine. *Acta Physiol Scand.* 1965;65:176–190.

42. Valencia FP, Munro RR. An electromyographic study of the lumbar multifidus in man. *Electromyogr Clin Neurophysiol.* 1985;25:205–221.

43. Floyd WF, Silver PHS. Function of erectores spinae in flexion of the trunk. *Lancet.* 1951;1:133–134.

44. Kippers V, Parker AW. Electromyographic studies of erectores spinae: symmetrical postures and sagittal trunk motion. *Aust J Physiother.* 1985;31:95–105.

45. Andersson BJ, Ortengren R. Lumbar disc pressure and myoelectric back muscle activity during sitting. II. Studies of an office chair. *Scand J Rehabil Med.* 1974;6:115–121.

46. Andersson BJ, Ortengren R, Nachemson AL, et al. The sitting posture: an electromyographic and discometric study. *Orthop Clin North Am.* 1975;6:105–120.

47. Nachemson AL. The lumbar spine. An orthopaedic challenge. *Spine.* 1976;1:59–71.

48. Nachemson A. Lumbar intradiscal pressure. In: Jayson MIV, ed. *The Lumbar Spine and Backache,* 2nd ed. London: Pitman; 1980:Ch. 12, 341–358.

49. Golding JSR. Electromyography of the erector spinae in low back pain. *Postgrad Med J.* 1952;28:401–406.

50. Koreska J, Robertson D, Mills RH. Biomechanics of the lumbar spine and its clinical significance. *Orthop Clin North Am.* 1977;8: 121–123.

51. Okada M. Electromyographic assessment of the muscular load in forward bending postures. *J Fac Sci (Tokyo).* 1970;8:311–336.

52. Pauly JE. An electromyographic analysis of certain movements and exercises. I. Some deep muscles of the back. *Anat Rec.* 1966;155: 223–234.

53. Andersson GBJ, Ortengren R, Herberts P. Quantitative electromyographic studies of back muscle activity related to posture and loading. *Orthop Clin North Am.* 1977;8:85–96.

54. Schulz A, Andersson GBJ, Ortengren R, et al. Analysis and quantitative myoelectric measurements of loads on the lumbar spine when holding weights in standing postures. *Spine.* 1982;7:390–397.

55. Kippers V, Parker AW. Posture related to myoelectric silence of erectores spinae during trunk flexion. *Spine.* 1984;7:740–745.

56. Andersson G. Loads on the lumbar spine: in vivo measurements and biomechanical analyses. In: Winter DA, Norman RW, Wells RP, et al, eds. *Biomechanics IX-B, International Series on Biomechanics.* Champaign: Human Kinetics; 1983:32–37.

57. Ortengren R, Andersson GBJ, Nachemson AL. Studies of relationships between lumbar disc pressure, myoelectric back muscle activity, and intra-abdominal (intragastric) pressure. *Spine.* 1981;6:98–103.

58. Andersson G, Ortengren R, Nachemson A. Quantitative studies of the load on the back in different working postures. *Scand J Rehabil Med Suppl.* 1978;6: 173–181.

59. Andersson BJ, Ortengren R, Nachemson A, et al. Lumbar disc pressure and myoelectric activity during sitting. I. Studies on an experimental chair. *Scand J Rehabil Med.* 1974;6:104–114.

60. Andersson BJ, Ortengren R, Nachemson A, et al. Lumbar disc pressure and myoelectric back muscle activity during sitting. IV. Studies on a car driver's seat. *Scand J Rehabil Med.* 1974;6:128–133.

61. Nachemson A. The load on lumbar disks in different positions of the body. *Clin Orthop.* 1966 45:107–122.

62. Nachemson AL, Elfstrom G. Intravital dynamic pressure measurements in lumbar discs. A study of common movements, manoeuvers and exercises. *Scand J Rehabil Med.* 1970;2 (suppl 1): 1–40.

63. Nachemson A, Morris JM. In vivo measurements of intradiscal pressure. *J Bone Joint Surg.* 1964;46:1077–1092.

64. Andersson GBJ, Ortengren R, Nachemson A. Quantitative studies of back loads in lifting. *Spine.* 1976;1:178–184.

65. Vakos JP, Nitz AJ, Threlkeld AJ, et al. Electromyographic activity of selected trunk and hip muscles during a squat lift: effect of varying the lumbar posture. *Spine.* 1994;19:687–695.

66. McNeill T, Warwick D, Andersson G, et al. Trunk strengths in attempted flexion, extension, and lateral bending in healthy subjects and patients with low-back disorders. *Spine.* 1980;5:529–538.

67. Jorgensen K, Nicholaisen T, Kato M. Muscle fiber distribution, capillary density, and enzymatic activities in the lumbar paravertebral muscles of young men: significance for isometric endurance. *Spine.* 1993;18: 1439–1450.

68. Bogduk N, Macintosh JE, Pearcy MJ. A universal model of the lumbar back muscles in the upright position. *Spine.* 1992;17:897–913.

69. Macintosh JE, Bogduk N, Pearcy MJ. The effects of flexion on the geometry and actions of the lumbar erector spinae. *Spine.* 1993;18:884–893.

70. Macintosh JE, Pearcy MJ, Bogduk N. The axial torque of the lumbar back muscles: torsion strength of the back muscles. *Aust NZ J Surg.* 1993;63:205–212.

71. Crossman K, Mahon M, Watson PJ, et al. Chronic low back pain – associated paraspinal muscle dysfunction is not the result of a constitutionally determined 'adverse' fibre-type composition. *Spine.* 2004;29:628–634.

72. Farfan HF. Muscular mechanism of the lumbar spine and the position of power and efficiency. *Orthop Clin North Am.* 1975;6:135–144.

73. Farfan HF. The biomechanical advantage of lordosis and hip extension for upright activity. Man as compared with other anthropoids. *Spine.* 1978;3: 336–342.

74. Bartelink DL. The role of abdominal pressure in relieving the pressure on the lumbar intervertebral discs. *J Bone Joint Surg.* 1957;39B:718–725.

75. Davis PR. Posture of the trunk during the lifting of weights. *BMJ.* 1959;1:87–89.

76. Davis PR. The use of intra-abdominal pressure in evaluating stresses on the lumbar spine. *Spine.* 1981;6:90–92.

77. Davis PR, Stubbs DA. Safe levels of manual forces for young males (1). *Appl Ergon.* 1977;8:141–150.

78. Davis PR, Troup JDG. Pressures in the trunk cavities when pulling, pushing and lifting. *Ergonomics.* 1964;7:465–474.

79. Stubbs DA. Trunk stresses in construction and other industrial workers. *Spine.* 1981;6:83–89.

80. Troup JDG. Relation of lumbar spine disorders to heavy manual work and lifting. *Lancet.* 1965;1: 857–861.

81. Troup JDG. Dynamic factors in the analysis of stoop and crouch lifting methods: a methodological approach to the development of safe materials handling standards. *Orthop Clin North Am.* 1977;8: 201–209.

82. Troup JDG. Biomechanics of the vertebral column. *Physiotherapy.* 1979;65:238–244.

83. McGill SM, Norman RW. Potential of lumbodorsal fascia forces to generate back extension moments during squat lifts. *J Biomed Eng.* 1988;10:312–318.

84. Leskinen TPJ, Stalhammar HR, Kuorinka IA, et al. Hip torque, lumbosacral compression, and intra-abdominal pressure in lifting and lowering tasks. In: Winter DA, Norman RW, Wells RP, et al, eds. *Biomechanics IXB, International Series on Biomechanics*. Champaign: Human Kinetics; 1983:55–59.

85. Nachemson AL, Andersson GBJ, Schultz AB. Valsalva maneuver biomechanics. Effects on trunk load of elevated intra-abdominal pressure. *Spine*. 1986;11:476–479.

86. Hemborg B, Moritz U. Intra-abdominal pressure and trunk muscle activity during lifting. II. Chronic low-back patients. *Scand J Rehabil Med*. 1985;17:5–13.

87. Hemborg B, Moritz U, Hamberg J, et al. Intra-abdominal pressure and trunk muscle activity during lifting – effect of abdominal muscle training in healthy subjects. *Scand J Rehabil Med*. 1983;15:183–196.

88. Hemborg B, Moritz U, Hamberg J, et al. Intra-abdominal pressure and trunk muscle activity during lifting. III. Effects of abdominal muscle training in chronic low-back patients. *Scand J Rehabil Med*. 1985;17:15–24.

89. Farfan HF, Gracovetsky S. The abdominal mechanism. Paper presented at the International Society for the Study of the Lumbar Spine Meeting, Paris; 1981.

90. Farfan HF, Gracovetsky S, Helleur C. The role of mathematical models in the assessment of task in the workplace. In: Winter DA, Norman RW, Wells RP, et al, eds. *Biomechanics IXB, International Series on Biomechanics*. Champaign: Human Kinetics; 1983:38–43.

91. Gracovetsky S, Farfan HF, Helleur C. The abdominal mechanism. *Spine*. 1985;10:317–324.

92. Bearn JG. The significance of the activity of the abdominal muscles in weight lifting. *Acta Anat*. 1961;45:83–89.

93. Gracovetsky S, Farfan HF, Lamy C. A mathematical model of the lumbar spine using an optimal system to control muscles and ligaments. *Orthop Clin North Am*. 1977;8:135–153.

94. Macintosh JE, Bogduk N, Gracovetsky S. The biomechanics of the thoracolumbar fascia. *Clin Biomech*. 1987;2:78–83.

95. Crock HV, Crock MC. A technique for decompression of the lumbar spinal canal. *Neuro-Orthopaedics*. 1988;5:96–99.

96. Mykelbust JB, Pintar F, Yoganandan N, et al. Tensile strength of spinal ligaments. *Spine*. 1988;13:526–531.

97. Cyron BM, Hutton WC. The tensile strength of the capsular ligaments of the apophyseal joints. *J Anat*. 1981;132:145–150.

98. Hukins DWL, Aspden RM, Hickey DS. Thoracolumbar fascia can increase the efficiency of the erector spinae muscles. *Clin Biomech*. 1990;5:30–34.

99. Aspden RM. Intra-abdominal pressure and its role in spinal mechanics. *Clin Biomech*. 1987;2:168–174.

100. Aspden RM. The spine as an arch. A new mathematical model. *Spine*. 1989;14:266–274.

101. Adams M. Letter to the editor. *Spine*. 1989;14:1272.

Chapter | **10** |

Nerves of the lumbar spine

The lumbar spine is associated with a variety of nerves, the central focus of which are the lumbar **spinal nerves**. These lie in the intervertebral foramina and are connected to the spinal cord by the **spinal nerve roots**, which occupy the vertebral canal. Peripherally (i.e. outside the vertebral column), the spinal nerves divide into their branches: the **ventral** and **dorsal rami**. Running along the anterolateral aspects of the lumbar vertebral column are the lumbar **sympathetic trunks**, which communicate with the ventral rami of the lumbar spinal nerves.

LUMBAR SPINAL NERVES

The lumbar spinal nerves lie in the intervertebral foramina and are numbered according the vertebra beneath which they lie. Thus, the L1 spinal nerve lies below the L1 vertebra in the L1–2 intervertebral foramen, the L2 spinal nerve lies below the L2 vertebra, and so on. Centrally, each spinal nerve is connected to the spinal cord by a dorsal and ventral **root**. Peripherally, each spinal nerve divides into a larger ventral ramus and a smaller dorsal **ramus**. The spinal nerve roots join the spinal nerve in the intervertebral foramen, and the ventral and dorsal rami are formed just outside the foramen. Consequently, the spinal nerves are quite short. Each is no longer than the width of the intervertebral foramen in which it lies (Fig. 10.1).

The medial (or central) end of the spinal nerve may be difficult to define, for it depends on exactly where the dorsal and ventral roots of the nerve converge to form a single trunk. Sometimes, the spinal nerve may be very short, less than 1 mm, in which case the roots distribute their fibres directly to the ventral and dorsal rami without really forming a spinal nerve. Otherwise, the roots generally form a short trunk whose length measures a few millimetres from the point of junction of the nerve roots to the point of division of the ventral and dorsal rami.

LUMBAR NERVE ROOTS

The **dorsal root** of each spinal nerve transmits sensory fibres from the spinal nerve to the spinal cord. The **ventral root** largely transmits motor fibres from the cord to the spinal nerve but may also transmit some sensory fibres.

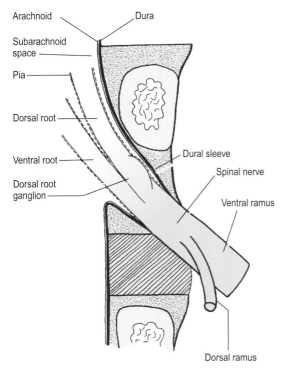

Figure 10.1 A lumbar spinal nerve, its roots and meningeal coverings. The nerve roots are invested by pia mater and covered by arachnoid and dura as far as the spinal nerve. The dura of the dural sac is prolonged around the roots as their dural sleeve, which blends with the epineurium of the spinal nerve.

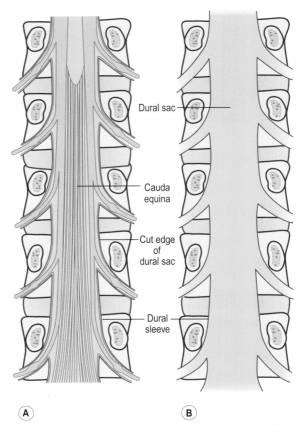

Figure 10.2 The lumbar nerve roots and the dural sac. (A) The posterior half of the dural sac has been removed to reveal the lumbar nerve roots as they lie within the dural sac, forming the cauda equina. (B) The intact dural sac is depicted, as it lies on the floor of the vertebral canal.

The ventral roots of the L1 and L2 spinal nerves additionally transmit preganglionic, sympathetic, efferent fibres.

The spinal cord terminates in the vertebral canal opposite the level of the L1–2 intervertebral disc, although it may end as high as T12–L1 or as low as L2–3.[1] Consequently, to reach the spinal cord, the lower lumbar (and sacral) nerve roots must run within the vertebral canal where they are largely enclosed in the dural sac (Fig. 10.2). Within the dural sac, the lumbar nerve roots run freely, mixed with the sacral and coccygeal nerve roots to form the **cauda equina**, and each root is covered with its own sleeve of pia mater, which is continuous with the pia mater of the spinal cord. All the roots of the cauda equina are bathed in cerebrospinal fluid (CSF), which percolates through the subarachnoid space of the dural sac.

For the greater part of their course, the nerve fibres within each nerve root are gathered into a single trunk, but near the spinal cord they are separated into smaller bundles called **rootlets**, which eventually attach to the spinal cord. The size and number of rootlets for each nerve root are variable but in general they are 0.5–1 mm in diameter and number between two and 12 for each root.[2]

The rootlets of each ventral root attach to the ventrolateral aspect of the cord, while those of the dorsal roots attach to the dorsolateral sulcus of the cord, and along the ventral and dorsal surface of the cord the rootlets form an uninterrupted series of attachments (Fig. 10.3).

A pair of spinal nerve roots leaves the dural sac just above the level of each intervertebral foramen. They do so by penetrating the dural sac in an inferolateral direction, taking with them an extension of dura mater and arachnoid mater referred to as the **dural sleeve** (see Fig. 10.2). This sleeve encloses the nerve roots as far as the intervertebral foramen and spinal nerve, where the dura mater merges with, or becomes, the epineurium of the spinal nerve (see Fig. 10.1). The pia mater of each of the nerve roots also extends as far as the spinal nerve, as does an extension of the subarachnoid space (see Fig. 10.1). Thus, the nerve roots are sheathed with pia mater and bathed in CSF as far as the spinal nerve.

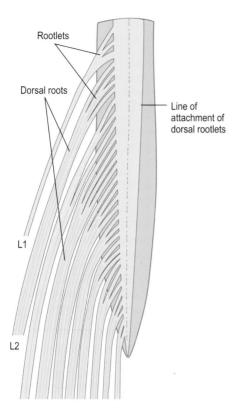

Rootlets

Dorsal roots

Line of
attachment of
dorsal rootlets

L1

L2

Figure 10.3 The lower end of the spinal cord and the pattern of attachment of the dorsal nerve roots and dorsal nerve rootlets.

Immediately proximal to its junction with the spinal nerve, the dorsal root forms an enlargement, the **dorsal root ganglion**, which contains the cell bodies of the sensory fibres in the dorsal root. The ganglion lies within the dural sleeve of the nerve roots and occupies the upper, medial part of the intervertebral foramen, but may lie further distally in the foramen if the spinal nerve is short.

The angle at which each pair of nerve roots leaves the dural sac varies from above downwards. The L1 and L2 roots leave the dural sac at an obtuse angle but the dural sleeves of the lower nerve roots form increasingly acute angles with the lateral margins of the dural sac (see Fig. 10.2). The angles formed by the L1 and L2 roots are about 80° and 70°, respectively, while the angles of the L3 and L4 roots are each about 60°, and that of the L5 roots is 45°.[3]

The level of origin of the nerve root sleeves also varies from above downwards. In general, the sleeves arise opposite the back of their respective vertebral bodies. Thus, the L1 sleeve arises behind the L1 body, the L2 sleeve behind the L2 body, and so on. However, successively lower sleeves arise increasingly higher behind their vertebral bodies until the sleeve of the L5 nerve roots arises behind the L4–5 intervertebral disc.[3]

Relations of the nerve roots

The relations of the nerve roots are of critical importance in the pathology of nerve root compression, for space-occupying lesions of any of the tissues intimately, or even distantly, related to the nerve roots may encroach upon them. In this regard, the majority of structures related to the nerve roots have already been described (see Ch. 5), although the anatomy of the spinal blood vessels is described in detail in Chapter 11.

The most intimate relation of the nerve roots are the meninges. The roots of the cauda equina are enclosed in the dural sac and bathed in CSF. Beyond the dural sac, individual pairs of roots are sheathed by pia, arachnoid and dura in the nerve root sleeves (Figs 10.1, 10.4). The relevance of this relationship is that tumours or cysts of the dura or arachnoid can at times form space-occupying lesions that compress the roots. Running within the root sleeves are the radicular arteries and veins (see Ch. 11), and the relevance of this relationship is described in Chapter 15.

As a whole, the dural sac rests on the floor of the vertebral canal (see Ch. 5). The anterior relations of the dural sac, therefore, are the backs of the vertebral bodies and the intervertebral discs, and covering these structures is the posterior longitudinal ligament (see Fig. 10.4). Running across the floor of the vertebral canal, and therefore anterior to the dural sac, are the anterior spinal canal arteries (see Ch. 11) and the sinuvertebral nerves (see below). Posteriorly, the dural sac is related to the roof of the vertebral canal, the laminae and ligamenta flava (see Ch. 5).

A space intervenes between the dural sac and the osseoligamentous boundaries of the vertebral canal; this space is referred to as the **epidural space**. This space, however, is quite narrow, for the dural sac is applied very closely to the osseoligamentous boundaries of the vertebral canal. It is almost a 'potential space', and the term 'epidural region' has been advocated as an alternative description to avoid the connotation of a wide, empty space (see Fig. 10.4).[4]

The epidural space is principally filled by a thin layer of areolar connective tissue, which varies from diaphanous to pseudomembranous in structure.[4] Some investigators, however, consider this to be a substantive structure which they call the **epidural membrane**.[5] The membrane surrounds the dural sac and lines the deep surface of the laminae and pedicles. Ventrally, opposite the vertebral bodies, the membrane lines the back of the vertebral body and then passes medially deep to the posterior longitudinal ligament, where it attaches to the anterior surface of the deep portion of the ligament.[5] The membrane does not cover the back of the anulus fibrosus; it is prevented

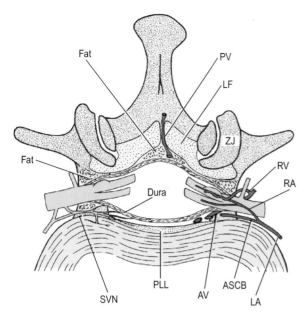

Figure 10.4 A transverse section through the vertebral canal and intervertebral foramina to demonstrate the relations of the lumbar nerve roots. The roots are enclosed in their dural sleeve, which is surrounded by epidural fat in the intervertebral foramina. Radicular veins (RV) and radicular arteries (RA) run with the nerve roots. Anteriorly, the roots are related to the intervertebral disc and posterior longitudinal ligament (PLL), separated from them by the sinuvertebral nerves (SVN), elements of the anterior internal vertebral venous plexus (AV) and the anterior spinal canal branches (ASCB) of the lumbar arteries (LA). Posteriorly, the roots are separated from the ligamentum flavum (LF) and zygapophysial joints (ZJ) by elements of the posterior internal vertebral venous plexus (PV) and epidural fat, which lodges in the recess between the ligamentum flavum of each side.

from doing so by the posterior longitudinal ligament as it expands laterally over the back of the disc. Consequently, the membrane blends with the upper and lower borders of the anulus fibrosus but in a plane just anterior to that of the posterior longitudinal ligament. Opposite the intervertebral foramen, the membrane is drawn laterally to form a circumneural sheath around the dural sleeve of the nerve roots and spinal nerve.[5]

Running within the areolar tissue of the epidural membrane are the anterior and posterior internal vertebral venous plexuses (see Ch. 11), and located within it are collections of fat. The epidural fat is not distributed uniformly throughout the epidural space but is concentrated around the nerve roots in the intervertebral foramina and in collections wrapped in areolar tissue and lodged in the midline recesses between the ligamenta flava at each segmental level.[4]

Individual pairs of nerve roots, enclosed in their dural sleeves, course to their intervertebral foramina along the radicular canals. Consequently, they are related laterally to a pedicle, and ventrally, from above downwards, they cross the back of a vertebral body to enter the upper portion of their intervertebral foramen. Dorsally, they are covered by a lamina and its ligamenta flava, which separate the root sleeve from the overlying zygapophysial joints.

Within the vertebral canal, the dural sac and the nerve root sleeves are tethered to the vertebral column by condensations of the epidural fascia that have been referred to as **dural ligaments** or **meningovertebral ligaments** or the ligaments of **Hofmann**.[4,6–8] Although the first term is the more traditional, the second is a better description, in that the tissue is not an extension of dura but a connection *between* the meninges and the vertebral column.

The ventral meningovertebral ligaments pass from the ventral surface of the dura to the posterior longitudinal ligament. They are most evident when the dura is drawn backwards and the ligaments are tensed. At rest, they are barely distinguishable from the epidural membrane. When tensed, they form a discontinuous septum in the median or paramedian plane. Individual ligaments may form single bands, bands that bifurcate in a Y shape towards the posterior longitudinal ligament, or two or more paramedian bands that skirt the posterior longitudinal ligament and attach to the periosteum of the lateral recesses.[6,7] These ligaments are variably developed at the L1–L4 levels but are well developed at L5.[8]

Lateral meningovertebral ligaments pass from the lateral surface of the dural sac to blend with the periosteum of the pedicles and with the capsule of the zygapophysial joint.[6] Posteriorly, the dural sac is attached to the roof of the vertebral canal by occasional, weak pseudoligamentous connections,[4] which represent dorsal meningovertebral ligaments.[6]

The nerve root sleeves are tethered both within the vertebral canal and in the intervertebral foramen. At the proximal end of the root sleeve, the meningovertebral ligaments tether the dura to the posterior longitudinal ligament and the periosteum of the adjacent pedicle.[8,9] In the intervertebral foramen, the root sleeve is surrounded by the circumneural sheath, which indirectly binds the nerve roots and spinal nerve to the margins of the foramen, but mainly to the capsule of the zygapophysial joint dorsally.[8,9] At the outer end of the intervertebral foramen, the spinal nerve may be related to a transforaminal ligament when one is present (see Ch. 4). As a rule, the spinal nerve lies below most forms of transforaminal ligaments but emerges above the inferior transforaminal variety (see Ch. 4).[10]

The relative size of the spinal nerve and nerve roots within the intervertebral foramen varies from level to level and is important with respect to the risk of spinal nerve and nerve root compression. As an approximate rule, the cross-sectional area of an intervertebral foramen increases from L1–2 to L4–5, but the L5–S1 foramen is conspicuously smaller than the rest,[11] yet, paradoxically, the L5 spinal nerve is the largest of the lumbar nerves.[11] Consequently, the L5 spinal nerve occupies about 25–30% of the available area in an intervertebral foramen, while the other lumbar nerves occupy between 7% and 22%, making the L5 nerve the most susceptible to foraminal stenosis.

Anomalies of the nerve roots

The clinically most significant anomalies of the lumbar nerve roots are aberrant courses and anastomoses between nerve roots;[12–18] the morphology of these anomalies is summarised in Figure 10.5.

Type 1 anomalies are aberrant courses. Two pairs of nerve roots may arise from a single dural sleeve (type 1A), or a dural sleeve may arise from a low position on the dural sac (type 1B). Type 2 anomalies are those in which the number of roots in an intervertebral foramen varies. A foramen may be unoccupied by a nerve (type 2A), in which case the foramen above or below contains two sets of roots, or a foramen may contain a supernumerary set of roots (type 2B). Type 3 anomalies are extradural anastomoses between roots in which a bundle of nerve

fibres leaves one dural sleeve to enter an adjacent one. This type of anomaly may be superimposed on a type 2 anomaly.

These anomalies, per se, do not produce symptoms. Patients with conjoined or aberrant nerve roots may pass their entire life without developing symptoms. However, doubled nerve roots occupy far more of the available space in the radicular canal or the intervertebral foramen than a single root. Therefore, if a space-occupying lesion develops, it is more likely to compress a double nerve root, and produce symptoms sooner than if a normal single root was present. Thus, although root anomalies do not render patients more likely to develop disorders of the lumbar spine, they do render them more likely to develop symptoms in the presence of space-occupying lesions.

The other clinical significance of anomalous roots relates to the interpretation of clinical signs. Clinical examination might indicate compression of a particular nerve root but if that root has an anomalous course, the structural lesion causing the compression may not be located at the expected site. For example, signs of L4 nerve root compression most often suggest compression in the L4 radicular canal or in the L4–5 intervertebral foramen; in the case of an anomalous L4 root being compressed,

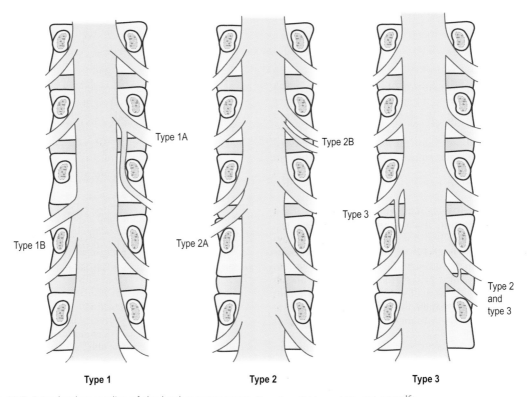

Type 1A
Type 1B
Type 1

Type 2B
Type 2A
Type 2

Type 3
Type 2 and type 3
Type 3

Figure 10.5 Extradural anomalies of the lumbar nerve roots. *(Based on Neidre and MacNab 1983.[16])*

the lesion could be at the L3 or perhaps the L5 vertebral level, depending on the type of anomaly. Alternatively, in the case of doubled nerve roots, a single compressive lesion could produce signs suggestive of two lesions compressing two consecutive nerve roots.

Fortunately, symptomatic nerve root anomalies are not common, and such confusing considerations do not regularly complicate clinical practice. The incidence of anomalies has been estimated at about 8.5%,[19] but when symptomatic the major types are readily recognised in myelograms.[2] Nonetheless, nerve root anomalies should be borne in mind and considered as a possibility in patients with unusual distributions of neurological signs.

The surgical significance of nerve root anomalies relates to the mobility of anomalous nerve roots, the care necessary when operating in their vicinity, and the types of procedures that can be carried out to decompress them. These issues are explored in the surgical literature.[2,16]

Another feature of nerve roots, which is not an anomaly but rather a variation, is intrathecal anastomoses. Within the dural sac, bundles of nerve fibres may pass from one nerve root to the next, and such communications have an incidence of 11–30%.[20] They usually occur close to the spinal cord and may vary in size from small filaments to substantial bundles.[20] Since they occur proximal to the regions where nerve roots are liable to compression, these anastomoses are not of diagnostic clinical significance, but they are of relevance to neurosurgeons operating on the proximal ends of nerve roots.[20,21]

DORSAL RAMI

The L1–L4 dorsal rami are short nerves that arise almost at right angles from the lumbar spinal nerves.[22] Each nerve measures about 5 mm in length[23] and is directed backwards towards the upper border of the subjacent transverse process. The L5 dorsal ramus differs, in that it is longer and travels over the top of the ala of the sacrum (Fig. 10.6).[23]

As they approach their transverse processes, the L1–4 dorsal rami divide into two or three branches (see Fig. 10.6). A **medial branch** and a **lateral branch** are always represented at every level. The variable, third branch is the **intermediate branch**. Although this branch is always represented, it frequently arises from the lateral branch instead of the dorsal ramus itself.[23] The L5 dorsal ramus forms only a medial branch and a branch that is equivalent to the intermediate branches of the other lumbar dorsal rami.

The lateral branches of the lumbar dorsal rami are principally distributed to the iliocostalis lumborum muscle, but those from the L1, L2 and L3 levels can emerge from the dorsolateral border of this muscle to become cutaneous. Cutaneous branches of these pierce the posterior layer

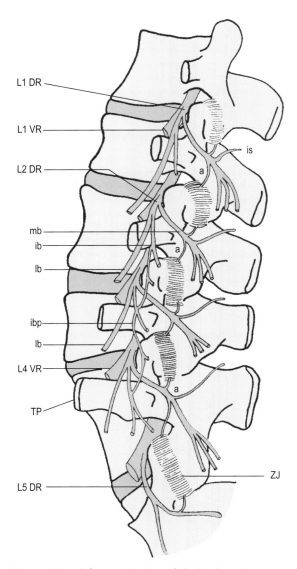

Figure 10.6 A left posterior view of the lumbar spine showing the branches of the lumbar dorsal rami. (Based on Bogduk et al. 1982.[23]) DR, dorsal ramus: ib, intermediate branch; ibp, intermediate branch plexus; lb, lateral branch; mb, medial branch. TP, transverse process; a, articular branch; is, interspinous branch. VR, ventral ramus. ZJ, zygapophysial joint.

of thoracolumbar fascia and descend inferolaterally across the iliac crest to innervate the skin of the buttock, over an area extending from the iliac crest to the greater trochanter.[24] When crossing the iliac crest, these nerves run parallel to one another with those from lower levels lying most medial.

Variations occur in the regularity with which branches of the L1, L2 and L3 dorsal rami become cutaneous.[25,26] In embryos and fetuses, the L1 lateral branch always becomes cutaneous, the L2 in 90% of cases, the L3 in 70%; the L4 lateral branch reaches the skin in 40%.[26] In dissections of adults a similar pattern emerges, except that cutaneous branches from L4 appear to be uncommon.[25] Most commonly, only the L1 lateral branch becomes cutaneous. This occurs in some 60% of individuals. Both L1 and L2 become cutaneous in about 27% of cases, and all three levels furnish cutaneous branches in only 13% of cases. Regardless of its segmental origin, the lowest and most medial nerve that crosses the iliac crest does so approximately 7–8 cm from the midline.[25]

The intermediate branches of the lumbar dorsal rami have only a muscular distribution to the lumbar fibres of the longissimus muscle and within this muscle they form an intersegmental plexus (see Fig. 10.6).[22,23] The intermediate branch of the L5 dorsal ramus supplies the lowest fibres of longissimus which arise from the L5 transverse process and attach to the medial aspect of the iliac crest (see Ch. 9).

It is the medial branches that are of paramount clinical relevance because of their distribution to the zygapophysial joints. The medial branches of the L1–L4 dorsal rami run across the top of their respective transverse processes and pierce the dorsal leaf of the intertransverse ligament at the base of the transverse process (see Fig. 4.7). Each nerve then runs along bone at the junction of the root of the transverse process with the root of the superior articular process (see Fig. 10.6). Hooking medially around the base of the superior articular process, each nerve is covered by the mamillo-accessory ligament (see Ch. 4). Finally, it crosses the vertebral lamina, where it divides into multiple branches that supply the multifidus muscle, the interspinous muscle and ligament, and two zygapophysial joints.

Each medial branch supplies the zygapophysial joints above and below its course (see Fig. 10.6).[22,23,27–30] An ascending **articular branch** arises from the nerve just beyond the mamillo-accessory ligament where the nerve starts to cross the lamina. A descending articular branch arises slightly more distally and courses downwards to the joint below.

The medial branch of the L5 dorsal ramus has a similar course and distribution to those of the L1 to L4 dorsal rami, except that instead of crossing a transverse process, it crosses the ala of the sacrum. It runs in the groove formed by the junction of the ala and the root of the superior articular process of the sacrum before hooking medially around the base of the lumbosacral zygapophysial joint. It sends an articular branch to this joint before ramifying in multifidus.

The muscular distribution of the medial branches of the lumbar dorsal rami is very specific. Each medial branch supplies only those muscles that arise from the lamina and

spinous process of the vertebra with the same segmental number as the nerve.[23,31] Thus, for example, the L1 medial branch supplies only those fibres from the L1 vertebra; the L2 nerve supplies only those muscles from the L2 vertebra, and so on. This relationship can be stated more formally as follows:

The muscles arising from the spinous process and lamina of a lumbar vertebra are innervated by the medial branch of the dorsal ramus that issues immediately below that vertebra.

The same applies for the interspinous ligaments. This relationship indicates that the principal muscles that move a particular segment are innervated by the nerve of that segment (see Ch. 9).

Histology

Histological studies have shown that capsules of the lumbar zygapophysial joints are richly innervated with encapsulated, unencapsulated and free nerve endings.[27,32,33] These joints are therefore endowed with the appropriate sensory apparatus to transmit proprioceptive and nociceptive information. Modern studies have ventured to characterise the nerve fibres in the zygapophysial joints according to their transmitter substance but this has yielded curious results. Nerves containing substance P and calcitonin gene-related peptide (CGRP) were encountered in very few specimens but nerves containing neuropeptide Y were often encountered.[34] This suggests either that the majority of nerves in the zygapophysial joints are sympathetic efferent fibres and not sensory fibres, or that technical problems still impede obtaining accurate profiles of neuropeptides in human material obtained at operation.

Nerve fibres and nerve endings also occur in the subchondral bone of the zygapophysial joints. They occur in erosion channels extending from the subchondral bone to the articular cartilage.[35] Such fibres might provide a pathway for nociception from these joints other than from their capsules.

Nerve fibres are distributed to the intra-articular inclusions of the zygapophysial joints.[36–38] These fibres contain substance P,[37,39] but it remains contentious whether these nerves are nociceptive[37] or predominantly vasoregulatory.[39]

Nerve fibres are plentiful in the interspinous ligaments,[40–43] where they give rise to Ruffini endings, paciniform endings and free nerve endings.[43] The Ruffini endings are sparse towards the centre of the ligament but more numerous towards its lateral surfaces.[40] These endings are mechanoreceptors and probably convey proprioceptive information from the ligament. Paciniform endings are uniformly distributed across the ligament but appear to be associated with blood vessels.[40] This intriguing juxtaposition requires an explanation for the function of the paciniform endings. Free nerve endings are located near the attachment of the ligament to the spinous processes.[43]

The supraspinous ligaments and adjacent thoracolumbar fascia are well innervated and contain nerve fibres, Ruffini endings and paciniform endings.[41,43,44] The ligamentum flavum appears to be sparsely innervated. Some studies have found no nerves,[34] or only a few nerves,[41] in this ligament. Others have found nerve endings only in the outermost layers of the dorsal surface of the ligament.[42]

Variations

Variations have been reported in the number and nature of branches of the lumbar dorsal rami that innervate the lumbar zygapophysial joints. Lazorthes and Juskiewenski[28] reported that, occasionally, an articular branch may arise from the dorsal ramus proper and innervate the ventral aspect of the adjacent joint. A similar branch was described by Auteroche,[45] who also described multiple articular branches arising from the spinal nerve, the lateral branch of the dorsal ramus, and from the entire length of the medial branch. Such a plethora of articular nerves has not been observed in any other study.[22,23,28–30] The study by Auteroche was based solely on dissection using magnifying glasses; the nature of the putative articular branches was not confirmed histologically. Under such conditions it is possible to mistake collagen fibres for articular nerves. Studies using a dissecting microscope and histological corroboration do not support his generous description of articular branches. Similarly, ascending articular branches from the root of the medial branch, as described by Paris,[46] have not been confirmed histologically nor have they been seen in previous studies,[21,22,27–29] and indeed they have been explicitly denied in subsequent studies.[47]

VENTRAL RAMI

The ventral rami of the lumbar spinal nerves emerge from the intervertebral foramen by piercing the ventral leaf of the intertransverse ligament (see Ch. 4). Therefore, they enter the space in front of the ligaments and lie within the substance of the psoas major muscle. Within the muscle, they enter into the formation of plexuses. The L1 to L4 ventral rami form the lumbar plexus, and the L4 and L5 ventral rami join to form the lumbosacral trunk, which enters the lumbosacral plexus. Because these plexuses are not particularly relevant to the pathology or physiology of lumbar spinal disorders, their anatomy will not be further explored. They are adequately described in other textbooks of anatomy.[48]

The one exception to this exclusion relates to the course of the L5 ventral ramus. This nerve crosses the ala of the sacrum, below the L5 transverse process, and in this location can be trapped between these two bones. This phenomenon has been called the 'far out syndrome' and is described fully elsewhere.[49]

DERMATOMES

The advent of fluoroscopically guided local anaesthetic blocks of the lumbar spinal nerves has enabled a reappraisal of classic data on the cutaneous distribution of the lumbar spinal nerves. Classically, dermatomes were defined on the basis of observations of patients with diseases or injuries of these nerves, such as herpes zoster or dorsal rhizotomies. Nerve root blocks have allowed dermatomes to be determined quantitatively under physiological conditions in individuals with no intrinsic neurological disease.

The dermatomes of the L4, L5 and S1 spinal nerves vary from individual to individual with respect to their total extent but nonetheless exhibit a consistent concentric pattern between individuals.[50] Each dermatome can extend from the posterior midline of the back, across the buttock and into the lower limb (Fig. 10.7). However, only a minority of individuals exhibits such an extensive distribution for L4 and L5. For L4, the majority of individuals exhibit an area centred on the medial aspect of the lower leg; for L5 the central area extends from the medial aspect of the foot, across the dorsum of the foot, and onto the lateral aspect of the lower leg (Fig. 10.7A,B). A more extensive distribution is characteristic for S1. Its area extends as a band from the posterior sacrum, along the entire length of the lower limb posteriorly to the lateral aspect of the foot (Fig. 10.7C).

The distal nature of each distribution indicates the cutaneous area supplied by branches of the ventral ramus of the particular spinal nerve. The distribution over the buttock, when it occurs, indicates a distribution from the dorsal ramus. Some 92% of individuals have a cutaneous distribution of the S1 dorsal ramus, 44% have a cutaneous distribution of the L5 dorsal ramus and 42% exhibit an L4 dorsal distribution.

These latter figures are inconsistent with traditional and contemporary anatomical data, which acknowledge a cutaneous distribution of the S1 dorsal ramus but deny such a distribution for L5. A 40% incidence of a cutaneous branch from L4 is consistent with embryological data[26] but not with dissection data.[25] The presence of a cutaneous distribution of L5 is inconsistent with both embryological and dissection data.

The results of nerve blocks indicate that traditional anatomical wisdom may need to be reappraised. Overtly, some 40% of individuals have either an L4 or L5 dorsal cutaneous branch, or both. A distribution from L5 might be expected from its communication with the dorsal sacral plexus,[26] but how branches of the L4 dorsal ramus get to

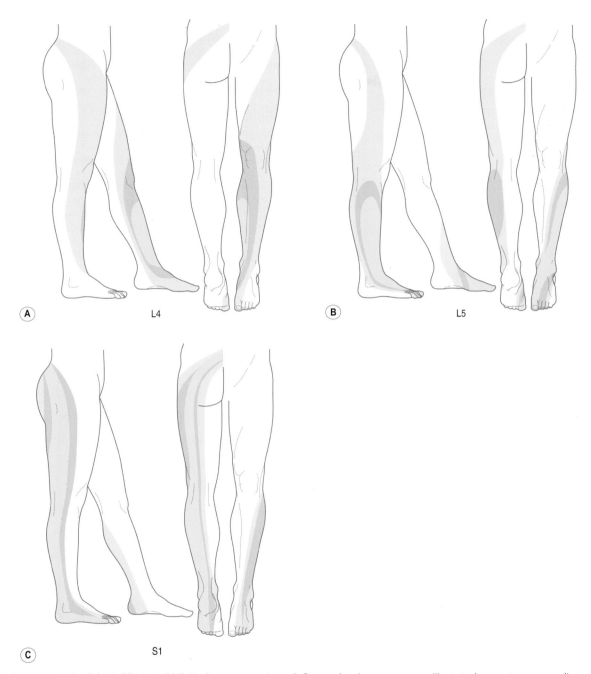

Figure 10.7 The (A) L4, (B) L5 and (C) S1 dermatomes. In each figure, the dermatomes are illustrated as contours according to the percentage of individuals who exhibit the particular pattern. The yellow zones are exhibited by at least 75% of the population, the blue zones by at least 50% and the purple zones by some 25% of individuals. *(Based on Nitta et al. 1993.[50])*

the skin remains a mystery. Nerve block data, however, stipulate that they do, in 40% of individuals.

SYMPATHETIC NERVES

The lumbar sympathetic trunks descend through the lumbar region along the anterolateral borders of the lumbar vertebral column. Each trunk is applied to the vertebral column next to the medial edge of the attachment of the psoas major muscle. The number of ganglia on the trunks varies from one to six,[51] but most commonly four are present.[52]

Branches of the lumbar sympathetic trunks are distributed to abdominal and pelvic blood vessels and viscera, and some direct branches pass into the psoas major muscle,[52] but the principal branches are the **rami communicantes** to the lumbar ventral rami. **White rami communicantes** are distributed to the L1 and L2 ventral rami, and **grey rami communicantes** are distributed to every lumbar ventral ramus. The number of rami communicantes to each lumbar nerve varies from one to three, and exceptionally may be as high as five.[52]

In general, the rami communicantes reach the ventral rami by passing through the tunnels deep to the psoas muscle that lie along the concave lateral surfaces of the lumbar vertebral bodies (see Ch. 9). These tunnels direct them to the lower borders of the transverse processes where the rami communicantes join the ventral rami just outside the intervertebral foramina. Rami communicantes may also reach the ventral rami by penetrating the substance of psoas.[52,53]

The efferent fibres of the rami communicantes are principally destined to be distributed to the blood vessels and skin in the territories supplied by the lumbar spinal nerves, but in the vicinity of the lumbar spine, rami communicantes are involved in the formation of the lumbar sinuvertebral nerves and in the innervation of the lumbar intervertebral discs.

SINUVERTEBRAL NERVES

The sinuvertebral nerves are recurrent branches of the ventral rami that re-enter the intervertebral foramina to be distributed within the vertebral canal.[27,28,53-56] They are mixed nerves, each being formed by a somatic root from a ventral ramus and an autonomic root from a grey ramus communicans. Although traditionally portrayed as a single nerve, the sinuvertebral nerve may be represented by a series of filaments that pass through the intervertebral foramen, or by an identifiable single trunk accompanied by additional fine filaments.[57] The filamentous sinu-

vertebral nerves may not be evident to the naked eye or even under a dissecting microscope.

In the intervertebral foramina the lumbar sinuvertebral nerves run across the back of the vertebral body, just below the upper pedicle (Fig. 10.8). Within the vertebral canal, each nerve forms an ascending branch which passes rostrally, parallel to the posterior longitudinal ligament, to which it sends branches, and ends in the next higher intervertebral disc, which it also supplies. A shorter descending branch ramifies in the disc and ligament at the level of entry of the parent nerve (see Fig. 10.8).

In addition to this skeletal distribution, each lumbar sinuvertebral nerve is distributed to the blood vessels of the vertebral canal and to the ventral aspect of the dura mater. In the dura mater each sinuvertebral nerve forms ascending and descending meningeal branches.[54,58] The descending branches are the longer, extending up to two

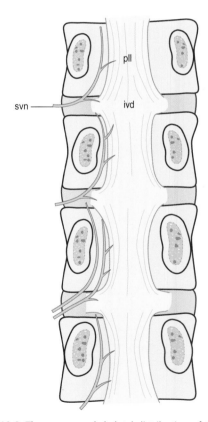

Figure 10.8 The course and skeletal distribution of the lumbar sinuvertebral nerves (svn). Each nerve supplies the intervertebral disc (ivd) at its level of entry into the vertebral canal, the disc above, and the intervening posterior longitudinal ligament (pll). In about one-third of cases, the nerve at a particular level may be represented by more than one filament.

segments caudally, while the ascending branch ascends up to one segment.[54] The dura mater is in fact covered with a dense plexus of nerves on its ventral surface.[59] This plexus extends around the lateral aspect of the dural sac but attenuates dorsally. The paramedian portion of the dorsal aspect of the dural sac is distinctly devoid of nerve fibres.[58,59]

INNERVATION OF THE LUMBAR INTERVERTEBRAL DISCS

Whether or not the lumbar intervertebral discs receive an innervation has long been a controversial issue. Early studies failed to demonstrate nerve fibres or nerve endings within the discs,[56,60,61] and the results of these studies have been used to promulgate the conclusion that the lumbar discs lack an innervation.[62–64] However, other studies identified nerve fibres in the superficial layers of the anulus fibrosus,[32,33,65,66] and in a painstaking study, Malinsky[67] demonstrated a variety of free and complex endings in the outer third of the anulus. Malinsky's findings have been confirmed in studies by Rabischong et al.[68] and by Yoshizawa et al.[69] The latter workers studied specimens of intervertebral discs removed at operation for anterior and posterior lumbar interbody fusion. They found abundant nerve endings with various morphologies throughout the outer half of the anulus fibrosus.

Histology

In the prenatal period, nerves are abundant in the anulus fibrosus, where they form simple free endings, and they increase in number in older fetuses.[67] During the postnatal period, various types of unencapsulated receptors emerge, and in adult material five types of nerve terminations can be found: simple and complex free nerve endings; 'shrubby' receptors; others that form loops and mesh-like formations; and clusters of parallel free nerve endings.[67] On the surface of the anulus fibrosus, various types of encapsulated and complex unencapsulated receptors occur. They are all relatively simple in structure in neonates, but more elaborate forms occur in older and mature specimens.

Within a given disc, receptors are not uniformly distributed. The greatest number of endings occurs in the lateral region of the disc, and nearly all the encapsulated receptors are located in this region.[67] Following postnatal development, there is a relative decrease in the number of receptors in the anterior region, such that in adults the greatest number of endings occurs in the lateral regions of the disc, a smaller number in the posterior region, and the least number anteriorly.

The varieties of nerve endings found in adult discs include free terminals, often ending in club-like or bulbous expansions or complex sprays and, less commonly, terminals forming convoluted tangles or glomerular formations that were occasionally demarcated by a 'capsule-like' condensation of adjacent tissue.[67–69] Modern immunohistochemical techniques have revealed endings resembling Golgi tendon organs, Ruffini endings and paciniform endings in the outer lamellae of the anulus fibrosus that contain CGRP, substance P and vasoactive intestinal polypeptide.[70] Nerve endings are also frequent in the anterior and posterior longitudinal ligaments,[32,61,66] many of which contain substance P.[71] In the anulus fibrosus, the substance P neurones are distributed with blood vessels that express NK1 receptors.[72] This suggests a vasoactive role for substance P in the disc.

Sources

The sources of the nerve endings in the lumbar discs are two extensive microscopic plexuses of nerves that accompany the anterior and posterior longitudinal ligaments. These plexuses cannot be discerned by dissection but are evident in whole mounts of human fetuses stained for acetylcholinesterase.[57]

The **anterior plexus** bridges the two lumbar sympathetic trunks and covers the anterior longitudinal ligament (Fig. 10.9). It is formed by branches of the sympathetic trunks and branches from the proximal ends of the grey rami communicantes. The **posterior plexus** is derived from the sinuvertebral nerves and accompanies the posterior longitudinal ligament (Fig. 10.10). Within the posterior plexus, the sinuvertebral nerves constitute the largest and most visible elements but they are not the only components; the majority of fibres are microscopic. The anterior and posterior plexuses are connected around the lateral aspects of the vertebral bodies and discs by way of a less pronounced **lateral plexus** that is formed by branches of the grey rami communicantes (Fig. 10.11).

The anterior and posterior plexuses supply superficial branches that innervate the periosteum of the vertebral bodies, and long penetrating branches that enter the intervertebral discs and vertebral bodies, the latter following blood vessels as far as the centre of the bone. Through these branches the vertebral bodies and intervertebral discs are innervated around their entire circumference (Figs 10.12, 10.13).

The discovery of the anterior and posterior plexuses explains and corrects certain previous descriptions of the source of nerves to the lumbar discs. It had previously been established, by dissection, that direct branches of the ventral rami enter the posterolateral corner of the discs.[53,73] It now appears that these are not isolated, special 'disc branches'. Rather they represent one of the several sources that contribute to the plexus that overlies the discs and vertebral bodies laterally. The other sources are the grey rami communicantes, which send branches to the discs across their lateral surface and at their posterolateral corner (see Fig. 10.11).

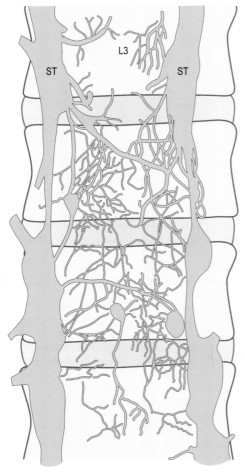

Figure 10.9 The nerve plexus accompanying the anterior longitudinal ligament at the levels of L3 and lower vertebrae, as seen in whole mounts of human fetuses. ST, lumbar sympathetic trunk. *(Based on Groen et al. 1990.[57])*

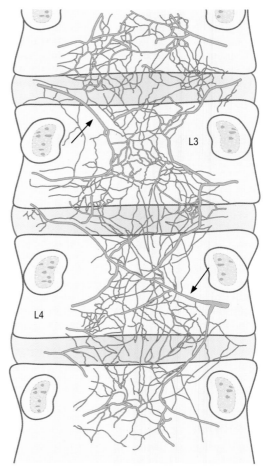

Figure 10.10 The nerve plexus accompanying the posterior longitudinal ligament at the levels of L3 and lower vertebrae, as seen in whole mounts of human fetuses. (Based on Groen et al. 1990.[57]) The large fibres arrowed represent what would be found, on dissection, to be the sinuvertebral nerves.

The fact that the lumbar intervertebral discs and their adjacent ligaments are innervated by branches of the sympathetic nervous system does not necessarily mean that afferent fibres from these structures return to the central nervous system via the sympathetic trunk. Rather, it has been suggested that somatic afferent fibres from the discs and ligaments simply use the course of the rami communicantes to return to the ventral rami.[53]

Within the vertebral body, nerve fibres consistently accompany the basivertebral veins and arteries, and ramify throughout the spongiosa along with the vessels.[74] These nerves extend to the vertebral endplates. Nerve endings are located on the endosteal surface of the endplate and underneath the cartilaginous endplate.[75] These latter endings endow the disc with an innervation additional to that in the anulus fibrosus.

Endplate innervation appears to be greater in discs that are painful, ostensibly because of a greater vascular supply.[75] However, the nerve endings contain substance P and CGRP, and they are often not related to blood vessels.[75] Both of these features indicate that they are sensory nerves not vasomotor nerves.

The presence of nerve endings in the lumbar intervertebral discs raises the question as to their function. Any free endings associated with blood vessels in the disc may reasonably be ascribed a vasomotor or vasosensory function[53,67] but because the anulus fibrosus contains so few blood vessels (see Ch. 11) this is unlikely to be the

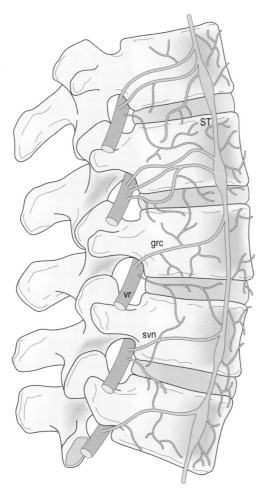

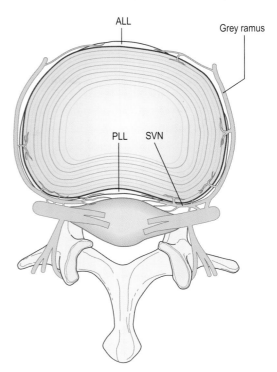

Figure 10.12 The nerve supply of a lumbar intervertebral disc depicted in a transverse view of the lumbar spine. Branches of the grey rami communicantes and the sinuvertebral nerves (SVN) are shown entering the disc and the anterior and posterior longitudinal ligaments (ALL, PLL). Branches from the sinuvertebral nerves also supply the anterior aspect of the dural sac and dural sleeve.

Figure 10.11 The lateral plexus of the lumbar spine and its sources. The plexus innervates the lateral aspects of the vertebral bodies and discs. The plexus is formed by branches of the grey rami communicantes (grc) and branches of the ventral rami (vr). Posteriorly, the lateral plexus is continued as the sinuvertebral nerves (svn) entering the intervertebral foramina. Anteriorly, the plexus blends with the anterior plexus and sympathetic trunks (ST).

function for the majority of the nerve fibres in the anulus fibrosus. For the encapsulated receptors on the surface of the disc, Malinsky[67] postulated a proprioceptive function. Theoretically, this would be a valid, useful role for these receptors but the only study that has addressed this contention failed to find any evidence in its favour.[76] However, this study was performed on cats, which are not a suitable model, for the cat is a quadrupedal animal whose vertebral column is not used for weight-bearing and may not be endowed with receptors and reflexes that would be appropriate for an upright vertebral column. Therefore, a proprioceptive role for the intervertebral disc has not been excluded.

In other tissues of the body, isolated free nerve endings are ascribed a nociceptive function, and it is presumably the case that they play a similar role in the lumbar intervertebral discs. Although there is no explicit evidence that disc pain can be ascribed to a particular type of nerve ending in the disc, there is abundant evidence that the disc can be painful. The issue of disc pain is addressed in Chapter 15.

Nerve ingrowth

In normal lumbar intervertebral discs, nerve fibres are only found in the outer third of the anulus fibrosus. They do not occur in the deeper anulus or nucleus pulposus.

Several studies have now shown that this pattern of innervation differs in certain discs. In discs shown to be painful by discography (see Ch. 15), and removed at operation, nerve fibers have been found in the deeper anulus and into the nucleus pulposus.[77–79]

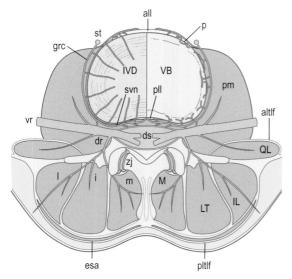

Figure 10.13 Innervation of the lumbar spine. A cross-sectional view incorporating the level of the vertebral body (VB) and its periosteum (p) on the right and the intervertebral disc (IVD) on the left. all, anterior longitudinal ligament; altlf, anterior layer of thoracolumbar fascia; dr, dorsal ramus; ds, dural sac; esa, erector spinae aponeurosis; grc, grey ramus communicans; i, intermediate branch; IL, iliocostalis lumborum; l, lateral branch; LT, longissimus thoracis; M, multifidus; m, medial branch; pll, posterior longitudinal ligament; pltlf, posterior layer of thoracolumbar fascia; pm, psoas major; QL, quadratus lumborum; st, sympathetic trunk; svn, sinuvertebral nerve; vr, ventral ramus; zj, zygapophysial joint.

The investigators referred to these as degenerated but it is probably more accurate to refer to them as damaged. The distinguishing feature of these discs was not that they were simply degenerated, in the sense that they were old (see Ch. 14). Rather they were discs that were painful, and sufficiently so, as to warrant surgical excision. Moreover, one study[78] compared discs from the same patients: the symptomatic one and an adjacent painless one. Nerve ingrowth was far more common in the painful disc even though the control disc was the same age.

Damage, rather than degeneration, also explains the origin of the nerves. It appears that they accompany blood vessels that grow in along fissures through the anulus fibrosus.[77-79] Fissuring, therefore, is a trigger for neovascularisation and neo-innervation of the disc. Fissuring is also the cardinal characteristic of internal disc disruption, which is an acquired traumatic disorder (see Ch. 15).

SUMMARY

The lumbar spine receives an extensive innervation (see Fig. 10.13). Posteriorly, the branches of the lumbar dorsal rami are distributed to the back muscles and the zygapophysial joints. Anteriorly, the ventral rami supply the psoas major and quadratus lumborum. The vertebral bodies and intervertebral discs are surrounded by extensive plexuses of nerves that accompany the longitudinal ligaments and which are derived from the lumbar sympathetic trunks. Within the posterior plexus, larger filaments constitute the sinuvertebral nerves. Short branches innervate the vertebral periosteum, and long penetrating branches enter the vertebral body from all aspects of its circumference. Nerves enter the outer third of the anulus fibrosus from the longitudinal plexuses anteriorly, laterally and posteriorly. The posterior plexus innervates the dura mater and nerve root sleeves along their anterior and lateral aspects.

REFERENCES

1. Louis R. Topographic relationships of the vertebral column, spinal cord, and nerve roots. *Anat Clin.* 1978;1:3–12.

2. Bouchard JM, Copty M, Langelier R. Preoperative diagnosis of conjoined roots anomaly with herniated lumbar disks. *Surg Neurol.* 1978;10:229–231.

3. Bose K, Balasubramaniam P. Nerve root canals of the lumbar spine. *Spine.* 1984;9:16–18.

4. Parkin IG, Harrison GR. The topographical anatomy of the lumbar epidural space. *J Anat.* 1985;141:211–217.

5. Wiltse LL, Fonseca AS, Amster J, et al. Relationship of the dura, Hofmann's ligaments, Batson's plexus, and a fibrovascular membrane lying on the posterior surface of the vertebral bodies and attaching to the deep layer of the posterior longitudinal ligament; an anatomical, radiologic, and clinical study. *Spine.* 1993;18:1030–1043.

6. Scapinelli R. Anatomical and radiologic studies on the lumbosacral meningovertebral ligaments of humans. *J Spinal Disord.* 1990;3:6–15.

7. Wadhwani S, Loughenbury P, Soames R. The anterior dural (Hofmann) ligaments. *Spine.* 2004;29:623–627.

8. Spencer DL, Irwin GS, Miller JAA. Anatomy and significance of fixation of the lumbosacral nerve roots in sciatica. *Spine.* 1983;8: 672–679.

9. Peretti F, Micalef JP, Bourgeon A, et al. Biomechanics of the lumbar spinal nerve roots and the first sacral root within the intervertebral foramina. *Surg Radiol Anat.* 1989;11:221–225.

10. Golub BS, Silverman B. Transforaminal ligaments of the lumbar spine. *J Bone Joint Surg.* 1969;51A:947–956.

11. Hasue M, Kikuchi S, Sakuyama Y, et al. Anatomic study of the interrelation between lumbosacral nerve roots and their surrounding tissues. *Spine.* 1983;8:50–58.

12. Cannon BW, Hunter SE, Picaza JA. Nerve root anomalies in lumbar disc surgery. *J Neurosurg.* 1962; 19:208–214.

13. Ethelberg S, Rishede J. Malformation of lumbar spinal nerve roots and sheaths in the causation of low backache and sciatica. *J Bone Joint Surg.* 1952;34B:442–446.

14. Keon-Cohen B. Abnormal arrangements of the lower lumbar and first sacral nerve roots within the spinal canal. *J Bone Joint Surg.* 1968;50B:261–266.

15. McElverry RT. Anomalies of the lumbar spinal cord and roots. *Clin Orthop.* 1956;8:61–64.

16. Neidre A, MacNab I. Anomalies of the lumbosacral nerve roots. *Spine.* 1983;8:294–299.

17. Postacchini F, Urso S, Ferro L. Lumbosacral nerve-root anomalies. *J Bone Joint Surg.* 1982;64A: 721–729.

18. Rask MR. Anomalous lumbosacral nerve roots associated with spondylolisthesis. *Surg Neurol.* 1977;8:139–140.

19. Hasner E, Schalintzek M, Snorrason E. Roentgenological examination of the function of the lumbar spine. *Acta Radiol.* 1952;37:141–149.

20. D'Avella D, Mingrino S. Microsurgical anatomy of lumbosacral spinal roots. *J Neurosurg.* 1979;51:819–823.

21. Pallie W. The intersegmental anastomoses of posterior spinal rootlets and their significance. *J Neurosurg.* 1959;16:187–196.

22. Bradley KC. The anatomy of backache. *Aust NZ J Surg.* 1974;44:227–232.

23. Bogduk N, Wilson AS, Tynan W. The human lumbar dorsal rami. *J Anat.* 1982;134:383–397.

24. Johnston HM. The cutaneous branches of the posterior primary divisions of the spinal nerves, and their distribution in the skin. *J Anat Physiol.* 1908;43:80–91.

25. Maigne JY, Lazareth JP, Surville HG, et al. The lateral cutaneous branches of the dorsal rami of the thoracolumbar junction. *Surg Radiol Anat.* 1989 11:289–293.

26. Pearson AA, Sauter RW, Buckley TF. Further observations on the cutaneous branches of the dorsal rami of the spinal nerves. *Am J Anat.* 1966;119:891–904.

27. Bogduk N. The innervation of the lumbar spine. *Spine.* 1983;8: 286–293.

28. Lazorthes G, Juskiewenski S. Etude comparative des branches postérieures des nerfs dorsaux et lombaires et leurs rapports avec les articulations interapophysaires vertébrales. *Bulletin de l'Association des Anatomistes, 49e Reunion.* 1964;1025–1033.

29. Lewin T, Moffet B, Viidik A. The morphology of the lumbar synovial intervertebral joints. *Acta Morphol Neerlando-Scand.* 1962;4:299–319.

30. Pedersen HE, Blunck CFJ, Gardner E. The anatomy of lumbosacral posterior rami and meningeal branches of spinal nerves (sinuvertebral nerves): with an experimental study of their function. *J Bone Joint Surg.* 1956;38A:377–391.

31. Macintosh JE, Valencia F, Bogduk N, et al. The morphology of the lumbar multifidus muscles. *Clin Biomech.* 1986;1:196–204.

32. Hirsch C, Ingelmark BE, Miller M. The anatomical basis for low back pain. *Acta Orthop Scand.* 1963;33: 1–17.

33. Jackson HC, Winkelmann RK, Bickel WH. Nerve endings in the human lumbar spinal column and related structures. *J Bone Joint Surg.* 1966;48A:1272–1281.

34. Ashton IK, Ashton BA, Gibson SJ, et al. Morphological basis for back pain: the demonstration of nerve fibres and neuropeptides in the lumbar facet joint capsule but not in ligamentum flavum. *J Orthop Res.* 1992;10:72–78.

35. Beaman DN, Graziano GP, Glover RA, et al. Substance P innervation of lumbar spine facet joints. *Spine.* 1993;18:1044–1049.

36. Giles LGF. Human lumbar zygapophyseal joint inferior recess synovial folds: a light microscope examination. *Anat Rec.* 1988;220: 117–124.

37. Giles LGF, Harvey AR. Immunohistochemical demonstration of nociceptors in the capsule and synovial folds of human zygapophyseal joints. *Br J Rheumatol.* 1987;26:362–364.

38. Giles LGF, Taylor JR. Innervation of lumbar zygapophyseal joint synovial folds. *Acta Orthop Scand.* 1987;58:43–46.

39. Gronblad M, Korkola O, Konttinen Y, et al. Silver impregnation and immunohistochemical study of nerves in lumbar facet joint plical tissue. *Spine.* 1991;16:34–38.

40. Jiang H, Russell G, Raso J, et al. The nature and distribution of the innervation of human supraspinal and interspinal ligaments. *Spine.* 1995;20:869–876.

41. Rhalmi S, Yahia L, Newman N, et al. Immunohistochemical study of nerves in lumbar spine ligaments. *Spine.* 1993;18:264–267.

42. Yahia LH, Newman NA. A light and electron microscopic study of spinal ligament innervation. *Z mikroskop anat Forsch Leipzig.* 1989;103: 664–674.

43. Yahia LH, Newman N, Rivard CH. Neurohistology of lumbar spine ligaments. *Acta Orthop Scand.* 1988;59:508–512.

44. Yahia LH, Rhalmi S, Isler M. Sensory innervation of human thoracolumbar fascia: an immunohistochemical study. *Acta Orthop Scand.* 1992;63:195–197.

45. Auteroche P. Innervation of the zygapophyseal joints of the lumbar spine. *Anat Clin.* 1983;5:17–28.

46. Paris SV. Anatomy as related to function and pain. *Orthop Clin North Am.* 1983;14:475–489.

47. Lynch MC, Taylor JF. Facet joint injection for low back pain. *J Bone Joint Surg.* 1986;68B:138–141.

48. Williams PL, ed. *Gray's Anatomy.* 38th ed. Edinburgh: Churchill Livingstone; 1995.

49. Wiltse LL, Guyer RD, Spencer CW, et al. Alar transverse process impingement of the L5 spinal nerve: the far-out syndrome. *Spine.* 1984;9:31–41.

50. Nitta H, Tajima T, Sugiyama H, et al. Study on dermatomes by means of selective lumbar spinal nerve block. *Spine.* 1993;18:1782–1786.

51. Bradley KC. Observations on the surgical anatomy of the thoracolumbar sympathetic system. *Aust NZ J Surg.* 1951;20:171–177.

52. Hovelacque A. *Anatomie des Nerfs Craniens et Rachidiens et du Système Grande Sympathique.* Paris: Doin; 1927.

53. Bogduk N, Tynan W, Wilson AS. The nerve supply to the human lumbar intervertebral discs. *J Anat.* 1981;132:39–56.

54. Kimmel DL. Innervation of spinal dura mater and dura mater of the posterior cranial fossa. *Neurology.* 1960;10:800–809.

55. Lazorthes G, Poulhes J, Espagno J. Etude sur les nerfs sinu-vertébraux lombaires. Le nerf de Roofe, existe-t-il? *Comptes Rendus de l'Association des Anatomistes.* 1947;34:317–320.

56. Wiberg G. Back pain in relation to the nerve supply of the intervertebral disc. *Acta Orthop Scand.* 1947;19:211–221.

57. Groen G, Baljet B, Drukker J. The nerves and nerve plexuses of the human vertebral column. *Am J Anat.* 1990;188:282–296.

58. Edgar MA, Nundy S. Innervation of the spinal dura mater. *J Neurol Neurosurg Psychiatry.* 1964;29:530–534.

59. Groen G, Baljet B, Drukker J. The innervation of the spinal dura mater: anatomy and clinical implications. *Acta Neurochir.* 1988;92:39–46.

60. Ikari C. A study of the mechanism of low-back pain. The neurohistological examination of the disease. *J Bone Joint Surg.* 1954;36A:195.

61. Jung A, Brunschwig A. Recherches histologiques des articulations des corps vertébraux. *Presse Med.* 1932;40:316–317.

62. Anderson J. Pathogenesis of back pain. In: Grahame R, Anderson JAD, eds. *Low Back Pain.* vol. 2. Westmount: Eden Press; 1980: Ch. 4, 23–32.

63. Lamb DW. The neurology of spinal pain. *Phys Ther.* 1979;59:971–973.

64. Wyke B. The neurology of low back pain. In: Jayson MIV, ed. *The Lumbar Spine and Back Pain.* 2nd ed. Tunbridge Wells: Pitman; 1980:Ch. 11, 265–339.

65. Ehrenhaft JC. Development of the vertebral column as related to certain congenital and pathological changes. *Surg Gynecol Obst.* 1943;76:282–292.

66. Roofe PG. Innervation of annulus fibrosus and posterior longitudinal ligament. *Arch Neurol Psychiatry.* 1940;44:100–103.

67. Malinsky J. The ontogenetic development of nerve terminations in the intervertebral discs of man. *Acta Anat.* 1959;38:96–113.

68. Rabischong P, Louis R, Vignaud J, et al. The intervertebral disc. *Anat Clin.* 1978;1:55–64.

69. Yoshizawa H, O'Brien JP, Thomas-Smith W, et al. The neuropathology of intervertebral discs removed for low-back pain. *J Path.* 1980;132:95–104.

70. Roberts S, Eisenstein SM, Menage J, et al. Mechanoreceptors in intervertebral discs: morphology, distribution, and neuropeptides. *Spine.* 1995;20:2645–2651.

71. Korkala O, Gronblad M, Liesi P, et al. Immunohistochemical demonstration of nociceptors in the ligamentous structures of the lumbar spine. *Spine.* 1985;10:156–157.

72. Ashton IK, Walsh DA, Polak JM, et al. Substance P in intervertebral discs: binding sites on vascular endothelium of the human annulus fibrosus. *Acta Orthop Scand.* 1994;65:635–639.

73. Taylor JR, Twomey LT. Innervation of lumbar intervertebral discs. *Med J Aust.* 1979;2:701–702.

74. Antonacci MD, Mody DR, Heggeness MH. Innervation of the human vertebral body: a histologic study. *J Spinal Dis.* 1998;11:526–531.

75. Brown MF, Hukkanen MVJ, McCarthy ID, et al. Sensory and sympathetic innervation of the vertebral endplate in patients with degenerative disc disease. *J Bone Joint Surg.* 1997;79B:147–153.

76. Kumar S, Davis PR. Lumbar vertebral innervation and intra-abdominal pressure. *J Anat.* 1973;114:47–53.

77. Coppes MH, Marani E, Thomeer RTWM, et al. Innervation of 'painful' lumbar discs. *Spine.* 1997;22:2342–2350.

78. Freemont AJ, Peacock TE, Goupille P, et al. Nerve ingrowth into diseased intervertebral disc in chronic back pain. *Lancet.* 1997;350:178–181.

79. Johnson WEB, Evans H, Menage J, et al. Immunohistochemical detection of Schwann cells in innervated and vascularised human intervertebral discs. *Spine.* 2001;26:2550–2557.

Blood supply of the lumbar spine

The blood supply of the lumbar spine is derived from the lumbar arteries, and its venous drainage is through the lumbar veins. The topographical anatomy of these vessels is described below, and more detailed descriptions of their distribution to the vertebral bodies, the spinal nerve roots and intervertebral discs are provided under separate headings.

THE LUMBAR ARTERIES

A pair of **lumbar arteries** arises from the back of the aorta in front of each of the upper four lumbar vertebrae.[1,2] Occasionally, the arteries at a particular level may arise as a single common trunk which rapidly divides into right and left branches. At the L5 level, the fifth lumbar arteries arise from the median sacral artery but otherwise they resemble the other lumbar arteries.

Each lumbar artery passes backwards around its related vertebral body (Fig. 11.1), lying in the concavity formed by the lateral surface of the vertebral body where it is covered by the tendinous arch of the psoas muscle. Upon reaching the level of the intervertebral foramen, the artery divides into several branches (Fig. 11.2).

Lateral branches pass through the psoas and quadratus lumborum muscles eventually to supply the abdominal wall. Others pass with the ventral ramus and dorsal ramus of the spinal nerve supplying the paravertebral muscles innervated by these nerves. A substantial posteriorly directed branch passes below the transverse process, running perpendicular to the lateral border of the pars interarticularis of the lamina, to enter the back muscles (see Fig. 11.2).[1,3] In addition to supplying the back muscles, the posterior branches of the lumbar arteries form anastomoses around the zygapophysial joints, which they supply, and plexuses that surround and supply the laminae and spinous processes.[1]

Opposite the intervertebral foramen, three medially directed branches arise from the lumbar artery (see Fig. 11.2). These are the **anterior spinal canal branch**, the **posterior spinal canal branch** and the **radicular branch**.[1,3] The radicular branches are described in detail later.

The anterior spinal canal branch at each level enters the intervertebral foramen and bifurcates into ascending and descending branches. The ascending branch crosses the intervertebral disc and circumvents the base of the pedicle above to anastomose with the descending branch from the next higher segmental level. In this way a series of arterial arcades is formed across the back of the lumbar vertebral bodies, i.e. along the floor of the vertebral canal (Fig. 11.3).

The posterior spinal canal branches also form arcades in a similar way but on the internal surface of the roof of the vertebral canal, i.e. along the laminae and ligamenta flava. Secondary branches of this arcade pass to the epidural fat and dural sac, and well-defined branches pass into the laminae and into the base of each spinous process. The branch to each lamina enters near its junction with the pedicle and bifurcates into branches that ascend and descend within the bone into the superior and inferior

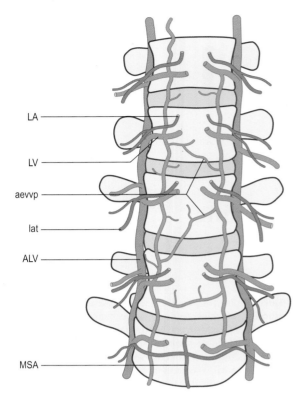

Figure 11.1 An anterior view of the lumbar spine showing its intrinsic blood vessels. aevvp, elements of the anterior external vertebral venous plexus; ALV, ascending lumbar vein; LA, lumbar artery; lat, lateral branches of the lumbar arteries; LV, lumbar vein; MSA, median sacral artery.

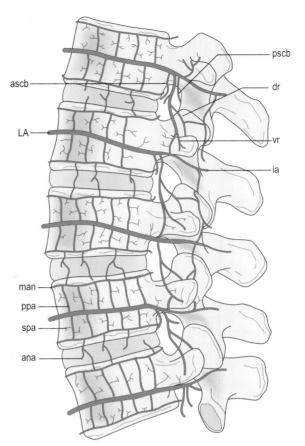

Figure 11.2 A lateral view of the lumbar spine showing the lumbar arteries and their branches. ana, anastomosis over the surface of the intervertebral disc; ascb, anterior spinal canal branch; dr, branches accompanying dorsal ramus of spinal nerve; ia, posterior branch related to the pars interarticularis of the lamina; LA, lumbar artery; man, metaphysial anastomosis; ppa, primary periosteal artery; pscb, posterior spinal canal branch; spa, secondary periosteal artery; vr, branches accompanying ventral ramus of spinal nerve.

articular processes. The branch to each spinous process penetrates the bone as far as its tip.

THE LUMBAR VEINS

Several veins surround and drain the lumbar spine. These are the lumbar veins, the ascending lumbar veins and several vertebral venous plexuses. The **lumbar veins** accompany the lumbar arteries in their course around the vertebral bodies, and drain into the inferior vena cava (see Fig. 11.1). Opposite the intervertebral foramina the lumbar veins on each side communicate with the **ascending lumbar vein**, a long channel that runs in front of the bases of the transverse processes (Fig. 11.4). Inferiorly on each side, the ascending lumbar vein communicates with the common iliac vein while, superiorly, the right ascending lumbar vein joins the azygos vein, and the left ascending lumbar vein joins the hemiazygous vein.

Over the anterolateral aspects of the lumbar spine, a variable series of vessels interconnect the lumbar veins to form the **anterior external vertebral venous plexus** (see Fig. 11.4). Within the vertebral canal, two other plexuses are formed. One covers the floor of the vertebral canal and is known as the **anterior internal vertebral venous plexus** (Fig. 11.5). The other lines the roof of the vertebral canal and is called the **posterior internal vertebral venous plexus**. Within the vertebral canal these plexuses extend superiorly to thoracic levels and inferiorly to sacral levels, and at each intervertebral foramen the two internal vertebral venous plexuses communicate with the ascending lumbar veins.

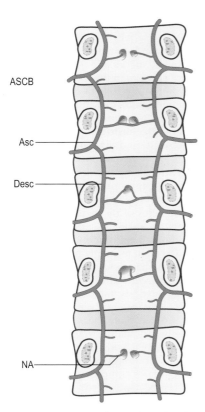

Figure 11.3 The anterior spinal canal branches (ASCB) of the lumbar arteries, their ascending (Asc) and descending (Desc) branches, and the nutrient arteries (NA) to the vertebral bodies.

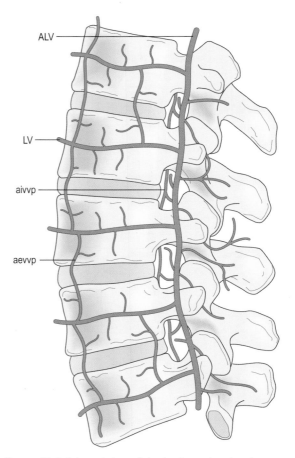

Figure 11.4 A lateral view of the lumbar spine showing the tributaries of the lumbar veins. aevvp, elements of the anterior external vertebral venous plexus; aivvp, elements of the anterior internal vertebral venous plexus; ALV, ascending lumbar vein; LV, lumbar vein.

Depending on local pressure changes, blood from the internal vertebral venous plexuses may drain to the ascending lumbar veins or may drain within the vertebral canal upwards to thoracic levels and higher, or downwards to sacral levels. Space-occupying lesions in the vertebral canal may therefore redirect flow in any of these directions, and raised intra-abdominal pressure may globally prevent drainage into the ascending lumbar veins and force blood to drain through the vertebral canal to thoracic levels.

Veins from the back muscles and from the external aspects of the posterior elements of the lumbar vertebrae drain towards the intervertebral foramina where they join the lumbar veins or the ascending lumbar veins. Internally, the posterior elements are drained by the posterior internal vertebral venous plexus. The venous drainage of the vertebral bodies and the spinal nerve roots is described below in conjunction with the arterial supply of these structures.

BLOOD SUPPLY OF THE VERTEBRAL BODIES

As each lumbar artery crosses its vertebral body, it gives off some 10–20 ascending and descending branches called the **primary periosteal arteries**.[2] Branches of these vessels supply the periosteum and outermost walls of the vertebral body (Figs 11.2, 11.6). Similar periosteal branches arise from the arcade of the anterior spinal canal arteries to supply the posterior wall of the vertebral body (see Figs 11.2, 11.6).

At the upper and lower ends of each vertebral body, terminal branches of the primary periosteal arteries form an anastomotic ring called the **metaphysial anastomosis**.[2] This ring runs parallel to the superior or inferior border of

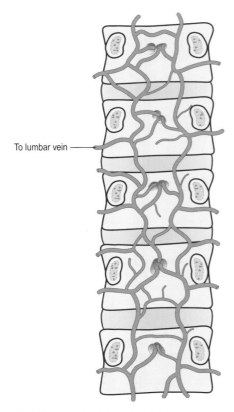

To lumbar vein —

Figure 11.5 The anterior internal vertebral venous plexus.

the vertebral body and surrounds its anterior and lateral aspects (see Figs 11.2, 11.6).

Branches from the metaphysial anastomosis and others from the lumbar arteries and the anterior spinal canal arteries penetrate and supply the internal parts of the vertebral body. The penetrating branches of the anterior spinal canal arteries pierce the middle of the posterior surface of the vertebral body and are known as the **nutrient arteries** of the vertebral body. They divide into ascending and descending branches that supply the central core of the vertebral body (see Fig. 11.6). Penetrating branches of the lumbar arteries, called the **equatorial arteries**, pierce the anterolateral surface of the vertebral body at its midpoint and divide into ascending and descending branches that join those of the nutrient arteries to supply the central core of the vertebra.

The peripheral parts of the upper and lower ends of the vertebral body are supplied by penetrating branches of the metaphysial anastomosis called **metaphysial arteries**. Several metaphysial arteries pierce the anterior and lateral surfaces of the vertebral body at its upper and lower ends, and each artery supplies a wedge-shaped region that points towards the central core of the vertebral body (see Fig. 11.6).

In the region of the vertebral endplate, terminal branches of the metaphysial arteries and the nutrient arteries form dense capillary plexuses in the subchondral bone deep to the endplate and in the base of the endplate cartilage.[1,4] Details of the morphology of this plexus are not known in humans, but in dogs, certain differences occur in different regions. Over the nucleus pulposus, the capillary terminations are sessile and discoid 'like the suckers on the tentacles of an octopus',[5] while over the anulus fibrosus the capillary terminals are less dense, smaller and simpler in appearance.[5] The functional significance of these differences, however, still remains obscure.

The principal veins of the vertebral body are the **basivertebral veins**. These are a series of long veins running horizontally through the middle of the vertebral body (Fig. 11.7). They drain primarily posteriorly, forming one or two large veins that pierce the posterior surface of the vertebral body to enter the anterior internal vertebral venous plexus. Anteriorly, the basivertebral veins drain to the anterior external vertebral venous plexus.

Within the vertebral body, the basivertebral veins receive vertically running tributaries from the upper and lower halves of the vertebral body. In turn these veins receive oblique tributaries from the more peripheral parts of the vertebral body. A large complement of vertical veins runs through the central core of the vertebral body and is involved in the drainage of the endplate regions.

In the region immediately adjacent to each vertebral endplate, the capillaries of the subchondral bone drain into a system of small veins that lies parallel to the disc–bone interface (see Fig. 11.7); this is the **subchondral postcapillary venous network**.[1,4] Short vertical veins drain this network into a larger venous system that again lies parallel to the vertebral endplate (see Fig. 11.7); this is the **horizontal subarticular collecting vein system**.[1,4] The veins in this system are arranged in a radial pattern that converges centrally opposite the nucleus pulposus. Here the veins turn towards the centre of the vertebral body and form the vertical veins that drain through the central core of the body to the basivertebral veins. Peripheral elements of the horizontal subarticular collecting vein system drain to the anterior external and anterior internal vertebral venous plexuses.

BLOOD SUPPLY OF THE SPINAL NERVE ROOTS

The lumbar spinal nerve roots receive their blood supply from two sources. Proximally, they are fed by vessels from the conus medullaris of the spinal cord. Distally, in the intervertebral foramina, they receive the radicular branches of the lumbar arteries.[6–8]

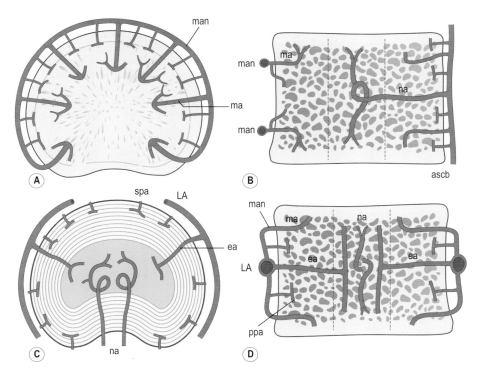

Figure 11.6 The intraosseous arteries of the lumbar vertebral bodies. (Based on Ratcliffe 1980.[2]) (A) Transverse section of upper or lower end of vertebral body showing the metaphysial anastomosis (man) and the sectors supplied by the metaphysial arteries (ma). (B) Midline, sagittal section showing the central distribution of the nutrient artery (na), and the peripheral distribution of the metaphysial arteries (ma) and the penetrating branches of the anterior spinal canal branches (ascb). (C) Transverse section through the middle of the vertebral body showing the central distribution of the nutrient arteries (na) augmented by equatorial branches (ea) of the lumbar artery (LA), and the superficial distribution of the secondary periosteal arteries (spa). (D) Frontal section through the middle of the vertebral body showing the central distribution of the nutrient arteries (na) and the equatorial arteries (ea), and the peripheral distribution of the metaphysial anastomosis (man), metaphysial arteries (ma) and the primary periosteal arteries (ppa) that arise from the lumbar artery (LA).

At their attachment to the conus medullaris, virtually each of the ventral and dorsal rootlets is supplied by a fine branch derived from the extra-medullary longitudinal vessels of the conus (Fig. 11.8) but the distribution of these small branches is limited to a few centimetres along the rootlets.[7] The rest of the proximal ends of the dorsal and ventral roots are supplied by the proximal, ventral and dorsal radicular arteries (see Fig. 11.8).

The **dorsal proximal radicular arteries** arise from the dorsolateral longitudinal vessels of the conus (derived from the posterior spinal arteries), and the **ventral proximal radicular arteries** arise from the 'accessory antero-lateral longitudinal channels' (derived from the anterior spinal artery).[7] Each proximal radicular artery travels with its root but is embedded in its own pial sheath, until several millimetres from the surface of the spinal cord, it penetrates the root.[7] Upon entering the root, the radicular artery follows one of the main nerve bundles along its entire length and gives off collateral branches that enter

and follow other nerve fascicles. Within a root there may be one to three substantial vessels that could be named as the proximal radicular artery.

At each intervertebral foramen, the **radicular branch** of the lumbar artery enters the spinal nerve and then divides into branches that enter the ventral and dorsal roots (see Fig. 11.8). These vessels may be referred to as the **distal radicular arteries**, to distinguish them from the proximal radicular arteries arising from the conus medullaris. Each distal radicular artery passes proximally along its root, giving off collateral branches, until it meets and anastomoses with its respective proximal radicular artery. En route, the dorsal distal radicular artery forms a plexus around the dorsal root ganglion.[8]

Within each root, collateral branches of the proximal and distal radicular arteries communicate with one another through transverse branches (Fig. 11.9), and a particular feature of these branches in the adult is that they are coiled.[7] Similarly, their parent vessels are coiled

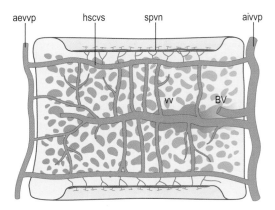

Figure 11.7 The intraosseous veins of the lumbar vertebral bodies. (Based on Crock et al. 1973.[4]) aevvp, anterior external vertebral venous plexus; aivvp, anterior internal vertebral venous plexus; BV, the basivertebral veins; hscvs, horizontal subchondral collecting vein system; spvn, subchondral postcapillary venous network; vv, vertical veins within the vertebral body.

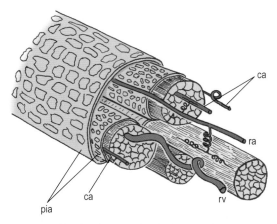

Figure 11.9 The distribution of radicular vessels in a nerve root. (Based on Parke and Watanabe 1985.[7]) The radicular artery (ra) runs with the nerve bundles in the nerve root, accompanied by several collateral arteries (ca) in adjacent nerve bundles. The arteries anastomose with one another through coiled junctions. The radicular vein (rv) has a sinuous course separate to that of the arteries. pia, pia mater.

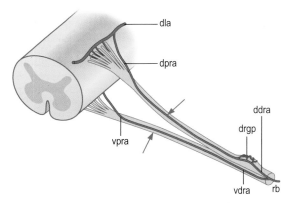

Figure 11.8 The arterial supply of a typical lumbar nerve root. The dorsal nerve rootlets are supplied by tiny branches of the dorsolateral artery (dla) of the spinal cord. The nerve roots are supplied by the dorsal and ventral proximal radicular arteries (dpra, vpra) and the dorsal and ventral distal radicular arteries (vdra, ddra). The proximal and distal arteries anastomose at the junction of the middle and medial thirds of the nerve root (arrows). The dorsal root ganglion is supplied by a plexus of small arteries (drgp). rb, radicular branch.

proximal and distal to the origin of each of these transverse communicating branches (see Fig. 11.9). These coils appear to be designed to accommodate the stretching of the nerve root that occurs during movements of the lumbar spine.[8] They are less developed in neonates because of the relatively shorter length of the lumbar spinal nerve roots, and hence there is a lesser propensity for them to stretch.

The point of anastomosis between the proximal and the distal radicular arteries lies in the proximal half of each root.[8] Consequently, the proximal radicular artery supplies the proximal one-third or so of the root, while the distal two-thirds are supplied by the distal radicular artery. Arterial supply, however, is neither the only nor the principal source of nutrition for the roots. Only some 35% of the glucose absorbed by a root comes from the radicular arteries. The rest is absorbed directly from the surrounding CSF.[7]

The veins of the nerve roots may be divided into proximal and distal radicular systems but are fewer in number than the corresponding arteries and run courses separate to those of the arteries.[7] The veins tend to lie deep in the nerve bundle and assume a spiralling course (see Fig. 11.9). The proximal veins drain towards the spinal cord, while the distal veins drain towards the intervertebral foramina where they join the tributaries of the lumbar veins and the ascending lumbar veins.

NUTRITION OF THE INTERVERTEBRAL DISC

The intervertebral disc is not an inert structure. The cartilage cells in the nucleus pulposus and the fibroblasts in the anulus fibrosus are biologically active, albeit at a low-grade level, but this activity is essential for the constant synthesis and replacement of proteoglycans and collagen.[9-12] To sustain this activity these cells require nutrition.[13] However, the intervertebral discs receive no major arterial branches.

The only vessels that actually enter the discs are small branches from the metaphysial arteries which anastomose over the outer surface of the anulus fibrosus (see Fig. 11.2) but these branches are restricted to the very outermost fibres of the anulus.[9] Consequently, for their nutrition, intervertebral discs are dependent on diffusion, and this diffusion takes place from the two closest available systems of vessels: those in the outer anulus, and the capillary plexuses beneath the vertebral endplates.

To reach the nucleus pulposus, nutrients like oxygen, sugar and other molecules must diffuse across the matrix of the vertebral endplate or through the anulus fibrosus. Subsequently, nutrients to the nucleus must permeate the proteoglycan matrix of the nucleus. The rate of diffusion of nutrients through these media is dependent on three principal factors: the concentration gradient of any particular substance; the resistance to diffusion offered by the endplate or the anulus fibrous; and the resistance to diffusion offered by the proteoglycans of the nucleus.[13]

In this respect, the permeabilities of the anulus fibrosus and the vertebral endplates differ. Virtually the entire anulus fibrosus is quite permeable to most substances but only the central portions of the vertebral endplates are permeable.[11-13] However, because the surface area of the endplates is greater than that of the anulus, the relative contributions to disc nutrition from the anulus and the endplates is approximately the same. This conclusion, however, holds only for uncharged molecules which are unaffected by other processes.[11-13] The diffusion of charged molecules is affected by the chemical properties of the nucleus pulposus.

The resistance to diffusion of charged molecules offered by the nucleus pulposus is a property of the high concentration of the negatively charged carboxyl and sulphate radicals in its mucopolysaccharides.[11,13] Uncharged molecules like glucose or oxygen permeate readily through the proteoglycan matrix of the nucleus, but negatively charged substances, like sulphate ions and chloride ions, meet great resistance once they cross the endplates and reach the matrix. On the other hand, positively charged ions like sodium and calcium pass readily from the endplates into the matrix.

Because the concentration of mucopolysaccharides in the anulus fibrosus is less than that in the nucleus pulposus, the anulus offers less resistance to the diffusion of negatively charged molecules, and most negatively charged solutes that reach the nucleus do so via the anulus.[13]

Although it is generally regarded that diffusion is the principal mechanism by which nutrients reach the inner parts of the intervertebral disc,[12,14] there has been some work to suggest that compression of the intervertebral disc tends to squeeze water out of it, and when the compression is released, the water returns. It is maintained by some authorities that this flux of water is capable of carrying nutrients with it.[15] In particular, it has been shown in animal experiments that spinal movements, over a long time, exert a positive nutritional effect on the disc.[16] It is presumable that a similar phenomenon occurs in humans but the extent to which exercise might benefit human discs, or whether it forestalls disc degeneration, still remains to be shown.

REFERENCES

1. Crock HV, Yoshizawa H. The blood supply of the lumbar vertebral column. *Clin Orthop.* 1976;115: 6–21.

2. Ratcliffe JF. The arterial anatomy of the adult human vertebral body: a microarteriographic study. *J Anat.* 1980;131:57–79.

3. Dommisse GF. *The Arteries and Veins of the Human Spinal Cord from Birth.* Edinburgh: Churchill Livingstone; 1975.

4. Crock HV, Yoshizawa H, Kame S. Observations on the venous drainage of the human vertebral body. *J Bone Joint Surg.* 1973; 55B:528–533.

5. Crock HV, Goldwasser M. Anatomic studies of the circulation in the region of the vertebral end-plate in adult greyhound dogs. *Spine.* 1984;9:702–706.

6. Dommisse GF, Grobler L. Arteries and veins of the lumbar nerve roots and cauda equina. *Clin Orthop.* 1976;115: 22–29.

7. Parke WW, Watanabe R. The intrinsic vasculature of the lumbosacral spinal nerve roots. *Spine.* 1985;10:508–515.

8. Parke WW, Gammell K, Rothman RH. Arterial vascularisation of the cauda equina. *J Bone Joint Surg.* 1981;63A:53–62.

9. Maroudas A, Nachemson A, Stockwell R, et al. Some factors involved in the nutrition of the intervertebral disc. *J Anat.* 1975;120:113–130.

10. Souter WA, Taylor TKF. Sulphated acid mucopolysaccharide metabolism in the rabbit intervertebral disc. *J Bone Joint Surg.* 1970;52B:371–384.

11. Urban J, Maroudas A. The chemistry of the intervertebral disc in relation to its physiological function. *Clin Rheum Dis.* 1980;6:51–76.

12. Urban JPG, Holm S, Maroudas A. Diffusion of small solutes into the intervertebral disc. *Biorheology.* 1978;15:203–223.

13. Maroudas A. Nutrition and metabolism of the intervertebral disc. In: Ghosh P, ed. *The Biology of*

the Intervertebral Disc. vol. II. Boca Raton: CRC Press; 1988:Ch. 9, 1–37.

14. Holm S, Maroudas A, Urban JPG, et al. Nutrition of the intervertebral disc: solute transport and metabolism. *Connect Tissue Res.* 1981;8:101–119.

15. Kraemer J, Kolditz D, Gowin R. Water and electrolyte content of human intervertebral discs under variable load. *Spine.* 1985;10:69–71.

16. Holm S, Nachemson A. Variations in the nutrition of the canine intervertebral disc induced by motion. *Spine.* 1983;8:866–874.

Chapter | 12 |

Embryology and development

After 15 days of development, the human embryo is in the form of a flat, ovoid disc which consists of two layers of cells: the **ectoderm** dorsally and the **endoderm** ventrally (Fig. 12.1). The ectoderm is that layer which principally will give rise to the skin and spinal cord. The endoderm forms the alimentary tract.[1] At the caudal end of the embryo, the cells of the ectoderm become rounded and heap up, forming an elevation known as the **primitive streak**.[1] Cells from the primitive streak migrate laterally and forwards, insinuating between the ectoderm and endoderm to form a third layer in the embryo called the **mesoderm** (Figs 12.1, 12.2). Just in front of the primitive streak, another thickening develops, known as **Hensen's node**. From this node, a cord of cells, known as the

notochord, migrates forwards between the ectoderm and endoderm (see Fig. 12.2). By about 28 days, the notochord fully demarcates the midline of the embryo[1] and induces the formation of the vertebral column around it. Dorsal to the notochord, the ectoderm forms the **neural tube**, which differentiates into the brain and spinal cord.

On each side of the notochord, the mesoderm of the embryo is thickened to form a longitudinal mass known as the **paraxial mesoderm**. By the 21st day of development, the paraxial mesoderm starts to be marked by transverse clefts across its dorsal surface. These clefts separate the paraxial mesoderm into segments called **somites** (Fig. 12.3). The first somites appear in the region of the head, and others appear successively caudally. By about the 30th day of embryonic development, a total of 42–44 somites are formed.[1]

The clefts demarcating the somites are actually indentations, so the segmentation they create is apparent only along the dorsal aspect of the paraxial mesoderm. Deeply, beneath the surface of the embryo, the paraxial mesoderm remains a single, longitudinally continuous mass.[2] Using the transverse clefts as a guide, however, the further development of each somite can be traced.

The 42–44 somites of the human embryo can be named as 4 occipital, 8 cervical, 12 thoracic, 5 lumbar, 5 sacral and 8–10 coccygeal. The first occipital and the last 7–8 coccygeal somites regress and give rise to no permanent structures.[1] The remaining three occipital somites are involved in the formation of the occipital region of the skull and the tongue. The other somites form the vertebral column and the trunk.

The cells in the somites are originally epithelial in nature but they gradually change into loosely arranged tissue called **mesenchyme** (Fig. 12.4). In transverse section, each somite is roughly triangular in outline,

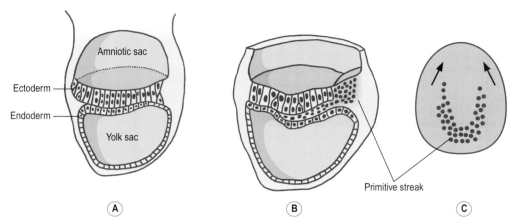

Figure 12.1 The development of the mesodermal layer of early human embryos. (A) A sagittal section of an early embryo consisting of only ectoderm and endoderm. The amniotic sac lies dorsal to the embryonic plate and the yolk sac is suspended from the endodermal layer. (B) Ectodermal cells at the caudal end of a 15-day embryo have heaped up to form the primitive streak, which gives rise to the mesodermal cells. (C) Top view of the embryo in (B) showing the forward migration of the mesodermal cells, either side of the midline, underneath the ectodermal layer.

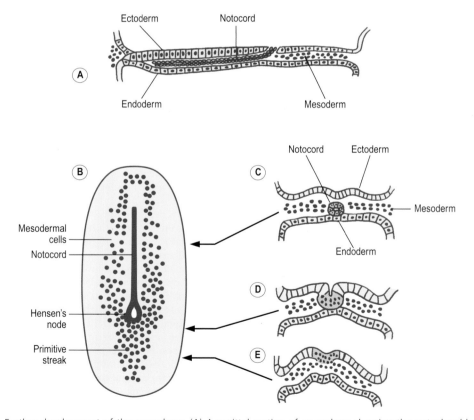

Figure 12.2 Further development of the mesoderm. (A) A sagittal section of an embryo showing the notochord having extended forwards between the ectoderm and endoderm, and behind it the mesoderm of the primitive streak. (B) A top view of the same embryo showing the notochord and mesoderm viewed through the ectoderm over the top of the embryo. (C–E) Transverse sections of the embryo through the notochord, Hensen's node and the primitive streak.

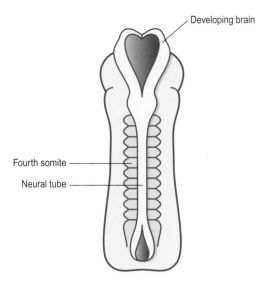

Figure 12.3 A dorsal view of an embryo with 10 somites.

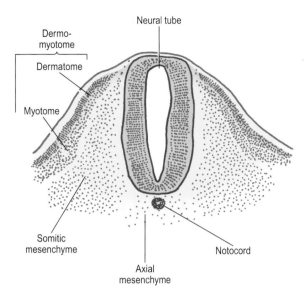

Figure 12.5 Transverse section of an early somite, showing the relationship of the mesenchyme to the neural tube and notochord, and its differentiation into the somitic mesenchyme and the dermomyotome.

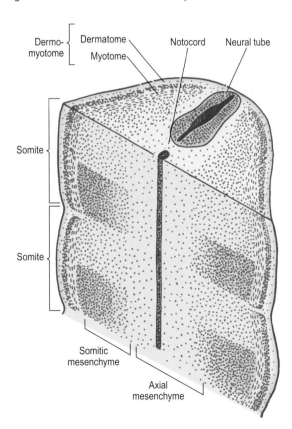

Figure 12.4 Combined coronal and transverse sections of the somites of an embryo. The somitic mesenchyme has differentiated into dense caudal halves and lighter cranial halves.

presenting ventral and dorsolateral borders, and a medial border facing the neural tube (Fig. 12.5).

Within the somite, two clusters of cells develop. Those cells in the ventral and medial regions of the somite rapidly multiply and form a mass, which, in the past, has been referred to as the **sclerotome**, but for reasons outlined elsewhere[2] the term **somitic mesenchyme** is used here. These cells are exclusively involved in the formation of the vertebral column. The remaining cells, along the dorsolateral border of the somite, give rise to the musculature and skin of the trunk and are collectively referred to as the **dermomyotome**.

The further development of the somitic mesenchyme and the dermomyotome is similar for every somite. Therefore, the development of the lumbar region, as described below, is in principle the same as that seen in the cervical and thoracic regions, the principal differences lying only in the particular segments of the vertebral column that are eventually formed.

THE FATE OF THE SOMITIC MESENCHYME

The somitic mesenchyme undergoes several changes that eventually result in the formation of a primitive model of the vertebral column, and this phase of development of the vertebral column is known as the **mesenchymal phase**.

143

The notochord lies between the aorta ventrally, and the neural tube dorsally. The neural tube is flanked by the somitic mesenchyme, but the somitic mesenchyme initially does not extend as far medially as the notochord. The notochord is surrounded separately by a continuous column of very loose-meshed mesenchyme called the **axial mesenchyme** (see Fig. 12.5).[2] The density of the axial mesenchyme gradually increases as these cells multiply and surround the notochord (Figs 12.6, 12.7). Meanwhile, a separate series of events occurs in the somitic mesenchyme.

In the caudal half of each somite, the density of nuclei increases, giving it a darker staining appearance (see Figs 12.4 and 12.7B). The cranial half of the somite remains less dense and is invaded by the developing spinal nerve (see Figs 12.6A and 12.7C). The nerve grows laterally to invade the dermomyotome, and as the nerve increases in length and thickness, the cells of the cranial half of the somite come to be arranged in concentric layers around the nerve.[2] In time, the developing nerve occupies most of the entire cranial half of the somite, which itself gives rise to little but perineural tissue. It is the denser, caudal half of each somite that participates in the formation of the vertebral column.

In the caudal half of each somite, two processes develop: a **dorsal process** and a **ventrolateral process**.[2] The dorsal process spreads dorsally to surround the neural tube and will give rise to the neural arch (see Fig. 12.6B). Hence, it is also referred to as the **arcual process**. The ventrolateral process extends laterally and gives rise to the costal element of the future vertebrae. Hence, it is also referred to as the **costal process** (see Fig. 12.6B). In the lumbar region, the costal elements of each vertebra are represented in the form of the transverse processes.

As the axial mesenchyme increases in density, its cells assume a concentric orientation around the notochord. These cells will form the greater part of the future vertebral body, and the portion of the body that they form is referred to as the **centrum** (see Fig. 12.7). Opposite the lower half of the cranial portion of the adjacent somite, a zone of higher density develops in the axial mesenchyme (see Fig. 12.7). This zone forms the predecessor to the future intervertebral disc.[2]

While these events take place in the axial mesenchyme, a third process develops in the somitic mesenchyme. This process, known as the ventral or **chordal process**, extends towards the notochord to blend with the axial mesenchyme just caudal to the zone of the future intervertebral disc.[2] In this way, the chordal process connects the somitic mesenchyme with the centrum of the vertebral body, and the vertebral body is eventually formed by the centrum and the terminal portions of the chordal processes from each side.

The dorsal processes of the somitic mesenchyme continue to extend around the sides of the neural tube, and

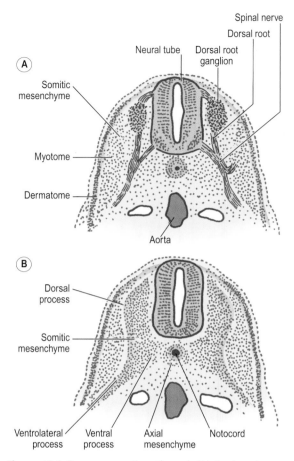

Figure 12.6 Transverse sections through (A) the less dense cranial half of a somite, and (B) the denser caudal half. In (A) the somitic mesenchyme surrounds the developing spinal nerve. In (B), the axial mesenchyme surrounds the notochord, and the somitic mesenchyme has formed dorsal, ventrolateral and ventral processes. *(Based on Verbout 1985.[2])*

just lateral to the developing dorsal root ganglion, the dorsal processes of adjacent somites blend with one another at the sites of the future zygapophysial joints.[2] Elsewhere, the neural arches of adjacent segments are bridged by less dense condensations of mesenchyme that will give rise to the ligaments of the neural arch.

By this stage of development, the shape of the future vertebra is outlined by mesenchymal tissue. Condensations of the axial mesenchyme have surrounded the notochord and have moulded the vertebral body. The future intervertebral disc has condensed in the axial mesenchyme opposite the lower half of the cranial portion of the somitic mesenchyme. The cranial half of each somite has condensed around the developing spinal nerve and will

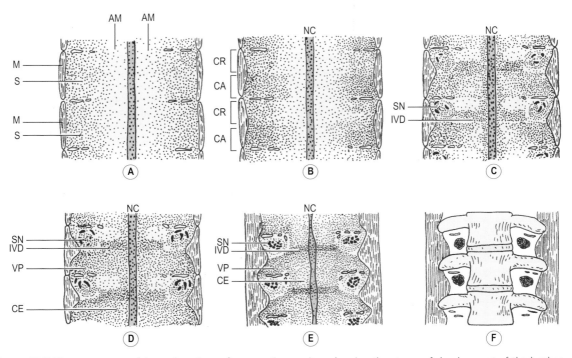

Figure 12.7 The appearance of coronal sections of consecutive somites, showing the stages of development of the lumbar vertebrae. (A) Early mesenchymal stage: AM, axial mesenchyme; M, myotome; NC, notochord; S, somitic mesenchyme. (B) The somites have differentiated into dense caudal (CA) and less dense cranial (CR) halves. (C) The cranial somitic mesenchyme has condensed around the developing spinal nerve (SN), and the future intervertebral disc (IVD) is marked as a zone of increased density in the axial mesenchyme opposite the lower end of the cranial half of the somite. (D) The ventrolateral process of the somitic mesenchyme (VP) extends between consecutive myotomes, and the ventral process blends with the axial mesenchyme to form the centrum (CE). (E) Mesenchymal cells have transformed into a cartilaginous model of the future vertebra, and the notochord is being squeezed out of the centrum. (F) The relative location of the definitive osseous vertebrae. *(Based on Verbout 1985.[2])*

form only perineural tissue. The condensed caudal half of the somitic mesenchyme has formed three processes. A ventral process blends with the axial mesenchyme below the intervertebral disc, while a dorsal process embraces the side of the neural tube. Together, the ventral and dorsal processes outline the future neural arch. The ventrolateral process radiates from the neural arch on each side to outline the future transverse process. At this stage of development, the left and right dorsal processes do not yet meet behind the neural tube and are united only by a membrane.[3,4] The neural arch is completed dorsally at a later stage of development.

The succeeding phases of development of the vertebrae involve the replacement of the mesenchymal model, first by cartilage, then by bone, and these phases are described later, after the description of the development of the dermomyotome.

THE FATE OF THE DERMOMYOTOME

Initially, two types of cells are evident in the dermomyotome. Epithelial cells cover the dorsolateral surface of the somite and can be recognised as the **dermatome**. Deep to these lie mesenchymal cells, collectively known as the **myotome**. Gradually, the cells of the dermatome lose their epithelial character and become incorporated into the myotomal mass, but they remain attached to the overlying ectoderm and give rise to the dermis and subcutaneous tissues.[1] The cells of the myotome give rise to muscular tissue.

The myotomal mass maintains its ventrolateral location in relation to the somitic mesenchyme. Opposite the condensed caudal half of the somite it is gradually displaced laterally by the developing ventrolateral process. Opposite

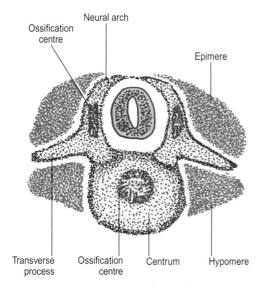

Figure 12.8 A transverse section of a cartilaginous lumbar vertebra showing the ossification centres in the centrum and neural arches, and the disposition of the myotomes into epimeres and hypomeres.

CHONDRIFICATION

As the mesenchymal models of the vertebrae are being completed, some of the mesenchymal cells change character and become cartilaginous. This occurs at about the 6th week of gestation[4] and heralds the onset of the **cartilaginous** phase of vertebral development.

A pair of **chondrification centres** appear in the centrum of each vertebra. They rapidly fuse into one centre, which expands to chondrify the entire centrum.[1] Chondrification centres also appear in each half of the neural arch. These expand dorsally through the dorsal process of the somitic mesenchyme on each side, and meet one another behind the neural tube to complete the neural arch. From the site of union, a cartilaginous spinous process develops dorsally. The neural arch centres also extend laterally to chondrify the transverse process, and ventrally along the ventral process of the somitic mesenchyme to blend with the chondrifying centrum.

As a consequence of these events, a cartilaginous model of the future vertebra is laid down, but even as chondrification of the vertebral column is being completed, these cartilaginous models start to be replaced by definitive, osseous vertebrae (see Fig. 12.8).

OSSIFICATION

Ossification is the third phase of development of the vertebral column. It commences during the 9th–10th weeks of intrauterine life,[6] but is not completed until adolescent life. The first process of ossification is called **primary ossification** and occurs at sites where blood vessels invade the cartilaginous models of the future vertebrae.

The cartilaginous neural arches are invaded from behind to form a **primary ossification centre** in each half of the neural arch (see Fig. 12.8). The cartilaginous vertebral body is invaded by blood vessels through its anterior and posterior surfaces. Some authorities maintain that these two sets of blood vessels give rise, respectively, to separate ventral and dorsal ossification centres, which rapidly fuse to form a single ossification centre in the middle of the future vertebral body,[7] but others maintain that this phenomenon is only a variation that occurs in about 5% of cases.[8,9] Another variant is to have two centres lying lateral to one another[8] but the most common pattern is to have one single centre.[8]

The onset of ossification differs according to vertebral level and the part to be ossified. Primary ossification centres in the neural arches first appear at cervicothoracic levels, followed by upper cervical and then thoracolumbar levels. Centres in the neural arches then appear progressively in cranial and caudal directions from these levels.[10] Primary centres in the vertebral bodies first appear at lower

the looser cranial half of the somite, it bulges towards the somite but is also indented by the developing spinal nerve (see Fig. 12.7).[2]

As the spinal nerve divides into a ventral and dorsal ramus at about the 40th day of development,[4] the myotome splits into two portions.[1] The division occurs along a plane depicted by the developing transverse processes, and the two portions are separated by a septum that forms the future intertransverse ligaments (Fig. 12.8). The dorsal portion of the myotome is known as the **epimere**, or **epaxial** portion, and is innervated by the dorsal ramus of the spinal nerve. The ventral portion is known as the **hypomere**, or **hypaxial** portion, and is innervated by the ventral ramus of the spinal nerve.

In the lumbar region, the hypomere will develop into those muscles ventral to the intertransverse ligaments. The lumbar myotomes largely give rise to the intertransversarii laterales, and the quadratus lumborum and psoas muscles. Most of the muscles of the abdominal wall develop from the hypomeres of the lower thoracic somites but the L1 hypomere contributes to the lower portions of these muscles.

The epimeres throughout the vertebral column divide further into medial and lateral divisions,[1,5] which are supplied by the medial and lateral branches of the dorsal rami, respectively. In the lumbar region, the medial division forms the multifidus muscle, while the lateral division forms the iliocostalis and longissimus muscles.

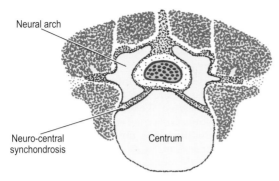

Figure 12.9 A neonatal lumbar vertebra showing the extent of ossification of the centrum and the neural arches.

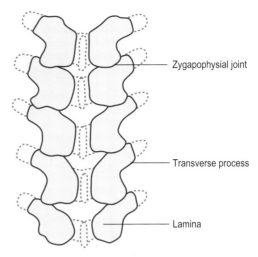

Figure 12.10 A dorsal view of a neonatal lumbar spine showing the extent of ossification of the neural arches.

thoracic and upper lumbar levels, and then progressively appear at levels above and below these.[10] In this way, ossification centres are established in the bodies and neural arches of the lumbar vertebrae by the 12th–14th week of gestation.

In the centrum of the vertebral body, the primary ossification centre expands radially and towards the intervertebral discs above and below. It reaches the anterior aspect of the centrum by about 22 weeks of antenatal life, and the posterior aspect by about 25 weeks,[11] but ossification does not reach the superior and inferior surfaces of the vertebral body, which remain cartilaginous and form the growth plates of the vertebral body. In the neural arches, ossification extends in all directions from the primary centre: ventrally towards the vertebral body; laterally into the transverse process; and dorsally around the neural tube.

At birth, the lumbar vertebrae are still not completely ossified (Figs 12.9, 12.10). The bulk of the centrum is ossified, and in lateral radiographs has the appearance of an ovoid block of bone with convex upper and lower surfaces.[12–14] Large vascular channels penetrate the anterior and posterior aspects of the centrum,[7] and on radiographs of neonatal spines these appear as areas of translucency.[14] The upper and lower surfaces of the vertebral body are still covered by the thick cartilage plates, and the combined height of these plates and the intervertebral disc is approximately the same as the height of the ossified lumbar vertebral bodies.[12–14] The pedicles and the proximal parts of the laminae and transverse processes are ossified but the spinous processes and the distal parts of the transverse processes are still cartilaginous. The articular processes are ossified for the most part but their distal ends remain cartilaginous.

After birth, ossification of the vertebrae continues as the vertebrae increase in size with growth. Ossification of the vertebral body extends radially and in the direction of the endplates. Further details of vertebral body growth are described separately in a later section.

Ossification continues to spread slowly through the neural arch and its processes. The laminae are fully ossified and unite dorsal to the spinal cord during the first postnatal year.[6,15] At this same time the bulk of the spinous process is ossified[14] but its dorsal edge remains cartilaginous until puberty, as do the tips of the transverse processes and the ends of the articular processes.

At puberty, **secondary ossification centres** appear in the cartilaginous tips of the spinous processes, the tips of the transverse processes and in the cartilaginous mamillary processes.[6,16] Secondary ossification centres may appear in the tips of the inferior articular processes but this phenomenon does not occur regularly; it is described further in the section on the zygapophysial joints.

The secondary ossification centres of each lumbar vertebra are separated from the rest of the vertebra by a narrow interval of cartilage and remain separated during the final periods of spinal growth. Gradually, this intervening cartilage is replaced by bone, and the secondary centres fuse with the rest of the vertebra by about the 25th year of life.[6]

THE FATE OF THE NOTOCHORD

During the mesenchymal phase of development of the vertebral column, the notochord persists as a central axis through the middle of the future vertebral bodies and intervertebral discs. The deepest mesenchymal cells gradually assume a concentric arrangement around the notochord, forming a **perichordal sheath**.

As chondrification of the vertebral bodies proceeds, the cells of the notochord appear to be squeezed out of the vertebral body into the intervertebral discs (see Fig. 12.7)[7,17,18] and the notochord is progressively narrowed until it forms little more than a streak of tissue on the vertebral body, known as the **mucoid streak**. Expansion of the ossification centre of the vertebral centrum destroys the mucoid streak, and in general, any vestige of the notochord in the vertebral body is obliterated.[7]

In about 7% of cases, ossification does not completely obliterate the region of the notochord, and a vertical canal may persist in the vertebral body.[19] These canals are most frequently filled with fibrocartilage or fibrous tissue, but rarely, pockets of notochordal cells may persist in parts of the canal.[19]

In the developing intervertebral disc, the fate of the notochord is entirely different, for instead of being obliterated, it participates in the formation of the nucleus pulposus.

DEVELOPMENT OF THE INTERVERTEBRAL DISC

In the primitive mesenchymal intervertebral disc, the cells gradually come to be arranged in concentric layers, lying in parallel rows between one vertebra and the next.[20] This arrangement foreshadows the future concentric structure of the lamellae of the anulus fibrosus (Fig. 12.11A).

Towards the centre of the disc, the cells are irregularly arranged around the notochord, and gradually the cells closer to the notochord take on the appearance of embryonic cartilage (Fig. 12.11B).[20] At about 55 days of development, the notochord expands in the centre of the disc, its cells being separated into strands and groups, called the **chorda reticulum**, embedded in an amorphous mucoid substance (Fig. 12.11B). The expanded notochord is surrounded by embryonic cartilage, and around the perimeter

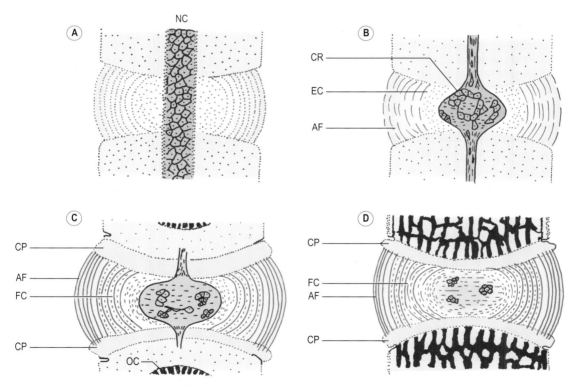

Figure 12.11 Stages in the development of the intervertebral disc. (Based on Peacock 1951.[20]) (A) A mesenchymal disc in which the central cells surround the notochord (NC), and the peripheral cells are arranged in a radial pattern indicative of the future lamellae of the anulus fibrosus. (B) The notochord has expanded and its cells form the chorda reticulum (CR). Mesenchymal cells surrounding the notochord have transformed into embryonic cartilage (EC), and the peripheral cells have formed the orientated collagen fibres of the anulus fibrosus (AF). (C) The disc consists of an expanded notochord with fewer cells, surrounded by fibrocartilage (FC) and the collagenous anulus fibrosus which attaches to the cartilaginous plates of the vertebrae (CP). Ossification centres (OC) are present in the centra. (D) A neonatal disc.

of the disc, collagen fibres appear to form the anulus fibrosus.

Collagen fibres are deposited in the anulus fibrosus as early as the 10th week of gestation,[21] and their orientation is the same as that in the adult.[22] Their ends are inserted into the cartilage plates that cover the superior and inferior aspects of the vertebral bodies. Fibres in the anulus fibrosus are quite evident in the 4th month and are well developed by 5–6 months.[7] Accompanying the development of the anulus fibrosus, the anterior and posterior longitudinal ligaments condense out of the perivertebral mesenchyme during the 7th–9th weeks.[7]

In the centre of the intervertebral disc, the notochord continues to expand radially, and the perichordal cartilage assumes a looser arrangement.[20] The cartilage cells closer to the anulus fibrosus undergo a transition to fibrocartilage, whose collagen fibres are arranged in parallel sheets like the fibres of the anulus fibrosus (Fig. 12.11C).

At birth, the notochordal area is formed essentially by an amorphous mucoid material that contains only a few small groups of notochordal cells. The notochordal area is surrounded by a capsule of fibrocartilage, and beyond this lies the collagenous anulus fibrosus. At this stage, the structure of the anulus resembles that seen in the adult (Fig. 12.11D).

After birth, some of the notochordal cells may persist in the disc, but eventually all notochordal cells undergo necrosis during infancy.[23,24] After the age of 4 years, no viable notochordal cells remain and the centre of the disc contains only the notochordal mucoid material and the perichordal fibrocartilage.

From this account, it is evident that the anulus fibrosus develops in situ from the mesenchyme of the primitive intervertebral disc, while the nucleus pulposus has a dual origin. Its central part is derived from the notochord, while its peripheral part is formed by fibrocartilage derived from the mesenchyme of the primitive disc. After birth, notochordal cells disappear, leaving only fibrocartilage and a proteoglycan matrix in the nucleus.

In the neonate and infant, the nucleus pulposus is wedge shaped in the median section, with its main mass located posteriorly in the disc.[11] By 2 years of age this shape is reversed, and the main mass lies anteriorly.[11] From the 4th to 8th years of life, the nucleus assumes an elliptical shape and occupies the centre of the disc. This final change in position occurs as the child masters upright weight-bearing and gait, and accompanies the development of the lumbar lordosis and a rapid increase in height of the lumbar vertebrae and discs.[11]

Between the ages of 2 and 7 years, the lumbar discs change their shape from a biconcave disc bounded by convex bony surfaces to a biconvex disc bounded by concave surfaces,[11] and throughout childhood the lumbar discs undergo a major increase in height. The L4–5 disc, for example, increases from 3 mm in height to about 10 mm, between birth and the age of 12.

GROWTH OF THE VERTEBRAL BODIES

After birth, the lumbar vertebral bodies lose their rounded, ovoid appearance and become rectangular in profile. However, they are still largely covered by cartilage. Superiorly and inferiorly they are capped by cartilage that forms the growth plates of the vertebrae and which will eventually form the endplates of the intervertebral discs. Posterolaterally on each side, the centrum is covered by a layer of cartilage that separates the centrum from the ossified ventral process of the neural arch, now the pedicle of the vertebra. Technically, this junction between the neural arch and the centrum forms a joint, which is known as the **neurocentral joint**, or more accurately as the **neurocentral synchondrosis**.

The neurocentral joints persist into childhood but gradually the cartilage is ossified and the pedicles fuse with the centrum by about the age of 6 years.[14] In fusing with the centrum, the pedicles contribute to the formation of the vertebral body, which is therefore formed largely by the ossified centrum but also by the ventral ends of the neural arches.

Horizontal growth

Horizontal growth of the vertebral body occurs by periosteal ossification,[12,13,25] and from birth to the age of 7 years the anteroposterior diameter of a typical lumbar vertebral body increases from 3 mm to about 22 mm[12] or 27 mm.[11] During the same period, the lateral diameter increases from 7 mm to about 36 mm.[11] By the age of 17 years, the anteroposterior diameter reaches 34 mm.[12] Between the ages of 5 and 13 years, the transverse diameter of the lumbar vertebral bodies in males increases by about 26% at the L1 and L3 levels, and by 30% at the L5 level. In females, the corresponding increases are about 15% and 22%.[26] From puberty to adulthood the transverse diameters increase by 5–10% in both males and females. The mean values for the L1, L3 and L5 vertebrae increase from 38, 42 and 48 mm to 42, 44 and 52 mm, respectively.[26]

Longitudinal growth

Longitudinal growth of the vertebral bodies occurs as a result of the proliferation and ossification of the cartilages remaining on the superior and inferior surfaces of the vertebral body.[13,27] These cartilages cover the entire superior and inferior surfaces, but also overlap onto the anterior, lateral and posterior margins of the vertebral body (Fig. 12.12).[7,14,28] On their discal aspect these cartilages blend with the developing intervertebral disc. They are directly confluent with the fibrocartilage of the developing nucleus, and they anchor the fibres of the anulus fibrosus (see Fig. 12.12). On the vertebral aspect of each plate, the

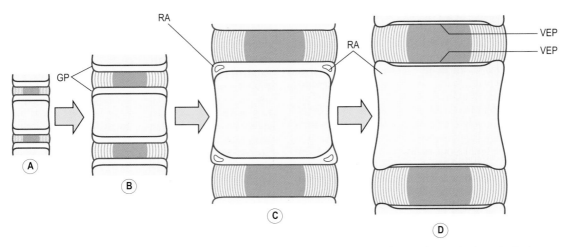

Figure 12.12 Stages in the growth of the vertebral bodies. (A) The vertebral bodies, discs and growth plates (GP) of a 1-year-old infant. (B) The same structures in a prepubertal child. (C) The appearance of the ring apophyses (RA) in adolescence. (D) Ossification of the ring apophyses and the formation of the vertebral endplates (VEP) in adulthood.

cartilage cells are arranged in vertical columns,[17,27] and ossification occurs by the same process seen in the metaphyses of long bones.[29]

The cells furthest away from the cartilage plate are surrounded by calcified matrix and undergo ossification, whereupon they are incorporated into the vertebral body. Longitudinal growth occurs as these cells are replaced by division of cells closer to the main body of the cartilage plate. Growth continues as long as this replacement continues, and the rate of growth appears to be equal at both the upper and lower growth plates.[25,30]

Between birth and the age of 5 years, a typical lumbar vertebra increases in height from 5 mm to about 15 mm[11,26] or 18 mm.[12] From the age of 5 to the age of 13, it increases to about 22 mm, and reaches 25 mm by adulthood.[26] Other studies estimate the sizes of the vertebrae at the age of 13 and at adulthood to be 26 mm and 34 mm, respectively.[12] The average vertical dimensions of all the lumbar vertebrae and intervertebral discs at various ages are shown in Table 12.1. The dramatic increase in size during childhood is readily apparent. During adolescence, females exhibit somewhat smaller average dimensions than males, but approach male dimensions more closely by adulthood.

The extent of longitudinal growth of the central region of the vertebral body appears to be genetically determined, but the longitudinal growth of the peripheral portions is dependent on activity associated with weight-bearing in the erect posture.[11] With assumption of the lumbar lordosis, the nucleus pulposus comes to be located in the centre of each intervertebral disc,[11] and this location of the nucleus acts as a stimulus for growth of the more peripheral parts of the vertebral body.[11] It is as if the peripheral parts grow to attempt to surround the nucleus, and this

differential growth accounts for the relatively concave shape of the superior and inferior surfaces of the developing vertebral bodies.

Longitudinal growth of the vertebral bodies continues throughout childhood and adolescence, but gradually the rate of growth slows down and is completed between the ages of 18 and 25.[16] As ossification ceases, the growth plates become thinner, and the vertebral surface of the growth plate is sealed off from the vertebral body by both a calcified layer of cartilage and the development of the subchondral bone plate at each end of the vertebral body. The hyaline and fibrocartilage remaining on the surfaces of the body then becomes the vertebral endplate of the intervertebral disc.

During vertebral growth the cartilaginous growth plates are nourished by blood vessels that ascend and descend along the outer surfaces of the vertebral body and enter the peripheral edges of the growth plates. They then run within the growth plate towards its centre, raising ridges in the cartilage over the upper and lower surfaces of the vertebral body. These ridges radiate from the centre of the growth plate to its perimeter and are more marked anteriorly. As growth slows down, the vessels in these ridges are gradually obliterated, and the ridges disappear.[28]

Ring apophysis

During the growth period, a separate series of events involve the perimeter of the cartilaginous growth plates but do not contribute to growth. These events relate to the formation of the ring apophyses of the vertebrae (see Ch. 1). In the edges of the cartilaginous plates, where they overlap the anterior, lateral and posterior margins of the vertebral body, foci of calcification appear, at the ages of

Table 12.1 Vertical dimension of lumbar vertebrae and intervertebral discs

Age (years)	Mean vertical dimension (mm)[a]				
	0–1.5	**1.5–12**	**13–19**	**20–35**	
L1 body	7.9	14.4	25.2 22.8	25.3 24.9	Males Females
L1–2 disc	2.6	5.7	7.1 7.0	6.0 6.2	
L2 body	8.0	15.0	25.1 22.4	25.8 25.3	
L2–3 disc	3.5	7.6	10.4 10.4	10.4 10.0	
L3 body	7.9	14.8	25.2 22.3	25.7 25.6	
L3–4 disc	4.0	7.9	10.7 11.3	11.0 10.5	
L4 body	7.6	14.5	25.1 22.6	25.5 25.0	
L4–5 disc	4.0	8.5	11.8 10.4	11.5 11.1	
L5 body	7.2	14.5	23.7 22.1	24.1 24.1	
L5–S1 disc	3.6	8.2	11.2 9.8	10.7 10.8	

[a]Based on direct measurements of the mid-vertical diameters of the vertebral bodies and intervertebral discs in 204 cadavers. (L. Twomey, unpublished data.)

6–8 years in girls and 7–9 years in boys.[14] These foci are subsequently ossified as a result of vascular infiltration. At first, many such foci surround the upper and lower margins of the vertebral body, but by about the age of 12 years they coalesce to form a single rim, or a ring. This ring surrounds the entire perimeter of the vertebral body but is better developed anteriorly and laterally. It remains separated from the rest of the vertebral body by a thin layer of hyaline cartilage but eventually fuses with the vertebra, some time between the ages of 14 and 15[14] or 16 and 21 (see Fig. 12.12).[31,32]

At no time does the ring apophysis contribute to growth, but its fusion with the rest of the vertebral body signals the cessation of longitudinal growth. One effect of the ring apophysis is that, because it develops as a result of ossification of the margins of the cartilage growth plate, it incorporates those fibres of the anulus fibrosus that insert into the perimeter of the plate (Fig. 12.12D). This explains why the peripheral fibres of the adult anulus have a bony attachment, while the more central fibres are inserted into the vertebral endplate.

DEVELOPMENT OF THE ZYGAPOPHYSIAL JOINTS

Compared to the embryology and development of the vertebral bodies, the development of the lumbar zygapophysial joints has received scant attention. There are few descriptions in the English language literature, although some major studies have been published in the continental literature.[33–36] Notwithstanding this relative neglect, there are some fascinating and clinically relevant aspects of the development of these joints.

The lumbar zygapophysial joints develop from the mesenchyme of the neural arches, rudimentary mesenchymal articular processes appear at about 32 days of development,[3] and the mesenchymal processes of consecutive vertebrae eventually meet one another at about 50 days.[34] The future joint space is initially surrounded and filled with mesenchyme but as the articular processes chondrify, this tissue gradually recedes to form the articular capsule,

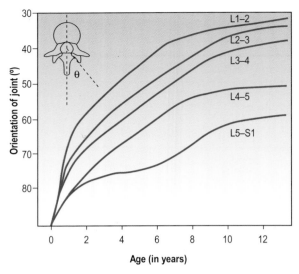

Figure 12.13 The orientation of the lumbar zygapophysial joints as a function of age during growth. *(Based on Lutz 1967.[34])*

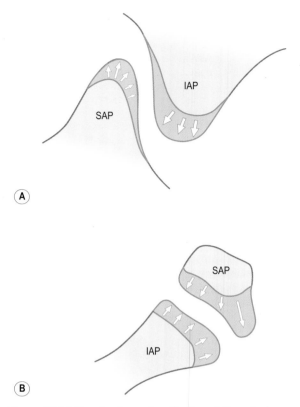

Figure 12.14 The directions of ossification of the articular processes. (A) Lateral view. (B) Top view. (Based on Reichmann 1971.[39]) IAP, inferior articular process; SAP, superior articular process. In the neonate only the basal regions of each articular process are ossified. Their tips are covered by cartilage into which ossification extends.

any intra-articular structures, and a joint space. Chondrification commences at about 50 days,[3] and ossification by about 100 days.

Although definitive joints are formed by the 9th month of gestation,[34,36] at birth the articular processes are incompletely ossified. They are flat and spatula-like, and their tips are still covered by cartilage.[15] The superior articular process is rudimentary and is about half the length of the inferior articular process, but undergoes extensive development during the first 2 years of life.

At birth, the lumbar zygapophysial joints are all orientated in a coronal plane, like the joints of the thoracic vertebrae, but during postnatal growth their orientation changes to that seen in adults by about the age of 11 years (Fig. 12.13).[34,36–38] Rotation is achieved by differential rates and extents of ossification of the articular processes.[39]

At birth, bone occurs in the medial and basal parts of both inferior and superior articular processes. Further ossification occurs in three directions: towards the apex of each articular process along the medial margins of the joint; towards the joint surface leaving a joint cartilage; and around the lateral aspects of each articular process (Fig. 12.14).[39] Medial growth occurs rapidly but ceases at the age of 6 months. After this age the medial margin of the joint is resorbed and remodelled as the neural arch expands to assume adult proportions.[39,40] Lateral ossification is more protracted as further cartilage is laid down as ossification proceeds. With medial ossification completed, continued lateral ossification brings about the apparent rotation of the joint (Fig. 12.15). The joints are fully ossified by about 7–9 years of age, by which time the adult orientation is virtually fully established (see Fig. 12.13).

Variations in the extent of developmental rotation account for the variations in orientation of the lumbar zygapophysial joints seen in adults (see Ch. 3). Joints with a more pronounced posterior, lateral growth would exhibit curvatures (see Fig. 12.15A); those with a more pronounced lateral growth and less dorsal growth would tend to remain planar (see Fig. 12.15B).

The cause of joint 'rotation' is unknown. It may be a genetically determined property of the lumbar zygapophysial joints but other explanations have been suggested. Because it occurs as the child learns to stand erect and begins to use the multifidus muscle in everyday activities, some authors[38] attribute rotation of the lumbar zygapophysial joints to the action of multifidus (see Ch. 9). By pulling on the mamillary processes, the multifidus swings the lateral extremity of the superior articular process to a more dorsal position, thereby rotating the plane of the joint or imparting a curvature to it.

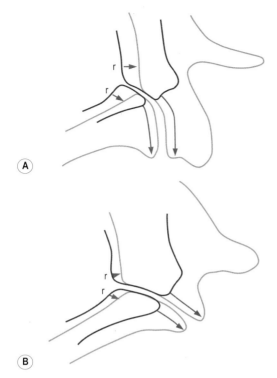

Figure 12.15 Relative directions of growth of a zygapophysial joint as seen in transverse sections. (A) Upper lumbar levels. (B) Lower lumbar levels. The darker outline represents the size and configuration of the neonatal joint. The lighter outline represents the size and configuration established by later childhood. The larger arrows indicate the direction of growth of the articular processes. The smaller arrows indicate areas where bone is resorbed (r) to allow the neural canal to enlarge with growth. *(Based on Reichmann 1971.[39])*

The articular processes continue to grow until about the age of 20;[41] infrequently, secondary ossification centres (epiphyses) may appear in the tip of the inferior articular processes at puberty. The exact incidence of these centres is unknown but, when formed, they fuse with the main part of the inferior articular process between 15 and 21 years of age.[14,42,43]

SIGNIFICANCE

Details of the development of the lumbar vertebral bodies and zygapophysial joints have been emphasised above not so much for academic purposes but to illustrate that the developing lumbar spine is plastic. The adult shape of the vertebrae and their joints is not established at birth, nor are the spines of children miniature versions of those of adults. The vertebrae are continually growing and moulding to the forces habitually exerted on them. The final adult form is as much a product of the postures and activities assumed during childhood as is it is a product of genetic programming. The implications of this relationship with respect to preventing possibly deleterious aberrations of the shape of vertebrae and joints have still to be explored.

DEVELOPMENTAL ANOMALIES

The developmental anomalies of the lumbar spine are vast and varied. In general they are thoroughly described in major textbooks of spinal morphology and radiology,[14,15,44,45] and in research papers specifically addressing this issue.[46–50]

Systematically, lumbar vertebral anomalies can be classified into:

- agenesis, or failure of development, of one or more parts of a vertebra
- failure of union of parts
- changes in number or identity.

Part or all of a vertebral body may fail to be formed. When this occurs, the body assumes a wedge shape, with the orientation of the wedge dependent on which part of the body fails: failure of the anterior half of the body leads to anterior wedging; failure of the posterior part causes posterior wedging; and lateral failure leads to lateral wedging. The embryological basis for these deformities is described in detail elsewhere.[14]

Individual components of the neural arches may fail to develop. In particular, a pedicle may be absent or not ossified,[51–53] and articular processes, mostly inferior articular processes, may fail to develop.[54–57]

The most common form of non-union is spina bifida, in which the laminae of a vertebra, most commonly L5, fail to unite dorsally behind the cauda equina. This may simply be a failure of ossification of an otherwise united cartilaginous neural arch, but spina bifida can be associated with minor and quite major abnormalities of the dural sac, cauda equina and spinal cord.[14,44,46]

The secondary ossification centres of the inferior articular processes may fail to unite with the articular process, or may be late in so doing. Under these circumstances, the isolated ossicle formed by the secondary centre may mimic a fractured articular process.[58,59] United epiphyses occur in asymptomatic[58–62] and symptomatic[58,59,61–64] individuals, and it is not clear under what circumstances they can cause symptoms. It seems possible that if they were detached from the articular process, they could interfere with the mechanics of the zygapophysial joint like a loose body;[15] compression of the underlying spinal nerve roots by a dislocated epiphysis has been described.[65] Estimates of the incidence of united epiphyses vary from 1.5%[60,65] to 14%.[66]

Alterations in vertebral number and identity affect principally the lumbosacral region, where the last lumbar vertebra may become incorporated into the sacrum (sacralisation), thereby reducing the number of lumbar vertebrae to four; or conversely the first sacral vertebra may be mobile (lumbarisation), in which case the number of lumbar vertebrae increases to six. Various intermediate states of these same processes occur, with vertebrae showing features of partial lumbarisation or sacralisation.[14,46,48,50] None of these anomalies, per se, are the cause of symptoms,[67] unless some other disease process or injury is superimposed.

However, anomalous vertebrae may form joints – with the sacrum below or with the ilium laterally – and these joints may be injured or strained, and become symptomatic. The diagnosis is made by anaesthetising the putatively painful joint.[68]

Articular tropism

One of the consequences of the rotation that the lumbar zygapophysial joints undergo is that the extent of rotation of the left and right joints at any segmental level may not be equal. Thus, the joints may be asymmetrically orientated, a condition referred to as **articular tropism**. The incidence of tropism is about 20% at all lumbar levels,[48,66] but may be as high as 30% at the lumbosacral level,[46] with 20% of lumbosacral zygapophysial joints showing an asymmetry greater than 10°.[69]

Early views suggested that articular tropism predisposed to the development of osteoarthritis in the more asymmetrical joint and to consequent narrowing of the related intervertebral foramen.[70] Others felt that asymmetry allowed unequal rotation of the intervertebral joint[70] and rendered it more susceptible to 'ligamentous injury' (although exactly which ligaments were likely to be injured was not specified).[49,69] Modern interest has focused on the significance of articular tropism in torsion injuries of the intervertebral disc, disc degeneration and disc herniation.

Biomechanical studies have shown that asymmetrical zygapophysial joints do not equally resist posteroanterior shear stresses applied to the intervertebral joint. The unequal load-sharing causes the intervertebral joint to rotate whenever it is subjected to shear stress, as in weight-bearing or flexion (see Ch. 8). The upper vertebra in the joint rotates towards the side of the more coronally orientated joint.[71] Consequently, the anulus fibrosus is subjected to inordinate stresses during weight-bearing and flexion movements of the lumbar spine. Repeated insults sustained in this way could damage the anulus fibrosus.

Post-mortem studies support this contention. Radial fissures in the anulus fibrosus are a sign of injury to the intervertebral disc (see Ch. 15), and post-mortem studies reveal that over 80% of unilateral fissures occur in intervertebral joints whose zygapophysial joints are asymmetrical by more than 10°. In 80% of these cases the fissure points towards the side of the more obliquely (coronally) orientated joint.[72] However, clinically, studies differ.

In one study, based on plain radiographs, articular tropism was found to occur in as many as 90% of patients presenting with low back pain and sciatica, with the symptoms occurring on the side of the more obliquely set joint.[73] Later studies, however, using CT scans, found no relationship between articular tropism and either the presence or side of protrusion.[74,75] On the other hand, another study did find a statistically significant relationship, not with disc herniation but between tropism seen on CT scans and disc degeneration seen on magnetic resonance imaging.[76] In that study tropism was defined as joint asymmetry greater than 5°.

An exhaustive study, based on CT discography, established the prevalence of tropism in 108 patients with back pain.[77] Joint asymmetry was normally distributed in that population, with a mean of 0°, a one standard deviation range of 7° and a two standard deviation range of 15°. No significant association was found between tropism and either disc degeneration or discogenic pain.

Thus, despite earlier enthusiasm, and despite the purported biomechanical significance of tropism, there is no clinically useful relationship between tropism and disc degeneration, disc herniation or discogenic pain. Whether or not tropism has a relationship to torsion injuries of the disc (see Ch. 15) has yet to be explored.

REFERENCES

1. Hamilton WJ, Boyd JD, Mossman HW. *Human Embryology*. 3rd ed. Cambridge: Heffer; 1962.

2. Verbout AJ. The development of the vertebral column. *Adv Anat Embryol Cell Biol*. 1985;90: 1–122.

3. O'Rahilly R, Meyer DB. The timing and sequence of events in the development of the human vertebral column during the embryonic period proper. *Anat Embryol*. 1979;157: 167–176.

4. O'Rahilly R, Muller F, Meyer DB. The human vertebral column at the end of the embryonic period proper. *J Anat*. 1980;131:565–575.

5. Winckler G. Les muscles profonds du dos chez l'homme. *Arch Anat Histol Embryol*. 1948;31:1–58.

6. Williams PL, ed. *Gray's Anatomy.* 38th ed. Edinburgh: Churchill Livingstone; 1995.

7. Ehrenhaft JC. Development of the vertebral column as related to certain congenital and pathological changes. *Surg Gynecol Obst.* 1943; 76:282–292.

8. Bagnall KM, Harris PF, Jones PRM. A radiographic study of variations of the human fetal spine. *Anat Rec.* 1984;208:265–270.

9. Cohen J, Currarino G, Neuhauser EBD. A significant variant in the ossification centers of the vertebral bodies. *Am J Roentgenol.* 1956;76: 469–475.

10. Bagnall KM, Harris PF, Jones PRM. A radiographic study of the human fetal spine. 2. The sequence of development of ossification centres in the vertebral column. *J Anat.* 1997;124:791–802.

11. Taylor JR. Growth of the human intervertebral discs and vertebral bodies. *J Anat.* 1975;120:49–68.

12. Brandner MF. Normal values of the vertebral body and intervertebral disc index during growth. *Am J Roentgenol.* 1970;110:618–627.

13. Caffey J. *Pediatric X-ray Diagnosis.* 6th ed. Chicago: Year Book Medical Publishers; 1972.

14. Schmorl G, Junghanns H. *The Human Spine in Health and Disease.* 2nd American ed. New York: Grune & Stratton; 1971:18.

15. Hadley LA. *Anatomico-roentgenographic Studies of the Spine.* Springfield: Thomas; 1964.

16. Carpenter EB. Normal and abnormal growth of the spine. *Clin Orthop.* 1961;21:49–55.

17. Coventry MB, Ghormley RK, Kernohan JW. The intervertebral disc: its microscopic anatomy and pathology. Part I. Anatomy, development and physiology. *J Bone Joint Surg.* 1945;27: 105–112.

18. Keyes DC, Compere EL. The normal and pathological physiology of nucleus pulposus of the intervertebral disc. *J Bone Joint Surg.* 1932;14:897–938.

19. Taylor JR. Persistence of the notochordal canal in vertebrae. *J Anat.* 1972;111:211–217.

20. Peacock A. Observations on the pre-natal development of the intervertebral disc in man. *J Anat.* 1951;85:260–274.

21. Hickey DS, Hukins DWL. Collagen fibril diameters and elastic fibres in the annulus fibrosus of human fetal intervertebral disc. *J Anat.* 1981;133: 351–357.

22. Hickey DS, Hukins DWL. X-ray diffraction studies of the arrangement of collagen fibres in human fetal intervertebral disc. *J Anat.* 1980;131:81–90.

23. Coventry MB. Anatomy of the intervertebral disk. *Clin Orthop.* 1969;67:9–15.

24. Meachim G, Cornah MS. Fine structure of juvenile human nucleus pulposus. *J Anat.* 1970;107:337–350.

25. Knuttson F. Growth and differentiation of the post-natal vertebrae. *Acta Radiol.* 1961;55: 401–408.

26. Taylor JR, Twomey LT. Sexual dimorphism in human vertebral body shape. *J Anat.* 1984;138: 281–286.

27. Bick EM, Copel JW. Longitudinal growth of the human vertebrae. *J Bone Joint Surg.* 1950;32A:803–814.

28. Donisch EW, Trapp W. The cartilage endplate of the human vertebral column (some considerations of postnatal development). *Anat Rec.* 1971;169:705–716.

29. Ham AW, Cormack DH. *Histology.* 8th ed. Philadelphia: Lippincott; 1979:373.

30. Gooding CA, Neuhauser EBD. Growth and development of the vertebral body in the presence and absence of normal stress. *Am J Roentgenol.* 1965;93:388–394.

31. Calvo LJ. Observations on the growth of the female adolescent spine and its relation to scoliosis. *Clin Orthop.* 1957;10:40–46.

32. Walmsley R. Growth and development of the intervertebral disc. *Edin Med J.* 1953;60:341–364.

33. Guntz E. Die Erkrankungen der Zwischenwirbelgelenke. *Arch Orthop Unfallchir.* 1933–1934;34: 333–355.

34. Lutz G. Die Entwicklung der kleinen Wirbelgelenke. *Z Orth.* 1967;104:19–28.

35. Tondury G. Beitrag zur Kenntnis der klein Wirbelgelenke. *Z Ant Entwickl Gesch.* 1940;110:568–575.

36. Tondury G. Anatomie fonctionelle des petits articulations du rachis. *Ann Med Phys.* 1972;15:173–191.

37. Huson A. Les articulations intervertébrales chez le foetus humain. *Comptes Rendus de l'Association des Anatomistes.* 1967;52:676–683.

38. Odgers PNB. The lumbar and lumbosacral diarthrodial joints. *J Anat.* 1933;67:301–317.

39. Reichmann S. The postnatal development of form and orientation of the lumbar intervertebral joint surfaces. *Z Anat Entwickl-Gesch.* 1971;133:102–121.

40. Reichmann S, Lewin T. Growth processes in the neural arch. *Z Anat Entwickl-Gesch.* 1971;133:89–101.

41. Lewin T. Osteoarthritis in lumbar synovial joints. *Acta Orthop Scand.* 1964;73(Suppl.):1–112.

42. Hadley LA. Secondary ossification centers and the intraarticular ossicle. *Am J Roentgenol.* 1956; 76:1095–1101.

43. McMurrich JP. *The Development of the Human Body.* 6th ed. Philadelphia: Blakiston; 1919:167.

44. Epstein BS. *The Spine. A Radiological Text and Atlas.* 4th ed. Philadelphia: Lea & Febiger; 1976.

45. McCulloch JA. Congenital anomalies of the lumbosacral spine. In: Genant HK, ed. *Spine Update 1984.* San Francisco: Radiology Research and Education Foundation; 1983:43–49 Ch. 6.

46. Brailsford JF. Deformities of the lumbosacral region of the spine. *Br J Surg.* 1929;16:562–627.

47. Pheasant HC, Swenson PC. The lumbosacral region. A correlation of the roentgenographic and anatomical observations. *J Bone Joint Surg.* 1942;24:299–306.

48. Southworth JD, Bersack SR. Anomalies of the lumbosacral vertebrae in five hundred and fifty individuals without symptoms referable to the low back. *Am J Roentgenol.* 1950;64:624–634.

49. Willis TA. An analysis of vertebral anomalies. *Am J Surg.* 1929;6: 163–168.

50. Willis TA. Anatomical variations and roentgenographic appearance of the low back in relation to sciatic pain. *J Bone Joint Surg.* 1941;23: 410–416.

51. De Boeck M, De Smedy E, Potvliege R. Computed tomography in the evaluation of a congenital absent lumbar pedicle. *Skeletal Radiol.* 1982;8:197–199.

52. Macleod S, Hendry GMA. Congenital absence of a lumbar pedicle. *Pediatr Radiol.* 1982;12:207–210.

53. Yousefzadeh DK, El-Khoury GY, Lupetin AR. Congenital aplastic–hypoplastic lumbar pedicle in infants and young children. *Skeletal Radiol.* 1982;7:259–265.

54. Arcamano JP, Karas S. Congenital absence of the lumbosacral articular process. *Skeletal Radiol.* 1982;8:133–134.

55. Keim HA, Keagy RD. Congenital absence of lumbar articular facets. *J Bone Joint Surg.* 1967;49A:523–526.

56. Klinghoffer LK, Muedock MM, Hermal MB. Congenital absence of lumbar articular facets. *Clin Orthop.* 1975;106:151–154.

57. Phillips MR, Keagy RD. Congenital absence of lumbar articular facets with computerized axial tomography documentation. *Spine.* 1988;13:676–678.

58. Bailey W. Anomalies and fractures of the vertebral articular processes. *JAMA.* 1937;108:266–270.

59. Rendich RA, Westing SW. Accessory articular process of the lumbar vertebrae and its differentiation from fracture. *Am J Roentgenol.* 1933;29:156–160.

60. Farmer HL. Accessory articular processes in the lumbar spine. *Am J Roentgenol.* 1936;36:763–767.

61. Nichols BH, Shiflet EL. Ununited anomalous epiphyses of the inferior articular processes of the lumbar vertebrae. *J Bone Joint Surg.* 1933;15:591–600.

62. Fulton WS, Kalbfleisch WK. Accessory articular processes of the lumbar vertebrae. *Arch Surg.* 1934;29:42–48.

63. King AB. Back pain due to loose facets of the lower lumbar vertebrae. *Bull Johns Hopkins Hosp.* 1955;97:271–283.

64. Pellegrini VD, Hardy JH. The absent lumbosacral articular process. A report of three cases and review of the literature. *Clin Orthop.* 1983;175:197–201.

65. Pou-Serradell A, Casademont M. Syndrome de la queue de cheval et présence d'appendices apophysaires vertébraux, ou apophyses articulaires accessoires, dans la région lombaire. *Rev Neurol.* 1972;126:435–440.

66. Horwitz T, Smith RM. An anatomical, pathological and roentgenological study of the intervertebral joints of the lumbar spine and of the sacroiliac joints. *Am J Roentgenol.* 1940;43:173–186.

67. Splithoff CA. Lumbosacral junction: roentgenographic comparisons of patients with and without backache. *JAMA.* 1953;152:199–201.

68. Jonsson B, Stromqvist B, Egund N. Anomalous lumbosacral articulations and low-back pain: evaluation and treatment. *Spine.* 1989;14:831–834.

69. Badgley CE. The articular facets in relation to low-back pain and sciatic radiation. *J Bone Joint Surg.* 1941;23:481–496.

70. Von Lackum HL. The lumbosacral region. An anatomic study and some clinical observations. *JAMA.* 1924;82:1109–1114.

71. Cyron BM, Hutton WC. Articular tropism and stability of the lumbar spine. *Spine.* 1980;5:168–172.

72. Farfan HF, Huberdeau RM, Dubow HI. Lumbar intervertebral disc degeneration. The influence of geometrical features on the pattern of disc degeneration – a post-mortem study. *J Bone Joint Surg.* 1972;54A:492–510.

73. Farfan HF, Sullivan JD. The relation of facet orientation to intervertebral disc failure. *Can J Surg.* 1967;10:179–185.

74. Cassidy JD, Loback D, Yong-Hing K, et al. Lumbar facet joint asymmetry: intervertebral disc herniation. *Spine.* 1992;17:570–574.

75. Hagg O, Wallner A. Facet joint asymmetry and protrusion of the intervertebral disc. *Spine.* 1990;15:356–359.

76. Noren R, Trafimow J, Andersson GBJ, et al. The role of facet joint tropism and facet angle in disc degeneration. *Spine.* 1991;16:530–532.

77. Vanharanta H, Floyd T, Ohnmeiss DD, et al. The relationship of facet tropism to degenerative disc disease. *Spine.* 1993;18:1000–1005.

Chapter | **13** |

Age changes in the lumbar spine

Textbook descriptions imply that the structure of the lumbar spine conforms to some sort of standard or even ideal form, and that a standard description is applicable to all individuals. However, such descriptions only reflect the average, healthy, young adult spine. Yet, even then the lumbar spine is subject to variations, e.g. in the shape and orientation of the zygapophysial joints (see Ch. 3), the shape of the lumbar lordosis (see Ch. 5) and the possible ranges of movement (see Ch. 8). What is considered the 'normal' lumbar spine is only a composite of the mean values, or most common form, of these and other possible variables.

In this regard, 'normal' is defined as the structure most commonly exhibited by individuals in a population. However, when defined in this way, normality is greatly influenced by age. As individuals age, their lumbar spines undergo changes that are fairly uniformly reflected by the population. Thus, what is 'normal' for a young adult population may not be 'normal' for an older population. Moreover, if changes uniformly exhibited by an older population are not associated with symptoms, then they cannot be regarded as pathological. They are simply part of the natural biological process of ageing. Each age group, therefore, defines its own normal standards, and in order that clinicians neither confuse age changes with pathological changes, nor misconstrue them as such, they should be aware of what constitutes the natural changes with age in the lumbar spine.

In this regard, the fundamental age changes of the lumbar spine occur at the biochemical level. In turn, these affect the microbiomechanical and overt biomechanical properties of the spine, which are ultimately reflected in the morphology of different components of the lumbar spine and its patterns of movement.

BIOCHEMICAL CHANGES

One of the most fundamental changes in the lumbar spine occurs in the nuclei pulposi. Changes in biochemistry are most dramatic from infancy to about the age of ten years.[1,2] These seem to be triggered by the regression in infancy of the meagre blood supply to the disc, and they set the trend that occurs through later life as the disc adapts to anaerobic metabolism.[1,2]

With ageing, the rate of synthesis of proteoglycans decreases[3] and the concentration of proteoglycans in the nucleus pulposus also decreases.[4–7] In early adult life, proteoglycans amount to about 65% of the dry weight of the nucleus (see Ch. 2) but by the age of 60 they constitute only about 30%.[8] Those proteoglycans that persist are smaller in size[9,10] and have a smaller molecular weight.[11,12] The proportion of aggregated proteoglycans decreases[3] and the number of large proteoglycan aggregates decreases such that, by adolescence, the nucleus pulposus consists largely of clusters of short aggrecan molecules and non-aggregated proteoglycans.[5] Associated with these latter changes is a decline in the concentration of functional link proteins.[5]

Apart from these changes in composition, the nature of the proteoglycans also changes. While the keratan sulphate content of the disc remains fairly constant, the concentration of chondroitin sulphate falls, and this results in a rise in the keratan sulphate/chondroitin sulphate (KS/CS) ratio.[6,12–15]

The other major change in the nucleus pulposus is an increase in its collagen content,[5,16] and an increase in collagen–proteoglycan binding.[9] The collagen content of the anulus fibrosus also increases[17] but the concentration of elastic fibres in the anulus drops, from 13% at the age of 26 to about 8% at the age of 62.[18]

The collagen of the intervertebral disc not only increases in quantity but also changes in nature. The fibril diameter of collagen in the nucleus pulposus increases,[5,19–22] such that the type II collagen of the nucleus starts to resemble the type I collagen of the anulus fibrosus. Reciprocally, the average fibril diameter in the anulus fibrosus decreases.[20] Consequently, there is less distinction between the collagen of the nucleus pulposus and the anulus fibrosus.

The changes in collagen are related not only to age but also to location.[23] While the collagen content of the anulus in general increases with age, there is a significant increase in the amount of type I collagen in the outermost laminae of the posterior quadrant of the anulus, and a reciprocal decrease in type II collagen. This suggests that some of the changes in collagen are not generalised age changes but are active metabolic responses to changes in the internal stresses of the anulus.[23]

The concentration of non-collagenous proteins in the nucleus pulposus increases,[24–28] and ageing is characterised by the appearance of certain distinctive non-collagenous proteins.[28] However, because the functions of non-collagenous proteins are not known (see Ch. 2), the significance of changes in these proteins remains obscure. In contrast, the changes in collagen, proteoglycans and elastic fibres have major biomechanical effects on the disc.

Because chondroitin sulphate is the major source of ionic radicals that bind water to proteoglycans (Ch. 2), it is tempting to expect that the change in the KS/CS ratio would result in a decrease in the water-binding capacity and the water content of the nucleus pulposus. Indeed, the water content of the nucleus does decrease with age.[16] At birth, the water content of the nucleus pulposus is about 88%, and this drops to about 65–72% by the age of 75 years.[6,29] However, most of this dehydration occurs during childhood and adolescence, and the water content of the nucleus pulposus decreases by only about 6% from early adult life to old age.[30]

Sophisticated biochemical studies indicate that it is not simply the loss of proteoglycans or the change in the KS/CS ratio that decreases water-binding in the nucleus. Rather, the increased collagen and increased collagen–proteoglycan binding leave fewer polar groups of the proteoglycans available to bind water,[16] and the decrease in water-binding capacity of the nucleus is a function of the complex way in which the ionic interactions between proteoglycans and proteins are altered.[10,11]

Regardless of the actual mechanism, the lumbar intervertebral discs become drier with age, and with the increase in collagen and the loss of elastin, they become more fibrous and less resilient. The increased collagen and increased collagen–proteoglycan binding render the discs stiffer, i.e. more resistant to deformation, and their decreased water-binding capacity renders them less able to recover from creep deformation. The clinical effect of these changes is expressed as changes in the mobility of the lumbar spine, and these are described in a later section below.

STRUCTURAL CHANGES IN THE INTERVERTEBRAL DISCS

As the disc ages, the number of viable cells in the nucleus decreases, and the proportion of cells that exhibit necrosis changes from 2% in infancy to 50% in young adults and 80% in elderly individuals.[5] Lipofuscin granules accumulate with advanced age.[31]

Macroscopically, as the intervertebral disc becomes more fibrous, the distinction between nucleus pulposus and anulus fibrosus becomes less apparent. The two regions coalesce and the nucleus pulposus appears to be encroached by the anulus fibrosus.[32] After middle life, the nucleus pulposus becomes progressively more solid, dry and granular.[32]

As the nucleus pulposus dries out and becomes more fibrous, it is less able to exert fluid pressure.[33,34] Thus, the nucleus is less able to transmit weight directly and less able to exert radial pressure on the anulus fibrosus (cf. Ch. 2). A greater share of any vertical load is therefore borne by the anulus fibrosus. Consequently, the anulus fibrosus is subject to greater stresses and undergoes changes reflecting the increasing and different strains it suffers.

With age, the collagen lamellae of the anulus increase in thickness and become increasingly fibrillated[35–38] and cracks and cavities may develop,[5,39] which may enlarge to become clefts and overt fissures.[32] The number of incomplete lamellae increases.[37] Such changes are not necessarily due to externally applied injuries to the spine but can simply be due to repeated minor insults sustained by the overloaded anulus fibrosus during trunk movements in the course of activities of daily living. Although the tensile strength of the anulus decreases with degeneration of the disc, there is no simple relationship between age and tensile properties.[40]

Narrowing of the intervertebral discs has previously been considered one of the signs of pathological ageing of the lumbar spine[32,41,42] but large-scale post-mortem studies have now refuted this notion. The dimensions of the lumbar intervertebral discs increase with age. Between the second and seventh decades, the anteroposterior diameter of the lumbar discs *increases* by about 10% in females and 2% in males,[30] and there is about a 10% increase in the height of most discs.[30] Furthermore, the upper and lower surfaces of the discs increase in convexity,[30] a change which occurs at the expense of the shape of the vertebral bodies (see below).

Maintenance of disc height is the 'normal' feature of ageing, and any loss of trunk stature with age is the result of decreases in vertebral body height.[43–46] Overt disc narrowing invites the consideration of some process other than ageing, and this is considered in Chapter 15.

CHANGES IN THE VERTEBRAL ENDPLATE

In the newborn, the vertebral endplate is part of the growth plate of the vertebral body. Towards the intervertebral disc, the articular region of the endplate is formed by fibrocartilage, while on the vertebral body side, columns of proliferating cells extend into the ossifying vertebral body (see Ch. 12). By the age of 10–15 years, the articular region of the endplate becomes relatively thicker, while the growth zone decreases in thickness, and proliferating cells become fewer.[47] As vertebral growth slows during the 17th–20th years, the vertebral endplate is gradually sealed off from the vertebral body by the development of the subchondral bone plate, and after the age of 20 only the articular region of the original growth plate persists.[47] Between the ages of 20 and 65, the endplate becomes thinner[47] and cell death occurs in the superficial layers of the cartilage.[38]

In the subchondral bone of the endplate, vascular channels are gradually occluded,[47] resulting in a decrease in the permeability of the endplate region for nutrients to the disc. This impaired nutrition may be one of the factors that cause the biochemical changes in the nucleus pulposus, but it seems to come too late in life to be the fundamental cause.

With age, the apparent strength of the vertebral endplate decreases,[34,48] but because the strength of the endplate depends on the strength of the underlying vertebral body, this change is better considered together with the other changes that affect the vertebral body.

CHANGES IN THE VERTEBRAL BODY

With age, there is an overall decrease in bone density in the lumbar vertebral bodies[43,44,49] and a decrease in bone strength.[34,50] These changes in density and strength correlate with changes in the size and pattern of trabeculae in the vertebral body.

Vertical trabeculae are slowly absorbed, although those that persist are said to be thickened.[51] On the other hand, horizontal trabeculae are absorbed and not replaced.[49,51] Consequently, ageing of the vertebral bodies is characterised by the loss of horizontal trabeculae[49,51] and this is most marked in the central portion of the vertebral body (that part overlying the nucleus pulposus).

The loss of horizontal trabeculae removes their bracing effect on the vertical trabeculae (see Ch. 1), and the load-bearing capacity of the central portion of the vertebral body decreases. Overall, with weakening of the trabecular system, a greater proportion of the compressive load on vertebral bodies is borne by cortical bone. Over the age of 40, the trabecular bone bears only 35% of the load.[34,50] However, cortical bone fails at only 2% deformation, whereas trabecular bone tolerates 9.5% deformation before failing.[34] Consequently, with greater reliance on cortical bone, the vertebral body becomes less resistant to deformation and injury.

Lacking support from the underlying bone, the vertebral endplates deform by microfracture[52] and gradually bow into the vertebral body, imparting a concave shape to the superior and inferior surfaces of the vertebral body.[30,49] Moreover, the central portion of the vertebral endplate is rendered more liable to fracture in the face of excessive compressive loads applied to the disc, and with increasing age microfractures can be found in the endplates and vertical trabeculae of vertebral bodies.[53–58]

Fractures in the vertebral endplates may be large enough to allow nuclear material to extrude into the vertebral body, forming so-called **Schmorl's nodes**. Schmorl's nodes, however, are more a feature of the lower thoracic and thoracolumbar spines and have a low incidence below the level of L2.[59,60] Per se, they are not symptomatic, nor are they related to age; their incidence is greatest in adolescence and they do not increase in frequency with age.[59,60] Nevertheless, smaller protrusions of disc material into the vertebral bodies are not without significance and this is described in Chapter 15.

CHANGES IN THE ZYGAPOPHYSIAL JOINTS

The subchondral bone of the lumbar zygapophysial joints increases in thickness during growth and reaches a maximum between the ages of 20 and 50 years.[61,62]

Thereafter, it gradually gets thinner.[61,63] The articular cartilage, on the other hand, steadily increases in thickness with age but exhibits certain focal changes that start in the fourth decade and which can be related to the stresses applied to these joints.

In the anteromedial third of curved zygapophysial joints, the cartilage exhibits cell hypertrophy (particularly in the midzone layer), which progresses to vertical fibrillation of the cartilage associated with sclerosis of the subchondral bone plate.[62] At any stage, these changes are more advanced in the concave, superior articular process than in the inferior articular process. It is the anteromedial, or backward-facing, portion of this facet that resists the forward shear stresses applied to the intervertebral joint during weight-bearing and flexion movements (see Chs 2 and 8), and it can be surmised that the fibrillation that develops with age in this region reflects the repeated stresses incurred in the course of normal activities of daily living.[62–64] Severe or repeated pressures may result in erosion and focal thinning of the cartilage, while other regions may exhibit swelling that accounts for the general increase in thickness of the articular cartilage.[63,64] Where cartilage is lost, fibro-fatty intra-articular inclusions may increase in size to fill the space vacated by the cartilage.[62]

The posterior section of the joint characteristically exhibits a different kind of splitting of cartilage – parallel to the joint surface. A split piece of cartilage may remain attached to the joint capsule and form a false intra-articular meniscoid.[62]

Cell hypertrophy is almost universal in the fourth decade, and minor fibrillation is common in the fourth and fifth decades. Older joints exhibit gross thickening and irregularity of the calcified zone of cartilage and increased collagen in the superficial layers. The cells are fewer and have smaller nuclei. The changes in cartilage are more severe in the polar regions of the joint than at its centre. In older joints, the distinction between changes in the anteromedial and posterior portions of the joint is lost.[62]

Other features exhibited by the joints are the development of osteophytes and 'wrap-around bumpers'. Osteophytes develop along the attachment sites of the joint capsule and ligamentum flavum to the superior articular process. Wrap-around bumpers are extensions of the edges of the articular cartilage curving around the dorsal aspect of the inferior articular process. Presumably, as a result of repeated stresses at these sites during rotatory movements, the articular cartilage spreads out to cover and protect the edges of the bony articular process.

CHANGES IN MOVEMENTS

The biochemical and structural changes in the joints of the lumbar spine have an inevitable effect on the mechanical properties, and therefore movements, of the spine. Older lumbar spines show a greater amount of creep and hysteresis, and a greater set after creep deformation,[65] but they show a decreased range of motion. A progressive decrease in range of motion with age has been demonstrated in cadavers[59,66–68] and in living subjects using both clinical[67] and radiographic[59,66,69] methods, and is evident in the ranges of motion both of the entire lumbar spine[67,68] and of individual intervertebral joints.[59,66,69]

Young children, strikingly, show the greatest lumbar mobility. At various segmental levels, they are between 50% and 300% more mobile than middle-aged subjects.[67,69] Mobility decreases considerably by adolescence, and beyond the age of 30 there is a gradual but definite decrease in mobility.[59,66,67,69]

Because 'release' experiments show that removing the posterior ligaments and zygapophysial joints does not greatly increase the range of flexion in older cadavers,[68] it appears that increased stiffness in the intervertebral discs is the principal cause of the reduction in mobility that develops with ageing. This can be readily ascribed to the dehydration and fibrosis of older intervertebral discs.

The greater hysteresis seen in older spines is probably due to the decreased water-binding capacity of their intervertebral discs.[65] Less able to attract water, these discs take longer to resume their original configuration and structure after deformation.

SPONDYLOSIS AND DEGENERATIVE JOINT DISEASE

It has been customary to describe certain changes in the intervertebral discs and zygapophysial joints as features of a disease. In the case of the intervertebral discs, the disease has been 'spondylosis', and in the case of the zygapophysial joints it has been called 'osteoarthrosis' or 'degenerative joint disease'.

The cardinal features of spondylosis are said to be the development of osteophytes (bony spurs) along the junction of vertebral bodies and their intervertebral discs.[70–72] However, when viewed in the context of other changes that occur with ageing, it is evident that the features of spondylosis are not those of some aggressive disease that seemingly attacks the body, but are the natural consequences of the stresses applied to the spine throughout life. Whether they should be called 'degenerative changes' or 'age changes' may appear simply to be semantics but the development of osteophytes can be viewed as a reactive and adaptive change that seeks to compensate for biomechanical aberrations. The process is active and purposeful, and does not warrant the description as a degenerative process.

As the nucleus pulposus dries out, the intervertebral disc becomes less resilient and stiffer, and the anulus fibrosus bears more of the loads applied to the disc. To sustain greater loads, the disc and the vertebral bodies adapt; the pattern of adaptation depends on the nature and direction of the particular stress being compensated.

Excessive compression can result in the ossification of the terminal ends of the collagen fibres of the anulus fibrosus. This can occur focally, along the anterior and posterior margins of the disc where compressive strains are concentrated during extension and flexion movements and postures. A more prolific development of osteophytes can occur around the entire margin of the vertebral body in response to excessive vertical load-bearing. This phenomenon can be viewed as if the vertebral body is trying to expand its articular surface area. By distributing axial loads over a wider area, the vertebral body lessens the stress applied to the anulus fibrosus during weight-bearing.

Interpreted in this way, the development of osteophytes is only a natural response to the altered mechanics of the lumbar spine in turn due to more fundamental biochemical changes in the intervertebral disc. Consequently, spondylosis should not be viewed as a disease but as an expected morphological change with age.

Similarly, osteoarthrosis is not a disease but an expression of the morphological consequences of stresses applied to the zygapophysial joints during life. The changes are concentrated at regions subject to the greatest and most repeated stresses. Adaptive changes occur when the stressed tissues are capable of remodelling and opposing the applied stresses, but in the face of severe or repeated stresses destructive features may develop.

Perhaps the most crucial argument against viewing spondylosis and spinal osteoarthrosis as diseases is that they are so irregularly (if not infrequently) associated with symptoms and disability. The incidence of spondylosis and osteoarthrosis is just as great in patients with symptoms as in patients without symptoms.[72-74]

This raises the great paradox in the field of spinal pain, namely that while some patients with spondylosis or osteoarthrosis may present with pain, there are others with the same age changes who do not have pain, and many patients with pain do not have a trace of spondylosis or osteoarthrosis. Consequently, spondylosis or osteoarthrosis cannot legitimately be viewed as a pathological diagnosis. Some other, or additional, factor must be the cause of pain, and the resolution of this problem is addressed in Chapter 15.

REFERENCES

1. Scott JE, Bosworth TR, Cribb AM, et al. The chemical morphology of age-related changes in human intervertebral disc glycosaminoglycans from cervical, thoracic and lumbar nucleus pulposus and annulus fibrosus. *J Anat.* 1994;184:73–82.

2. Taylor JR, Scott JE, Cribb AM, et al. Human intervertebral disc acid glycosaminoglycans. *J Anat.* 1992;180:137–141.

3. Johnstone B, Bayliss MT. The large proteoglycans of the human intervertebral disc. *Spine.* 1995;20:674–684.

4. Beard HK, Stevens RL. Biochemical changes in the intervertebral disc. In: Jayson MIV, ed. *The Lumbar Spine and Backache.* 2nd ed. London: Pitman; 1980:407–436, Ch. 14.

5. Buckwalter JA. Spine update. Aging and degeneration of the human intervertebral disc. *Spine.* 1995; 20:1307–1314.

6. Gower WE, Pedrini V. Age-related variation in protein polysaccharides from human nucleus pulposus, annulus fibrosus and costal cartilage. *J Bone Joint Surg.* 1969;51A:1154–1162.

7. Sylven B, Paulson S, Hirsch C, et al. Biophysical and physiological investigations on cartilage and other mesenchymal tissues. *J Bone Joint Surg.* 1951;33A:333–340.

8. Badgley CE. The articular facets in relation to low-back pain and sciatic radiation. *J Bone Joint Surg.* 1941;23:481–496.

9. Adams P, Muir H. Qualitative changes with age of human lumbar disks. *Ann Rheum Dis.* 1976;35:289–296.

10. Bushell GR, Ghosh P, Taylor TKF, et al. Proteoglycan chemistry of the intervertebral disks. *Clin Orthop.* 1977;129:115–123.

11. Comper WD, Preston BN. Model connective tissue systems. A study of the polyion-mobile ion and of excluded volume interactions of proteoglycans. *Biochem J.* 1974;143:1–9.

12. Urban J, Maroudas A. The chemistry of the intervertebral disc in relation to its physiological function. *Clin Rheum Dis.* 1980;6: 51–76.

13. Adams P, Eyre DR, Muir H. Biochemical aspects of development and ageing of human lumbar intervertebral discs. *Rheumatol Rehab.* 1977;16:22–29.

14. Naylor A. Intervertebral disc prolapse and degeneration. The biochemical and biophysical approach. *Spine.* 1976;1:108–114.

15. Naylor A, Shental R. Biochemical aspects of intervertebral discs in ageing and disease. In: Jayson MIV, ed. *The Lumbar Spine and Backache.* New York: Grune & Stratton; 1976:317–326, Ch. 14.

16. Hirsch C, Paulson S, Sylven B, et al. Biophysical and physiological investigation on cartilage and other mesenchymal tissues: characteristics of human nuclei pulposi during aging. *Acta Orthop Scand.* 1953;22:175–183.

17. Brinckmann P. Injury of the annulus fibrosus and disc protrusions: an in vitro investigation on human lumbar discs. *Spine.* 1986;11:149–153.

18. Johnson EF, Berryman H, Mitchell R, et al. Elastic fibres in the anulus fibrosus of the human lumbar intervertebral disc. A preliminary report. *J Anat.* 1985;143:57–63.

19. Bailey AJ, Herbert CM, Jayson MIV. Collagen of the intervertebral disc. In: Jayson MIV, ed. *The Lumbar Spine and Backache.* New York: Grune & Stratton; 1976:327–340, Ch. 12.

20. Happey F. A biophysical study of the human intervertebral disc. In: Jayson MIV, ed. *The Lumbar Spine and Backache.* New York: Grune & Stratton; 1976:293–316, Ch. 13.

21. Naylor A, Happey F, MacRae TP. The collagenous changes in the intervertebral disc with age and their effect on elasticity. *BMJ.* 1954;2:570–573.

22. Naylor A, Happey F, Turner RL, et al. Enzymic and immunological activity in the intervertebral disc. *Orthop Clin North Am.* 1975;6:51–58.

23. Brickley-Parsons D, Glimcher MJ. Is the chemistry of collagen in intervertebral discs an expression of Wolff's law? A study of the human lumbar spine. *Spine.* 1984;9:148–163.

24. Blakely PR, Happey F, Naylor A, et al. Protein in the nucleus pulposus of the intervertebral disc. *Nature.* 1962;195:73.

25. Dickson IR, Happey F, Pearson CH, et al. Variations in the protein components of human intervertebral disk with age. *Nature.* 1967;215:52–53.

26. Ghosh P, Bushell GK, Taylor TFK, et al. Collagen, elastin, and non-collagenous protein of the intervertebral disk. *Clin Orthop.* 1977;129:123–132.

27. Naylor A. The biochemical changes in the human intervertebral disc in degeneration and nuclear prolapse. *Orthop Clin North Am.* 1971;2:343–358.

28. Taylor TKF, Little K. Intercellular matrix of the intervertebral disk in ageing and in prolapse. *Nature.* 1965;208:384–386.

29. Puschel J. Der Wassergehalt normaler und degenerierter Zwischenwirbelscheiben. *Beitr path Anat.* 1930;84:123–130.

30. Twomey L, Taylor J. Age changes in lumbar intervertebral discs. *Acta Orthop Scand.* 1985;56:496–499.

31. Yasuma T, Arai K, Suzuki F. Age-related phenomena in the lumbar intervertebral discs: lipofuscin and amyloid deposition. *Spine.* 1992;17:1194–1198.

32. Vernon-Roberts B, Pirie CJ. Degenerative changes in the intervertebral discs of the lumbar spine and their sequelae. *Rheumatol Rehab.* 1977;16:13–21.

33. Kulak RF, Belytschko TB, Schultz AB, et al. Non-linear behaviour of the human intervertebral disc under axial load. *J Biomech.* 1976;9:377–386.

34. White AA, Panjabi MM. *Clinical Biomechanics of the Spine.* Philadelphia: Lippincott; 1978.

35. Bernick S, Walker JM, Paule WJ. Age changes to the anulus fibrosus in human intervertebral discs. *Spine.* 1991;16:520–524.

36. Harris RI, MacNab I. Structural changes in the lumbar intervertebral discs. Their relationship to low back pain and sciatica. *J Bone Joint Surg.* 1954;36B:304–322.

37. Marchand F, Ahmed AM. Investigation of the laminate structure of lumbar disc anulus fibrosus. *Spine.* 1990;15:402–410.

38. Pritzker KPH. Aging and degeneration in the lumbar intervertebral discs. *Orth Clin North Am.* 1977;8:65–77.

39. Hirsch C, Schajowicz F. Studies on structural changes in the lumbar annulus fibrosus. *Acta Orthop Scand.* 1952;22:184–189.

40. Acaroglu ER, Iatridis JC, Setton LA, et al. Degeneration and aging affect the tensile behaviour of human lumbar anulus fibrosus. *Spine.* 1995;20:2690–2701.

41. Lawrence JS. Disc degeneration, its frequency and relationship to symptoms. *Ann Rheum Dis.* 1969;28:121–138.

42. Schmorl G, Junghanns H. *The Human Spine in Health and Disease.* 2nd American ed. New York: Grune & Stratton; 1971:18.

43. Ericksen MF. Ageing changes in the shape of the human lumbar vertebrae. *Am J Phys Anthropol.* 1974;41:477.

44. Ericksen MF. Some aspects of ageing in the lumbar spine. *Am J Phys Anthropol.* 1975;45:575–580.

45. Nachemson AL, Schultz AB, Berkson MH. Mechanical properties of human lumbar spinal segments. *Spine.* 1979;4:1–8.

46. Twomey LT, Taylor JR. The effects of ageing on the lumbar intervertebral discs. In: Grieve G, ed. *Modern Manual Therapy.* Edinburgh: Churchill Livingstone; 1986:129–137, Ch. 12.

47. Bernick S, Cailliet R. Vertebral end-plate changes with aging of human vertebrae. *Spine.* 1982;7:97–102.

48. Perey O. Fracture of the vertebral end-plate in the lumbar spine. *Acta Orthop Scand.* 1957; Suppl. 25:1–101.

49. Twomey L, Taylor J, Furniss B. Age changes in the bone density and structure of the lumbar vertebral column. *J Anat.* 1983;136:15–25.

50. Rockoff SE, Sweet E, Bleustein J. The relative contribution of trabecular and cortical bone to the strength of human lumbar vertebrae. *Calcif Tissue Res.* 1969;3:163–175.

51. Atkinson PJ. Variations in trabecular structure of vertebrae with age. *Calcif Tissue Res.* 1967;1:24–32.

52. Hansson T, Roos B. Microcalluses of the trabeculae in lumbar vertebrae and their relation to the bone mineral content. *Spine.* 1981;6:375–380.

53. Brown T, Hansen RJ, Yorra AJ. Some mechanical tests on the lumbosacral spine with particular reference to the intervertebral discs. *J Bone Joint Surg.* 1957;39A:1135–1164.

54. Coventry MB, Ghormley RK, Kernohan JW. The intervertebral disc: its microscopic anatomy and pathology. Part I. Anatomy, development and physiology. *J Bone Joint Surg.* 1945;27:105–112.

55. Keyes DC, Compere EL. The normal and pathological physiology of nucleus pulposus of the intervertebral disc. *J Bone Joint Surg.* 1932;14:897–938.

56. Saunders JB, de CM, Inman VT. Pathology of the intervertebral disk. *Arch Surg.* 1940;40:380–416.

57. Vernon-Roberts B, Pirie CJ. Healing trabecular microfractures in the

bodies of lumbar vertebrae. *Ann Rheum Dis*. 1973;32:406–412.

58. Whitehouse WJ, Dyson ED, Jackson CK. The scanning electron microscope in studies of trabecular bone from a human vertebral body. *J Anat*. 1971;108:481–496.

59. Hilton RC. Systematic studies of spinal mobility and Schmorl's nodes. In: Jayson MIV, ed. *The Lumbar Spine and Backache*, 2nd ed. London: Pitman; 1980:115–134, Ch. 5.

60. Hilton RC, Ball J, Benn RT. Vertebral end-plate lesions (Schmorl's nodes) in the dorsolumbar spine. *Ann Rheum Dis*. 1976;35:127–132.

61. Taylor JR, Twomey LT. Age changes in the subchondral bone of human lumbar apophyseal joints. *J Anat*. 1985;143:233.

62. Taylor JR, Twomey LT. Age changes in lumbar zygapophyseal joints. *Spine*. 1986;11:739–745.

63. Twomey LT, Taylor JR. Age changes in the lumbar articular triad. *Aust J Physiother*. 1985;31:106–112.

64. Taylor JR, Twomey LT. Vertebral column development and its relation to adult pathology. *Aust J Physiother*. 1985;31:83–88.

65. Twomey L, Taylor J. Flexion creep deformation and hysteresis in the lumbar vertebral column. *Spine*. 1982;7:116–122.

66. Hilton RC, Ball J, Benn RT. In-vitro mobility of the lumbar spine. *Ann Rheum Dis*. 1979;38:378–383.

67. Taylor J, Twomey L. Sagittal and horizontal plane movement of the human lumbar vertebral column in cadavers and in living. *Rheumatol Rehab*. 1980;19:223–232.

68. Twomey LT, Taylor JR. Sagittal movements of the human lumbar vertebral column: a quantitative study of the role of the posterior vertebral elements. *Arch Phys Med Rehab*. 1983;64:322–325.

69. Tanz SS. Motion of the lumbar spine: a roentgenologic study. *Am J Roentgenol*. 1953;69:399–412.

70. Epstein BS. *The Spine. A Radiological Text and Atlas*, 4th ed. Philadelphia: Lea & Febiger; 1976.

71. Resnick D. Common disorders of the aging lumbar spine: radiographic-pathologic correlation. In: Genanat HK, ed. *Spine Update 1984*. San Francisco: Radiology Research and Education Foundation; 1983:35–42, Ch. 5.

72. Torgerson WR, Dotter WE. Comparative roentgenographic study of the asymptomatic and symptomatic lumbar spine. *J Bone Joint Surg*. 1976;58A:850–853.

73. Lawrence JS, Bremner JM, Bier F. Osteoarthrosis: prevalence in the population and relationship between symptoms and X-ray changes. *Ann Rheum Dis*. 1966;25:1–24.

74. Magora A, Schwartz A. Relation between the low back pain syndrome and X-ray findings. 1. Degenerative osteoarthritis. *Scand J Rehab Med*. 1976;8:115–125.

Chapter | **14** |

The sacroiliac joint

The sacrum has two unique roles. In a longitudinal direction, it lies at the base of the vertebral column and therefore supports the lumbar spine. Consequently, all longitudinal forces delivered to the lumbar spine are ultimately transmitted to the sacrum. Meanwhile, in a transverse direction, the sacrum is an integral part of the pelvic girdle. It is wedged between the two iliac bones and constitutes the posterior wall of the pelvis. This relationship enables it to transmit forces from the vertebral column sideways into the pelvis and thence into the lower limbs. Conversely, forces from the lower limbs can be transmitted through the pelvis to the sacrum and thence to the vertebral column.

The sacrum, however, is not fused with the rest of the pelvis. Rather, it forms a joint on each side with the corresponding ilium; but although the structure of the sacroiliac joint is well known, its purpose has been a source of contention.

At one extreme, conservative authorities have essentially dismissed the joint as having no functional significance on the grounds that it exhibits little or no movement. On the other hand, others have portrayed the joint as having important primary movements that can and should be assessed clinically like any other joint of the body.

Both views are in error. Despite its size, the sacroiliac joint cannot be considered like any other major joint of the body. Its ranges of movement are very small and it is not endowed with muscles that execute active movements of the joint. Structurally and functionally, the sacroiliac joint is more like the intertarsal joints of the foot, which do not exhibit active movements but which, nonetheless, move passively.

The essence of the sacroiliac joint is that it is a stress-relieving joint. This can be appreciated by imagining what would happen if the sacroiliac joint did not exist.

If the sacrum was fused with the rest of the pelvis, the pelvis would be a solid ring of bone. But this ring would be exposed daily to large twisting forces, particularly during walking. When the right lower limb is extended, the pelvis on that side would tend to twist forwards. For example, tension in the iliofemoral ligament would draw the anterior ilium downwards, thereby rotating the right pelvis clockwise, if viewed from the right. Meanwhile, if the left lower limb was flexed, the left half of the pelvis would be twisted backwards. For example, tension in the hamstrings would draw the ischium forwards, causing the left pelvis to rotate anticlockwise, if viewed from the right. As gait continues, the alternating flexion and extension of the lower limbs would impart alternating twisting forces on the pelvis around its transverse axis.

This effect can be modelled by holding a pretzel in two hands and twisting it around its long axis in alternating directions. Eventually the pretzel will snap. The same occurs clinically. Insufficiency fractures of the sacrum occur in elderly individuals, particularly females, in whom the sacroiliac joint is relatively ankylosed and in whom the sacrum has been weakened by osteoporosis. Under these conditions the torsional stresses, normally buffered by the sacroiliac joint, are transferred to the sacrum, which fails by fracture. Conspicuously and strikingly, these fractures run vertically through the ala of the sacrum parallel to the sacroiliac joint.[1-8]

This phenomenon indicates the need for, and role of, the sacroiliac joint. The joint is placed strategically in the pelvic ring at the site of maximum torsional stress in order to relieve that stress. In teleological terms, a solid ring of bone will not work; it will crack, and the sacroiliac joint is there in anticipation of that crack.

From these observations, the design features of the sacroiliac joint emerge. On the one hand, it must allow movements imposed on the pelvis by twisting forces from the lower limbs, but the movements need not be major in amplitude; it need only be that the twisting forces are absorbed into ligaments and thereby reduce the tendency of the pelvic ring to fracture. At the same time, the sacroiliac joint must be strong and stable in order to transmit the forces from the vertebral column to the lower limbs. A loose joint dependent on ligaments would simply creep under static body weight, let alone under the forces incurred during movements of the trunk. To this end, a bony locking mechanism can be used so as to spare the ligaments from static and longitudinal loads.

The structure of the sacroiliac joint can, therefore, be anticipated. For its longitudinal functions, it will exhibit osseous features that lock it into the pelvic ring. For its antitorsion functions it will exhibit, in a parasagittal plane, a planar surface that can allow gliding movements, but it will be strongly reinforced by ligaments that both retain the locking mechanism and absorb twisting forces.

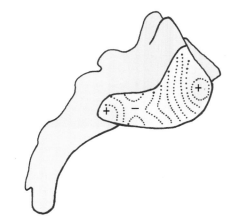

Figure 14.1 A lateral view of the sacrum showing the contours of its articular surface. '+' denotes an elevation; '−' denotes a depression.

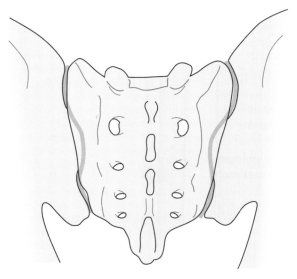

Figure 14.2 A posterior view of the sacroiliac joints showing the sinuous shape of the joint cavities.

STRUCTURE

Bones

The first design imperative is to lock the sacrum into the pelvis. To this end, the articular surface of the sacrum presents an irregular contour, marked by ridges, prominences, troughs and depressions (Fig. 14.1). These are matched by reciprocal depressions, troughs, prominences and ridges on the ilium, so that the bones can lock into one another. This gives the sacroiliac joint a sinuous appearance in frontal view (Fig. 14.2).[9]

Particularly evident is a major depression on the sacral surface, on the S2 segment, which receives a major prominence from the ilium, the latter being known as Bonnaire's tubercle.[10]

A further feature, noted in textbooks of anatomy[11] but not verified by modern quantitative studies, pertains to the plane of the joint. The articular surface of the sacrum is twisted from above downwards. Opposite the S1 segment, the dorsal edge of the articular surface projects slightly further laterally than the ventral edge. Conversely, at the S3 segment, the ventral edge projects slightly more laterally than the dorsal edge. Because of this, when viewed in transverse section, the sacrum is wedge shaped but in opposite directions at opposite ends of the sacroiliac joint. At the S1 segment, the posterior width of the sacrum is greater than its anterior width. Conversely, at the S3 segment, the anterior width is greater than its posterior width (Fig. 14.3).

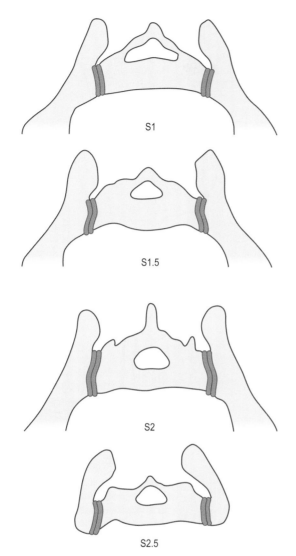

Figure 14.3 Transverse sections of the sacrum showing how, at upper sacral levels (S1), the sacrum is wider posteriorly than anteriorly, but at lower sacral levels (S2.5) the sacrum is wider anteriorly than posteriorly.

Cartilage

The cartilages differ on the sacrum and ilium. The sacral articular cartilage is normally white and smooth, and has the features of typical hyaline cartilage.[12] Its thickness ranges from 1 to 3 mm.[13] The iliac cartilage is duller in appearance and is marked by dense bundles of collagen, which give it the appearance of fibrocartilage,[12] but histologically and biochemically it is nonetheless hyaline in nature.[14] It is usually less than 1 mm thick. Its cell density, however, is greater than that of the sacral cartilage.[15]

Meanwhile, the subchondral plate of the ilium is some 50% thicker than that of the sacrum.[15]

The reasons for these differences between the sacral and iliac cartilages has not been established. One contention, however, is that the sacral cartilage is designed for transmitting forces (from the spine to the pelvis) whereas the iliac cartilage is designed to absorb them.[15]

Articulation

When articulated between the two ilia, the sacrum is held firmly in place by bony locking mechanisms. The interlocking contours of the sacrum and ilium prevent downward gliding of the sacrum under body weight. Indeed, the friction coefficient of the sacroiliac joint is larger than that of the knee and is considerably greater in proportion to the prominence of the ridges and depressions of the articular surface.[16]

Furthermore, the sacrum is set obliquely between the ilia such that its anterior end leans forwards. Consequently, under vertical loads it tends to tilt forwards and downwards, rotating around Bonnaire's tubercle; the wedge shape of the sacrum opposes this. If the sacrum rotates forwards, the wider posterior end of the S1 segment will move inferiorly and will tend to separate the ilia. Meanwhile, the wider anterior end of the S3 segment will move upwards and also will tend to separate the ilia.

None of these movements will occur, however, if the sacrum remains clamped between the two ilia. If the ilia press against the sacrum, the engaged corrugations will prevent the sacrum from sliding downwards. If the ilia are prevented from separating, the wedge shape of the sacrum will not allow it to rotate forwards. Critical to keeping the ilia locked against the sacrum are the ligaments of the sacroiliac joint.

Ligaments

The most important ligament of the sacroiliac joint is the **interosseous sacroiliac ligament**. This ligament is a dense, thick collection of short collagen fibres that connect the ligamentous surface of the sacrum with that of ilium. It lies deep in the narrow recess between the sacrum and ilium dorsal to the cavity of the joint. The full thickness of the ligament is most clearly evident in transverse sections of the sacrum and ilium (Fig. 14.4). *Gray's Anatomy*[11] recognises deep and superficial parts of this ligament, each divided into superior and inferior bands. The superior superficial band connects the superior articular processes and lateral crest of the first two sacral segments to the neighbouring ilium, and is highlighted as the **short posterior sacroiliac ligament**.

The cardinal function of the interosseous sacroiliac ligament is to bind the ilium strongly to the sacrum, thereby securing the bony interlocking mechanism.

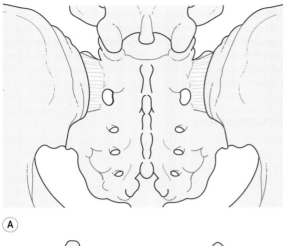

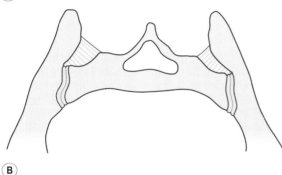

Figure 14.4 The interosseous sacroiliac ligament.
(A) Posterior view. (B) Axial view.

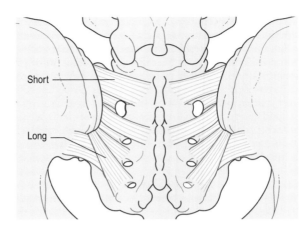

Figure 14.5 The short and long posterior sacroiliac ligaments.

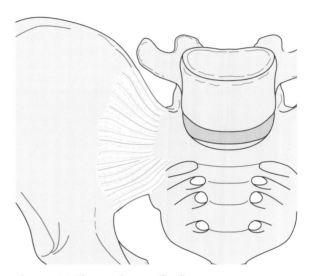

Figure 14.6 The anterior sacroiliac ligaments.

Behind the interosseous ligament lies the **posterior sacroiliac ligament** proper. This consists of several fascicles of different lengths which connect the intermediate and lateral crests of the sacrum to the posterior superior iliac spine and the posterior end of the inner lip of the iliac crest. Those fibres from the third and fourth sacral segments are longer than the others and constitute the **long posterior sacroiliac ligament** (Fig. 14.5).[11]

The short posterior sacroiliac ligament is disposed to act in concert with the interosseous ligament to bind the ilium to the sacrum. Moreover, its posterior location allows it to prevent posterior flaring or diastasis of the joint. The long posterior sacroiliac ligament has a more longitudinal orientation and prevents backward rocking (counternutation) of the sacrum with respect to the ilium.[17]

The **anterior sacroiliac ligament** covers the ventral aspect of the joint. It consists of long, transversely orientated fibres that extend from the ala and anterior

surface of the sacrum to the anterior surface of the ilium.

The fibres are attached to these bones for considerable distances beyond the margins of the joint (Figs 14.4, 14.6). Like the interosseous ligament, this ligament binds the ilium to the sacrum but its anterior location enables it to prevent anterior diastasis of the joint.

Remote from the joint proper are the **sacrospinous** and **sacrotuberous** ligaments. These ligaments are orientated to prevent upward tilting of the lower end of the sacrum (nutation) by anchoring it to the ischium.

The sacrospinous ligament takes a broad origin from the lateral edge of the sacrum below the sacroiliac joint. Its fibres converge on the ischial spine. The sacrotuberous ligament arises from the posterior superior iliac spine, where it blends with the long posterior sacroiliac ligaments; from the transverse tubercles of the lower sacral segments; and from the lateral margin of the sacrum, where it blends with the sacrospinous ligament. From this broad origin, the ligament narrows but broadens again to attach to the medial margin of the ischial tuberosity. The superficial fibres of the ligament are continuous with the tendon of the biceps femoris.[11]

Capsule

There is scant mention in the literature of the structure of the capsule of the sacroiliac joint. This is because the joint is so intimately surrounded by thick ligaments. Under these circumstances, it is difficult, if not impossible, to discern where a ligament ends and a capsule begins. For this reason, authors report that the posterior capsule is rudimentary or absent[18] and that the anterior sacroiliac ligament is a thickening of the anterior capsule.[11]

Innervation

Various descriptions but few data have been published on the innervation of the sacroiliac joint. Even with modern studies, it is unclear the extent to which the joint is innervated from the front and from the back and which neural segments are involved.

In 1936, Pitkin and Pheasant[19] lamented the lack of any description of the innervation of the sacroiliac joint in textbooks of anatomy. Indeed, this situation has still not changed.[11] Instead, Pitkin and Pheasant relied on the 19th-century German literature to assert that the joint was innervated anteriorly by direct branches of the lumbosacral trunk, the superior gluteal nerve and the obturator nerve; posteriorly it was innervated by branches of the S1 and S2 dorsal rami.

Modern authors have endorsed this pattern, reporting a posterior innervation from the lateral branches of the posterior rami of L4 to S3, and an anterior innervation from the L2 to the S2 segments.[18] However, the literature that they cite to this effect does not consist of authoritative anatomical studies. Others, referring to the same literature, describe a posterior innervation from L3 to S3 but emphasise that the principal segments are L5 to S2 but without citing any literature to this effect.[20]

Formal, modern anatomical studies provide conflicting conclusions. A German study[21] stipulated a posterior innervation exclusively from the S1 and S2 dorsal rami but expressly denied an anterior innervation from either the sacral plexus or the obturator nerve. A Japanese study, however, reported a posterior innervation from the L5 and sacral dorsal rami and an anterior innervation from the L5 ventral ramus and S2 ventral ramus.[22]

AGE CHANGES

The future sacroiliac joint becomes apparent during the second month of fetal development, as a strip of mesenchyme between the cartilages of the future ilium and sacrum.[23] Cavitation of this mesenchyme proceeds progressively and achieves its full extent by the seventh month. A synovial membrane appears by 37 weeks.[12]

In embryos, the articular surfaces remain smooth and flat. The anterior capsule is thin and lax, but the interosseous ligament is well developed.[12]

During the first 10 years of life, the joint enlarges in size but its surfaces remain flat; the anterior capsule thickens.[12] Corrugation of the joint surfaces starts to develop during the second decade, starting with a depression along the articular surface of the sacrum matched by a reciprocal ridge along the ilium.[12]

With increasing age, the prominence of the iliac ridge increases but the surfaces of the articular cartilages start to exhibit superficial fibrillation and erosion, particularly on the iliac side.[12] At the joint margins, the capsule and synovium become thicker and more fibrous, and osteophytes start to appear. By the fifth and sixth decades these changes are more marked. The articular cartilage loses its thickness and becomes fibrillated and eroded. Debris and fibrous tissue connecting the bones fill the joint cavity.[12] Sinuous corrugations along the joint are established by the sixth decade[9] but it is not clear when these start to develop.

By the eighth decade, osteophytes are large and interdigitate. Intra-articular fibrous adhesions are plentiful. The thickness of the articular cartilage is reduced to less than 1 mm on the sacrum and less than 0.5 mm on the ilium.[12]

These developmental changes predicate the nature and ranges of possible movements of the sacroiliac joint. By retaining a flat surface, young joints are able to glide in all directions. The advent of depressions on the sacral surface restricts possible movements to nodding movements along the longitudinal axis of the curved auricular surface. The range of available movement, however, decreases as fibrous ankylosis increases in the joint and as osteophyte formation increases.

BIOMECHANICS

A variety of difficulties have faced investigators intent on studying sacroiliac movement. One has been 'generalisability'. Studies on cadavers allow selected movements to be studied, but these movements may not be ones that occur in vivo. Studying a single isolated sacroiliac joint exaggerates the possible movements because the clamping effect of the other ilium has been removed. Fixing the entire pelvis in order to study pure sacroiliac motion eliminates the effects of pubic movement or deformation of the ilium when the sacrum is loaded.

For a realistic appreciation of sacroiliac movement, studies need to be conducted in living individuals but then technical difficulties obtain. Radiographically, the sacroiliac region is very complicated: the few landmarks are restricted to the sagittal plane and most margins of the bones under study are curved transversely. This makes landmark recognition essentially impossible. What appears to be the same point in lateral X-ray views is not necessarily the same point in a second view of a new position of the sacrum and pelvis. Errors in landmark recognition subsequently propagate into large errors in the geometry used to measure angular movement and the location of axes of rotation.

A further problem is sample size. A study of one specimen is inadequate, for it is not evident whether the specimen studied is typical or an extreme example.

Because of these problems, studies based on plain radiographs[24] or single specimens[25] are, in principle, unreliable and, at best, only indicative of what might be found using more reliable techniques or larger numbers of specimens. To ensure accurate landmark recognition, implanted devices are required. These establish unique landmarks. However, even then the implanted landmarks must be three-dimensional and multiple, lest rotations out of the plane of view exaggerate or reduce the apparent movement in the plane of view.

In this regard, studies using single wires or rods implanted into each of two moving bones[26] are unreliable because they do not account for three-dimensional movement. Furthermore, thin rods are subject to deformation and displacement by overlying skin, fascia and muscles.[27]

The most reliable results are obtained either by implanting tiny tantalum spheres into the bones of the pelvis and studying their relative movements by biplanar radiography, or by rigidly fixing onto the bones external devices that bear markers whose three-dimensional orientation can be determined.

The first study to use implanted spheres examined four patients moving from supine and prone positions to positions of standing, standing on one leg, and standing with maximum lumbar lordosis.[28] In essence, the range of sacroiliac motion observed in these manoeuvres, whether around a transverse, longitudinal or anteroposterior axis, was less that 2°, and was less than 1° in most cases. A later study of 25 patients, using the same technology confirmed these results.[29] Mean rotations were less than 2° and ranges were less than 4°. The same picture has been borne out in studies of intact pelvises in cadavers.[30,31]

A study using rigidly fixed external devices in 21 volunteers examined the range of motion of the sacroiliac joint during forward flexion of the trunk, during maximum extension of the trunk and standing on one leg.[32] The mean ranges of motion reported were less than 1°, with

standard deviations of not more than 0.9°. However, these results are somewhat illusory. They constitute the mean magnitude of the motion, irrespective of direction. During flexion of the trunk, the sacrum was just as likely to flex as to extend around its transverse axis.[32] Consequently, in a sample of individuals, the true mean range of motion of the sacroiliac joint is 0°, with as many individuals exhibiting up to 1° of rotation of the sacrum backwards as forwards, for the same excursion of the trunk. Thus, although the sacroiliac joints move, their direction of movement is irregular.

Subsequent, more recent, studies have examined the movements of the sacroiliac joint in a variety of postures and movements, such as the reciprocal straddle position,[33] and standing hip flexion.[34] They show that the range of movement is essentially only about 1°. Furthermore, even after therapeutic manipulation, the joint shows no change in position or movement.[35]

None of these data makes anatomical sense if one looks to the sacroiliac joint for primary movements. Its movements are feeble in magnitude and irregular in direction. Moreover, there are no muscles designed to act on the sacroiliac joint to produce active, physiological movements. All muscles that cross the joint are designed to act on the hip or the lumbar spine.

However, the nature of sacroiliac movements makes perfect sense in terms of the joint being a stress-relieving joint. In this regard the studies of Lavignolle et al. although not definitive, are nonetheless indicative.[36]

These investigators obtained biplanar radiographs of the sacroiliac region in individuals lying prone and alternatively flexing one hip while extending the other. The radiographs were used to determine the location of the instantaneous axes of rotation of the sacroiliac joint.

Instead of conventional axes passing transversely, longitudinally or sagittally through the joints, these investigators found that the axes of movement of the sacroiliac joints passed obliquely across the pelvis. For flexion, the axis passed backwards from the pubic symphysis to the greater sciatic notch. For extension, the axis passed from the pubic symphysis through the pelvis between the ischium and coccyx (Fig. 14.7). Given these axes, it is evident that during flexion and extension of the lower limbs, the sacrum undergoes complex movements. During flexion of the hip the ipsilateral ilium glides backwards and downwards across the sacrum and compresses against it, pivoting at the pubic symphysis. During extension, the ilium glides forwards and flares away from the sacrum.

None of these movements is produced by active movements of the sacrum. They are imposed on the sacroiliac joint by the mass of the trunk acting on the sacrum and tension exerted on the ilium from the muscles of the lower limbs. The nature of movements at the sacroiliac joint is fully consistent with the pelvis being distorted in three dimensions, and with the sacroiliac joint being designed to relieve the stress on the pelvic ring.

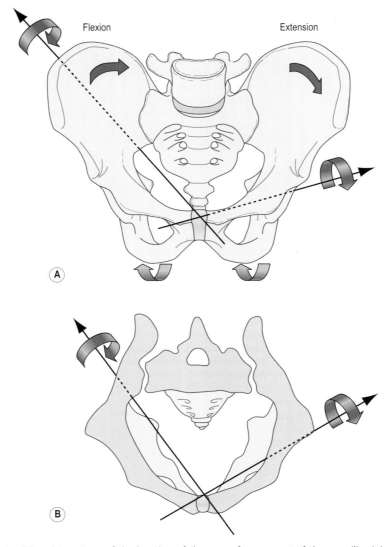

Figure 14.7 (A) Anterior (B) and top views of the location of the axes of movement of the sacroiliac joints during flexion and extension of the lower limbs. *(Based on Lavignolle et al. 1983.[36])*

REFERENCES

1. Cooper KL, Beabout JW, Swee RG. Insufficiency fractures of the sacrum. *Radiology*. 1985;156:15–20.

2. Cotty P, Fouquet B, Mezenge C, et al. Insufficiency fractures of the sacrum. *J Neuroradiol*. 1989;16: 160–171.

3. Davies AM, Evans NS, Struthers GR. Parasymphyseal and associated insufficiency fractures of the pelvis and sacrum. *Br J Radiol*. 1988;61: 103–108.

4. De Smet AA, Neff JR. Pubic and sacral insufficiency fractures: clinical course and radiologic findings. *Am J Roentgenol*. 1985;145:601–606.

5. Lourie H. Spontaneous osteoporotic fracture of the sacrum: an unrecognized syndrome of the elderly. *JAMA*. 1982;248:715–716.

6. Peris P, Guanabens N, Pons F, et al. Clinical evolution of sacral stress fractures: influence of additional pelvic fractures. *Ann Rheum Dis.* 1993;52:545–547.

7. Ries T. Detection of osteoporotic fractures with radionuclides. *Radiology.* 1983;146:783–785.

8. Weber M, Hasler P, Gerber H. Insufficiency fractures of the sacrum. Twenty cases and review of the literature. *Spine.* 1993;18: 2507–2512.

9. Vleeming A, Stoeckhart R, Volkers ACW, et al. Relation between form and function in the sacroiliac joint. Part I. Clinical anatomical aspects. *Spine.* 1990;15:130–132.

10. Wilder DG, Pope MH, Frymoyer JW. The functional topography of the sacroiliac joint. *Spine.* 1980;5: 575–579.

11. Williams PL, ed. *Gray's Anatomy.* 38th ed. Edinburgh: Churchill Livingstone; 1995.

12. Bowen V, Cassidy JD. Macroscopic and microscopic anatomy of the sacroiliac joint from embryonic life until the eighth decade. *Spine.* 1981;6:620–628.

13. Bellamy N, Park W, Rooney PJ. What do we know about the sacroiliac joint? *Semin Arthritis Rheum.* 1983;12:282–313.

14. Paquin JD, van der Rest M, Marie PJ, et al. Biochemical and morphologic studies of cartilage from the adult sacroiliac joint. *Arthritis Rheum.* 1983;26:887–895.

15. McLauchlan GJ, Gardner DL. Sacral and iliac articular cartilage thickness and cellularity: relationship to subchondral bone end-plate thickness and cancellous bone density. *Rheumatology.* 2002;41: 375–380.

16. Vleeming A, Volkers ACW, Snijders CJ, et al. Relation between form and function in the sacroiliac joint. Part II. Biomechanical aspects. *Spine.* 1990;15:133–135.

17. Vleeming A, Pool-Goudzwaard AL, Hammudoghlu D, et al. The function of the long dorsal sacroiliac ligament: its implication for understanding low back pain. *Spine.* 1996;21:556–562.

18. Bernard TN, Cassidy JD. The sacroiliac joint syndrome. Pathophysiology, diagnosis, and management. In: Frymoyer JW, ed. *The Adult Spine. Principles and practice.* New York: Raven Press; 1991:2107–2130.

19. Pitkin HC, Pheasant HC. Sacrarthogenetic telalgia I. A study of referred pain. *J Bone Joint Surg.* 1936;18:111–133.

20. Cole AJ, Dreyfuss P, Pauza K. Sacroiliac joint injection techniques. In: Vleeming A, Mooney V, Snijders C, et al, eds. *Second Interdisciplinary World Congress on Low Back Pain: the Integrated Function of the Lumbar Spine and Sacroiliac Joints.* Rotterdam: European Conference Organizers; 1995:569–597.

21. Grob KR, Neuhuber WL, Kissling RO. Innervation of the human sacroiliac joint. *Z Rheumatol.* 1995;54:117–122.

22. Ikeda R. Innervation of the sacroiliac joint: macroscopical and histological studies. *Nippon Ika Daigaku Zasshi.* 1991;58:587–596.

23. Schunke GB. The anatomy and development of the sacro-iliac joint in man. *Anat Rec.* 1938;72:313–331.

24. Weisl H. The movements of the sacroiliac joints. *Acta Anat.* 1955;80–91.

25. Frigerio NA, Stowe RR, Howe JW. Movement of the sacro-iliac joint. *Clin Orthop.* 1974;100:370–377.

26. Colachis SC, Worden RE, Bechtol CO, et al. Movement of the sacroiliac joint in the adult male. *Arch Phys Med Rehab.* 1963;44:490–498.

27. Vleeming A, Stoeckhart R, Snijders CJ. General introduction. In: Vleeming A, Mooney V, Snijders C, et al, eds. *First Interdisciplinary World Congress on Low Back Pain and its Relation to the Sacroiliac Joint.* Rotterdam: European Conference Organizers; 1992:3–64.

28. Egund N, Olsson TH, Schmid H, et al. Movements in the sacroiliac joints demonstrated with roentgen stereophotogrammetry. *Acta Radiol.* 1978;19:833–846.

29. Sturesson B, Selvik G, Uden A. Movements of the sacroiliac joints: a roentgen stereophotogrammetric analysis. *Spine.* 1989;14:162–165.

30. Miller JAA, Schultz AB, Andersson GB. Load–displacement behaviour of sacroiliac joints. *J Orthop Res.* 1987;5:92–101.

31. Vleeming A, van Wingerden JP, Dijkstra PF, et al. Mobility in the sacroiliac joints in the elderly: a kinematic and radiologic study. *Clin Biomech.* 1992;7:170–176.

32. Jacob HAC, Kissling RO. The mobility of the sacroiliac joints in healthy volunteers between 20 and 50 years of age. *Clin Biomech.* 1995;10:352–361.

33. Sturesson B, Uden A, Vleeming A. A radiostereometric, analysis of the movements of the sacroiliac joints in the reciprocal straddle position. *Spine.* 2000;25:214–217.

34. Sturesson B, Uden A, Vlemming A. A radiostereometric analysis of movements of the sacroiliac joints during the standing hip flexion test. *Spine.* 2000;25:364–366.

35. Tulberg T, Blomberg S, Branth B, et al. Manipulation does not alter the position of the sacroiliac joint. A Roentgen stereophotogrammetric analysis. *Spine.* 1998;23:1124–1129.

36. Lavignolle B, Vital JM, Senegas J, et al. An approach to the functional anatomy of the sacroiliac joints in vivo. *Anat Clin.* 1983;5:169–176.

Chapter | 15 |

Low back pain

Virtually every structure in the lumbar spine has at one time or another been implicated as a possible source of back pain. Throughout the 20th century, various structures were periodically popularised as the leading source of back pain. Some conjectures have lapsed, others persist, while still others have waxed and waned in popularity almost seasonally.

The reason for this sustained but erratic behaviour is that back pain demands an explanation, and the futility of conventional therapy renders practitioners susceptible to conjecture – when old ideas have proved unsatisfactory, any new theory that is in any way promising is readily adopted, even if it has been incompletely tested. As a result, controversy outweighs conviction in the field of low back pain. There is, however, information that sheds light on this field.

DEFINITIONS

Back pain

In an effort to standardise the use of terms and to set standards of diagnostic practice, the International Association for the Study of Pain (IASP) published the second edition of its taxonomy.[1] This document provides definitions of clinical terms used to describe pain and sets criteria for the diagnosis of specific entities.

With respect to presenting complaints, the taxonomy defines spinal pain topographically. It recognises 'lumbar spinal pain' and 'sacral spinal pain'.[1] Lumbar spinal pain is defined as pain perceived within a region bounded laterally by the lateral borders of the erector spinae, superiorly by an imaginary transverse line through the T12 spinous process, and inferiorly by a line through the S1 spinous process. Sacral spinal pain is defined as pain perceived within a region overlying the sacrum, bounded laterally by imaginary vertical lines through the posterior superior and posterior inferior iliac spines, superiorly by a transverse line through the S1 spinous process, and inferiorly by a transverse line through the posterior sacrococcygeal joints.

Low back pain can then be defined as pain perceived as arising from either of these two areas or from a combination of both. Whether or not the pain radiates elsewhere is another matter. The cardinal feature is that it appears to arise in these areas.

This definition does not presuppose the cause of pain, nor does it imply that the source of pain actually lies in the lumbar spine or sacrum. It is simply a definition based essentially on where a patient points to when they indicate where they *feel* their pain is stemming from.

Somatic pain

Somatic pain is pain that results from noxious stimulation of one of the musculoskeletal components of the body.[1,2] Neurophysiologically, the essential feature is that it arises as a result of the stimulation of nerve endings in a bone, ligament, joint or muscle.

'Somatic pain' is a term that stands in contrast to 'visceral pain', in which the noxious stimulus occurs in a body organ, and in contrast to 'neurogenic pain' in which the nociceptive information arises as a result of irritation or damage, not to nerve endings but to the axons or cell bodies of a peripheral nerve.

Referred pain

Referred pain is pain perceived in a region innervated by nerves other than those that innervate the actual source of pain.[1,2] As such, referred pain may be perceived in areas relatively remote from the source of pain, but often the distinction is blurred when the regions of local pain and referred pain are contiguous and the two pains appear to be confluent. A knowledge of the innervation of the affected regions, however, serves to make the distinction.

An example is low back pain associated with pain in the buttock. In this case, the low back pain appears to spread (i.e. radiate) into the buttock, but although the lumbosacral region and the buttock share a similar segmental nerve supply (L4, L5, S1), the back is innervated by the dorsal rami of these nerves, whereas the deep tissues of the buttock are innervated by the ventral rami (represented in the superior gluteal and inferior gluteal nerves). The buttock pain is therefore an example of referred pain.

The physiological basis for referred pain is convergence.[1] Within the spinal cord and in the thalamus, sensory neurones that subtend different peripheral sites converge onto common neurones that relay to higher centres. In the absence of any additional sensory information, the brain is unable to determine whether activity in the common neurone was initiated by one or the other of its peripheral inputs.

When the source of pain lies in a viscus, referred pain may be perceived in those parts of the body wall with a similar segmental nerve supply as the viscus. This type of referred pain may be described as **visceral referred pain**. In contrast, when the source of pain lies in skeletal or muscular structures, the referred pain may be described as **somatic referred pain** to emphasise its somatic, as opposed to visceral, origin.

Clinically, the characteristic features of somatic referred pain are that it is perceived deeply, it is diffuse and hard to localise and it is aching in quality.[2] Physiologically, the critical feature is that it is evoked by the stimulation of nerve endings in the structure that is the primary source of pain. The sensory nerves that innervate the region of referred pain are not activated by the primary stimulus, nor do they convey the referred pain. Referred pain occurs because of a misperception of the origin of the signal which reaches the brain by a convergent sensory pathway. These features underlie the distinction between somatic referred pain and radicular pain.

RADICULOPATHY

Radiculopathy is a neurological condition in which conduction is blocked in the axons of a spinal nerve or its roots.[1,2] Conduction block in sensory axons results in numbness; conduction block in motor axons results in weakness. Radiculopathy can be caused by compression or ischaemia of the affected axons. Systematically, these causes are outlined in Table 15.1.

Table 15.1 The causes of radiculopathy

Condition	Cause
Foraminal stenosis	Vertical subluxation of vertebrae[3,4]
	Osteophytes from disc[5–10]
	Osteophytes from zygapophysial joint[11–13]
	Buckled ligamentum flavum[14]
	Cyst of ligamentum flavum[15]
	Slipped inferior articular epiphysis[16]
	Ganglion[17–21]
	Synovial tumour[22]
	Infections and tumours of vertebrae[11,12]
	Paget's disease[11,23]
	Zygapophysial lipoma[24,25]
Epidural disorders	Lipoma; angioma[11,12]
	Infections[11]
Meningeal disorders	Cysts of the nerve root sleeve[11,26–29]
	Intradural ossification[30]
Neurological disorders	Diabetes[31]
	Cysts and tumours[11]
	Infections; tabes dorsalis[11]
Disc herniation	

An important realisation is that radiculopathy does not cause pain, either in the back or in the lower limbs. Explicitly, it is a state of neurological loss. If radiculopathy is associated with pain, the mechanism of that pain may not necessarily be the same as the cause of the radiculopathy. Radiculopathy may be associated with somatic referred pain, in which case the mechanisms of pain and the cause of radiculopathy will be distinctly different. On the other hand, radiculopathy may be associated with radicular pain, in which case the aetiology may be the same for both features, but the mechanisms of each will not be exactly the same.

RADICULAR PAIN

Radicular pain is pain that arises as a result of irritation of a spinal nerve or its roots.[1,2] Radicular pain may be associated with radiculopathy but not necessarily so. Radicular pain may occur without radiculopathy and radiculopathy may occur without radicular pain.

It was once believed that radicular pain was due to compression of nerve roots. This is patently untrue. Neurophysiological experiments have shown that compression of a nerve root does not evoke nociceptive activity; at best it evokes a brief discharge at the time of application of the compression stimulus, but thereafter the root becomes silent.[32,33] It is only when dorsal root ganglia are compressed that sustained activity is evoked, but this activity occurs not only in nociceptive axons but also in β fibres.[32,33] The sensation, therefore, must be more than just pain. This is borne out in clinical experiments.

Clinical experiments have shown that compressing normal nerve roots with urinary catheters evokes paraesthesia and numbness but not pain.[34] Similarly, traction on a normal nerve root does not evoke pain.[35] It is only when previously damaged nerve roots are squeezed by forceps[36] or pulled with sutures,[35] or when nerve roots are stimulated electrically,[37] that a characteristic pain is evoked. The pain is shooting or lancinating in quality and travels down the lower limb along a band no more than 50 mm (2 inches) wide.[35]

In quality and distribution, this type of pain is distinct from somatic referred pain. Radicular pain is shooting and band like, whereas somatic referred pain is constant in position but poorly localised and diffuse, and is aching in quality.

In the face of this evidence, it is pertinent to consider the term 'sciatica'. The implied basis for sciatica is nerve root compression or nerve root irritation, whereupon sciatica must be considered a form of radicular pain. However, the available physiological evidence dictates that radicular pain has a characteristic quality and distribution, and therefore the term sciatica should be restricted to this type of pain in the lower limb. The only type of pain that has ever been produced experimentally by stimulating nerve roots is shooting pain in a band-like distribution.[2] There is no physiological evidence that constant, deep aching pain in the lower limb arises from nerve root irritation. This latter type of pain constitutes somatic referred pain and there is no justification for misrepresenting it as 'sciatica', or for inferring that it arises from nerve root irritation. Moreover, there is no evidence that back pain can be caused by nerve root irritation, especially in the absence of neurological signs indicative of nerve root irritation. Indeed, on clinical grounds it has been estimated that fewer than 30%, and perhaps as few as 5% or 1%, of presentations of low back pain are associated with nerve root irritation due to disc herniation.[38–40] A formal survey in the USA established that no more than 12% of patients with low back pain had any clinical evidence of disc herniation.[41]

Disc herniation is the single most common cause of radicular pain, and there is increasing evidence that this condition causes pain by mechanisms other than simple compression. The evidence against compression is twofold. On myelography, CT or MRI, individuals can exhibit root compression by disc herniation but have no symptoms.[42–45]

Conversely, patients previously symptomatic can still exhibit root compression on medical imaging despite resolution of their symptoms.[46,47] These observations indicate that some factor in addition to, or quite apart from, root compression operates to produce symptoms. The current evidence implicates some form of inflammation.

Inflammation was implicated initially on the grounds that surgeons have often seen signs of nerve root inflammation when operating on herniated discs.[48,49] Some early post-mortem studies reported signs of inflammation around nerve roots obtained at autopsy,[50] but others found no such signs.[51,52] Subsequently, a variety of studies suggested that nuclear material was inflammatory[49,53-55] and perhaps capable of eliciting an autoimmune response.[56-62] However, clinical studies failed to reveal features of a classic autoimmune diathesis in patients with prolapsed discs.[63] Nevertheless, belief in some form of inflammation has persisted and has been explored.

In animal studies, compression of lumbar nerve roots causes oedema and increased intraneural pressure,[64,65] and application of nucleus pulposus to nerve roots induces inflammatory changes in the form of increased vascular permeability, oedema, and intravascular coagulation.[66-69] The inflammation damages the nerve roots, blocks nerve conduction,[67,70-73] and produces hyperalgesia and pain behaviour.[74-76] The mediators of this inflammatory response are phospholipase A_2, nitric oxide and tumour necrosis factor alpha (TNF-α).[70,75-82]

Studies in human patients have shown that herniated disc material attracts macrophages, fibroblasts and lymphocytes[83-90]; and that a variety of inflammatory chemicals are produced by these cells or the disc material itself. These chemicals include: phospholipase A_2;[91,92] metalloproteinases;[93,94] prostaglandin E_2;[89,93,94] leukotriene B_4 and thrombaxane;[95] nitric oxide;[80,81,93,94] interleukin 8;[96,97] interleukin 12 and interferon γ;[88] and TNF-α.[96] The disc material stimulates the production of IgM and IgG antibodies,[98] particularly to the glyco-sphingolipid of the nerve roots.[99] These inflammatory changes are more pronounced in patients in whom disc material has penetrated the anulus fibrosus and posterior longitudinal ligament, i.e. when it has become exposed in the epidural space.

The evidence is, thus, abundant that disc material evokes a chemical inflammation. The resulting nerve root oedema causes conduction block and the features of radiculopathy. Ectopic impulses generated in the dorsal root ganglia are responsible for the radicular pain,[100-102] and are probably produced by ischaemia.[65]

Yet, these processes are not restricted to the nerve roots. Unavoidably, perineurial inflammation must involve the dural sleeve of the affected nerve roots. Since the dura is innervated by the sinuvertebral nerves, pain may result from the epiduritis. But this pain is neither radicular nor neurogenic. Because it stems from irritation of nerve endings in the dura, it is a form of somatic pain.

Accordingly, nerve root inflammation may be associated not only with radicular pain but also with somatic referred pain from the inflamed dura of the nerve root sleeve.

BACK PAIN

Notwithstanding the exact mechanism of radicular pain, what is quite clear is that back pain and sciatica are not synonymous. Radicular pain is felt in the lower limb, not in the back. Back pain and somatic referred pain cannot be ascribed to disc herniation or nerve root irritation. Back pain implies a somatic origin for the pain and invites a search for its source among the skeletal elements of the lumbar spine.

Postulates

From a philosophical perspective, the status of any conjecture concerning the possible causes of back pain can be evaluated by adopting certain criteria analogous to Koch's postulates for bacterial diseases. For any structure to be deemed a cause of back pain:

1. The structure should have a nerve supply, for without access to the nervous system it could not evoke pain.
2. The structure should be capable of causing pain similar to that seen clinically. Ideally, this should be demonstrated in normal volunteers, for inferences drawn from clinical studies may be compromised by observer bias or poor patient reliability.
3. The structure should be susceptible to diseases or injuries that are known to be painful. Ideally, such disorders should be evident upon investigation of the patient but this may not always be possible. Certain conditions may not be detectable using currently available imaging techniques, whereupon the next line of evidence stems from post-mortem studies or biomechanical studies which can provide at least prima facie evidence of the types of disorders or injuries that might affect the structure.
4. The structure should have been shown to be a source of pain in patients, using diagnostic techniques of known reliability and validity. From such data, a measure of the prevalence of the condition in question can be obtained to indicate whether the condition is a rarity or oddity, or a common cause of back pain.

In the shadow of these postulates, the possible sources and causes of back pain can be determined by reviewing the anatomy of the lumbar spine and sacrum. The credibility of any source or of any cause can be measured by determining how well it satisfies the postulates.

Sources of back pain

VERTEBRAE

There is no doubt that the vertebral bodies of the lumbar vertebrae are innervated.[103–105] Nerve fibres, derived from the plexuses of the anterior longitudinal ligament and posterior longitudinal ligament, supply the periosteum of the bones and penetrate deep into the vertebral bodies where they provide a possible substrate for bone pain. However, it is not known whether the intraosseous nerves are exclusively vascular (either vasomotor or vasosensitive) or whether the bone of the vertebral body itself receives a sensory innervation.

For understandable logistic reasons, no experiments have demonstrated whether back pain can be evoked directly from bone in the vertebral body, but like periosteum in general[106] the vertebral periosteum is clearly pain sensitive. Needling the periosteum in the course of procedures such as lumbar sympathetic blocks is regularly associated with pain.

The vertebral body may be affected by painful, metabolic bone diseases such as Paget's disease[107] or osteitis fibrosa,[108] and it may be the site of primary or secondary tumours[109,110] or infections.[111,112] There is no dispute that such conditions can be painful, but how they actually cause pain is not known.

It may be that bone itself can hurt but no experimental data substantiate this belief. Irritation of perivascular sensory nerves within the bone is only a conjectural mechanism. Periosteal irritation as a result of either inflammation or distension by a space-occupying lesion is a plausible mechanism and has the attraction of being consistent with an early, silent phase for lesions like tumours or infections; pain ensues only when the periosteum is stretched.

Fractures of the vertebral body may or may not be painful,[113,114] and it is difficult to determine whether the pain stems from the fracture itself or arises from abnormal stresses applied to adjacent joints, muscles or ligaments as a result of the accompanying deformity. There is no evidence that fractures, anywhere in the body, are intrinsically painful, especially when stable. On the other hand, tissue deformation as a result of post-traumatic haematoma or oedema is readily viewed as a potent source of pain, particularly if this causes distension or inflammation of the periosteum. Such a model conveniently explains why acute vertebral fractures might be painful, but why old or healed fractures are not. Surrounding tissue swelling would be expected early in the history of a fracture, but in due course would subside. Persistent pain following a healed vertebral body fracture suggests a source beyond the fracture site and probably secondary to the resultant deformity.

The most common disease that affects lumbar vertebral bodies is osteoporosis but there is no evidence that this condition is painful, in the absence of fracture. The temptation is to infer that pain could arise directly from stresses applied to the weakened vertebral body, or that microfractures mechanically irritate perivascular sensory nerves within the vertebral spongiosa[115] but in the absence of even remote evidence about the physiology of bone pain, such explanations are purely speculative.

Citing the literature on vertebroplasty and its claims of success, some authors have argued that the pain of osteoporosis fractures is mediated by intraosseous nerves, and is relieved by a neurolytic effect of cement injected into the fractured vertebral body.[116] However, this argument is circular because it presupposes that the relief of pain reported from vertebroplasty can be attributed to a local effect of treatment at the fracture site. Others dispute this argument on the grounds that nerve fibres in the vertebral body are too irregularly present and too sparse to explain the relief of pain by vertebroplasty.[117] There is also evidence that the pain of osteoporotic fractures of vertebral arises, not from the affected vertebral body but from the posterior elements behind that vertebral body.[118]

A revolutionary, though now not new, concept concerning vertebral pain is that of intraosseous hypertension.[119,120] The notion is that, if obstructed, intraosseous veins become distended and stimulate sensory nerves in their adventitia. The cause of obstruction is suggested to be bony sclerosis, such as that which occurs in spondylosis and which narrows the bony channels through which the veins pass. This hypothesis is consistent with the presence of perivascular nerves in the vertebral bodies and is analogous to the pain of congestive venous disorders of the lower limb. However, while this is an attractive theory for the pain of spondylosis, manometric studies of vertebral intraosseous pressure have been limited in number and have not compared symptomatic with asymptomatic individuals to provide convincing statistical evidence in support of the theory.[119,120]

Regardless of how they might cause pain, disorders of the lumbar vertebrae are relatively easy to diagnose; they are readily apparent on radiographs and other medical imaging. Their prevalence is not explicitly known but appears to be very low. Infections, tumours and fractures of the vertebral bodies are rare amongst patients presenting with back pain under the age of 50 years.[121] Even in older patients they are uncommon.

Posterior elements

The posterior elements of the lumbar vertebrae may be affected by disorders such as secondary tumours in the pedicle and fractures of the transverse processes, and the mechanisms of pain in these disorders are understandable in terms similar to those applied for tumours and fractures of the vertebral body. Otherwise, there are several distinctive lesions of the posterior elements of the lumbar vertebrae.

Kissing spines

The lumbar spinous processes may be affected by Baastrup's disease,[122] otherwise known as 'kissing spines'.[123] This arises as a result of excessive lumbar lordosis or extension injuries to the lumbar spine in which adjacent spinous processes clash and compress the intervening interspinous ligament. The resultant pathology is perhaps best described as a periostitis of the spinous processes or inflammation of the affected ligament. Given that the periosteum of the spinous processes and the interspinous space are innervated by the medial branches of the lumbar dorsal rami,[124,105,125–127] it is understandable that such a condition would constitute a source of pain.

However, clinical studies suggest that this condition has been overrated. In one study, only 11 out of 64 patients with kissing spines responded to surgical excision of the lesion.[128]

Lamina impaction

A condition analogous to kissing spines can affect an inferior articular process. In some lumbar motion segments, extension is limited by impaction of an inferior articular process onto the lamina below (see Ch. 8). In such segments, repeated extension injuries can result in irritation of the periosteum of the lamina and, indeed, such lesions have been demonstrated at post-mortem.[129–131] This disorder is attractive as an explanation for some forms of back pain affecting athletes such as gymnasts accustomed to excessive forceful extension, but no clinical studies have yet provided evidence for its occurrence in living, symptomatic patients.

Spondylolysis

Spondylolysis was originally considered to be a defect due to failure of union of two ossification centres in the vertebral lamina. Modern evidence, however, clearly shows that it is an acquired defect caused by fatigue fracture of the pars interarticularis.[132–134] Anatomically, the defect is filled with fibrous scar tissue riddled with free nerve endings and nerve fibres containing calcitonin gene-related peptide, vasoactive intestinal peptide and neuropeptide Y.[135,136] Nominally, therefore, it could be a source of pain.

However, pars defects are not necessarily painful. In a survey of radiographs of 32 600 asymptomatic individuals, a pars defect was present in 7.2%.[137] Amongst 936 asymptomatic adults, a unilateral defect was present in 3% and a bilateral defect in a further 7%.[138] The corresponding figures in patients with back pain were 0.3% and 9%, respectively. In children aged 6 years, the prevalence of a defect was found to be 4.4%, and rose to 6% by adulthood.[139]

These population data indicate that it is not possible to incriminate a pars defect as the source of back pain on the basis of radiographic findings. The condition is as prevalent amongst patients with back pain as it is in the normal community. If the pars defect is to be incriminated, some other form of evidence is required. That comes in the form of diagnostic blocks.

The pars defect can be infiltrated with local anaesthetic under fluoroscopic control.[140] Relief of pain constitutes prima facie evidence that the defect is the source of pain. However, precautions need to be taken to ensure that the local anaesthetic has not anaesthetised an adjacent structure (such as a zygapophysial joint, which might be an alternative source of pain) and to ensure that the response to a single diagnostic injection is not due to a placebo effect. Nevertheless, relief of pain following infiltration of a pars defect is a good predictor of successful outcome following fusion of the defect and failure to obtain relief predicts poor response to fusion.[140]

Alternative sources of pain are an important consideration in view of the biomechanics of a bilateral pars defect. In the presence of a bilateral pars fracture, the spinous process and laminae of the affected vertebra constitute a flail segment of bone (the so-called 'rattler') to which fibres of the multifidus muscles still attach. It is therefore conceivable that during flexion movements of the lumbar spine, the multifidus would pull on the flail segment, but this affords no resistance to displacement of the vertebral body because it is disconnected from the spinous process on which the muscle is acting. Instead, the rattler is drawn further into extension as the vertebral body flexes. This extension could strain the zygapophysial joint to which the rattler remains attached. Pain could arise because of excessive movement either at the fracture site or at the zygapophysial joints. However, no published studies have addressed this hypothesis.

Bone scans are used by some practitioners to diagnose symptomatic pars fractures but the relationships between positive bone scans and either radiological evidence of a fracture or pain are imperfect.[141] Bone scans are most useful before a fracture has actually occurred, when the scan detects the stress reaction in the pars interarticularis. Once fracture has occurred the scan may or may not be positive, and tends to be negative in patients with chronic pain.[141]

MUSCLES

The muscles of the lumbar spine are well innervated. Quadratus lumborum and psoas are supplied by branches of the lumbar ventral rami,[142] while the back muscles are supplied by the dorsal rami.[124] The intertransverse muscles are variously supplied by the dorsal rami and ventral rami.[143]

There is no question that the back muscles can be a source of back pain and somatic referred pain. This has been demonstrated in experiments on normal volunteers in whom the back muscles were stimulated with injections of hypertonic saline.[144,145] These injections produced low back pain and various patterns of somatic referred pain in the gluteal region.

What remains contentious is the nature of disorders that can affect the muscles of the lumbar spine. Notwithstanding uncommon diseases such as polymyositis, which do not selectively affect the lumbar spine alone, the cardinal conditions that allegedly can affect the back muscles are sprain, spasm, imbalance and trigger points.

Sprain

A belief in the concept of muscle sprain stems from everyday experience and sports medicine where it is commonplace for muscles of the limbs to become painful following severe or sustained exertion, or after being suddenly stretched. It is therefore easy to postulate that analogous injuries might befall the back muscles, but what remains contentious is the pathology of such injuries.

Animal studies have shown that when muscles are forcibly stretched against contraction, they characteristically fail at the myotendinous junction.[146–148] The resulting lesion would presumably evoke an inflammatory repair response, which is easily accepted as a source of pain. In the case of the back muscles, such lesions could be incurred during lateral flexion or combined flexion–rotation injuries of the trunk and would be associated with tenderness near the myotendinous junctions of the affected muscles. Some of these sites are superficial and accessible to clinical examination, but others are deep. Deep sites lie near the tips of the transverse and accessory processes of the lumbar vertebrae. Accessible myotendinous junctions lie just short of the ribs near the insertions of the iliocostalis lumborum.

More diffuse muscle pain following exertion is theoretically explicable on the basis of ischaemia. One can imagine that during sustained muscle contraction the endomysial circulation is compressed, on the one hand obstructing washout of metabolites such as lactic acid and ADP which are algogenic, or on the other hand reducing arterial blood flow and causing muscle cell death, the breakdown products of which are also algogenic. Such mechanisms probably underlie some cases of exertional back pain, but this pain should be self-limiting as in the case of muscular pains of the limbs following severe exercise or unaccustomed activity.

Conspicuously, what is lacking in the case of back muscle injuries is any direct evidence of the responsible lesion. The only data that might be invoked come from experiments in animals in which the muscles of the limbs, not the back muscles, were studied. Biopsy data in humans or imaging data have not been published. For this reason a workshop sponsored by the American Academy of Orthopedic Surgeons and the National Institutes of Health was circumspect and inconclusive in its approach to the notion that sprained back muscles were a common cause of pain.[149] However, the advent of MRI may now provide a suitable non-invasive tool with which traumatic lesions of the back muscles might be identified.[150]

Spasm

Although myotendinous tears might underlie cases of acute back pain stemming from muscle, it is more difficult to explain chronic back pain in terms of muscle pain. A popular belief is that of muscle 'spasm'.[151] The implication is that as a result of some postural abnormality, or secondary to some articular source of pain, muscles become chronically active and therefore painful. If it occurs, such pain can only be explained on the basis of ischaemia, but the greatest liability of this model of muscular pain is that the purported evidence for its existence is inconclusive.[151] Electromyographic data are inconsistent, and it is unclear what so-called muscle spasm constitutes in objective physiological terms: whether it is tonic contraction or simply hyperreflexia. Further research data are required before this notion can become more acceptable, together with an explanation of whether the pain arises as a result of ischaemia, strain on the muscle attachments or some other mechanism.

Imbalance

Another concept is that of 'muscle imbalance'.[152] It is believed that aberrations in the balance of tone between postural and phasic muscles, or between flexors and extensors, can give rise to pain. In the case of the lumbar spine, the imbalance is said to occur between the trunk extensors and psoas major on the one hand, and the trunk flexors and hip extensors on the other. While attractive to some, this theory is without proper foundation. In the first instance, it is unclear how the imbalance comes to be painful: whether the pain arises from one or other of the muscles involved or whether the imbalance somehow stresses an underlying joint. Belief in the theory is founded on the clinical detection of muscle imbalance, but the reliability and validity of the techniques used have never been determined, and so-called muscle imbalances have been pronounced as abnormal without proper comparison to normal biological variation. Objective corroborating evidence is required before this theory attracts more widespread credibility.

Trigger points

Trigger points are tender areas occurring in muscle capable of producing local and referred pain. They are characterised by points of exquisite tenderness located within palpable bands of taut muscle fibres. Clinically, they are distinguished from tender areas by the presence of the palpable band of fibres, which, when snapped, elicits a localised twitch response in the muscle, and which when pressed reproduces the patient's referred pain.[153] The pain is relieved if the trigger point is injected with local anaesthetic.

Trigger points are believed to arise as a result of acute or chronic repetitive strain of the affected muscle,[153] or 'reflexly' as a result of underlying joint disease.[154] Histological and biochemical evidence as to the nature of trigger points are incomplete or inconclusive,[153] but they are believed to represent areas of hypercontracted muscle cells that deplete local energy stores and impair the function of calcium pumps, thereby perpetuating the contraction.[153–155] Pain is said to occur as a result of obstruction of local blood flow and the accumulation of algogenic metabolites such as bradykinin.[153]

Trigger points have been reported to affect the multifidus, longissimus and iliocostalis muscles,[156] and the quadratus lumborum.[157] However, it is not known how often they are a cause of back pain as the diagnostic criteria are so hard to satisfy.

For the diagnosis of trigger points in the iliocostalis and longissimus muscles, the kappa scores for two observers agreeing ranged from 0.35 to 0.46, which is less than satisfying.[158] Similar scores obtain for trigger points in the quadratus lumborum and gluteus medius.[159] It is only if the diagnostic criteria for trigger points are relaxed, to exclude palpable band and twitch response, that acceptable kappa scores are achieved,[159] but this changes the diagnosis from one of 'trigger point' to one of 'tender point' in the muscle.

Without reliable criteria for diagnosis, it is not possible to estimate the prevalence of trigger points as a cause of back pain. If classic criteria are used strictly, trigger points seem to be uncommon.[159] Tenderness, on the other hand, seems to be quite common but does not constitute a diagnosis.

THORACOLUMBAR FASCIA

Compartment syndrome

At its attachment to the supraspinous ligaments, the thoracolumbar fascia is well innervated.[126,127,160] However, little is known about the innervation of its central portions. There is only a mention in one study that it contains nociceptive nerve endings.[161] Nevertheless, it would appear that the fascia is appropriately innervated to be a source of pain if excessively stretched.

Since the thoracolumbar fascia encloses the back muscles, it forms a compartment surrounding them, and this has attracted the proposal that the back may be affected by a compartment syndrome.[162,163] The concept is that, in susceptible patients, the back muscles swell during and following activity but their expansion is restricted by the thoracolumbar fascia. Pain presumably arises as a result of excessive strain in the fascia.

The clinical marker of such a compartment syndrome would be raised intracompartmental pressure, but clinical studies have yielded mixed results. In one study, a series of 12 patients was investigated for suspected compartment syndromes. Only one patient exhibited sustained, elevated pressures in the compartment on the side of pain.[164] In another study, however, seven patients were identified whose compartment pressure rose above normal upon flexion and was associated with the onset of back pain; fasciotomy reportedly relieved their pain.[165] However, while offering intriguing results, this study did not rigorously report the variance of pressures in the control group and other diagnostic groups who also exhibited raised pressures. Therefore, it is not evident how unique the feature of raised pressure is to compartment syndrome.

Fat herniation

The posterior layer of thoracolumbar fascia is fenestrated to allow the transmission of the cutaneous branches of the dorsal rami. These sites may be associated with painful herniations of fat.[166–173] It is unclear exactly how these herniations actually cause pain, but reportedly the pain can be relieved by infiltrating the site with local anaesthetic. In this regard, painful fat herniations resemble trigger points, but are distinguished clinically from trigger points by their extramuscular, subcutaneous location. Their prevalence is unknown.

DURA MATER

The dura mater is innervated by an extensive plexus derived from the lumbar sinuvertebral nerves. The plexus is dense over the ventral aspect of the dural sac and around the nerve root sleeves, but posterolaterally the innervation is sparse, and is entirely lacking over the posterior aspect of the dural sac.[103,174] Clinical experiments have shown that the dura is sensitive both to mechanical and chemical stimulation.[35,175] In both cases, stimulation invokes back pain and somatic referred pain into the buttock. This raises the possibility that dural irritation could be a source of back pain.

Back pain is well known in the context of neurological diseases in which the dura mater becomes inflamed in response to intrathecal blood or infection.[176] This establishes that the dura *can* be a source of back pain. Whether it is or not, in the context of musculoskeletal diseases, is subject to conjecture.

Since it is known that disc herniation can elicit a chemical inflammation of the nerve roots and perineurial tissues,[55,67,68,70,72] and that disc material contains high concentrations of phospholipase A_2,[91] which is highly inflammatory,[92] it seems reasonable to expect that the dural sleeve of the nerve roots could be irritated chemically by this inflammation. Such irritation would elicit somatic pain, perhaps with referred pain, in addition to, and quite apart from, any pain stemming from the inflamed nerve roots. This conjecture raises the spectre that what has been traditionally interpreted as 'root pain' associated with disc herniation may not be purely radicular pain but a mixture of radicular and dural pain. However, no studies have yet ventured to dissect dural pain from radicular pain in cases of disc herniation.

It has been inferred that dural tethering can be a cause of pain. This is consistent with the sensitivity of the dura to mechanical stimulation. Presumably, adhesions could develop as a result of chronic epidural inflammation following disc herniation. However, despite its popularity, this model for dural pain has not been formally explored. No correlations have yet been demonstrated between the presence of pain, the presence of positive dural tension signs and evidence of epidural fibrosis either on CT scans or at operation.

In a similar vein, it has been proposed that the normally occurring epidural ligaments can tether nerve roots and be a source of somatic pain superimposed on radicular pain.[177] However, as with dural 'adhesions' appropriate clinicopathological correlations have yet to be demonstrated.

Seductive evidence for dural pain comes from neurosurgical studies that report relief of post-laminectomy pain following resection of the nerves to the dura sleeve of the symptomatic nerve root.[178,179] Ostensibly, the pain was due to stimulation of the nerves by fibrosis of the dura.

However, no studies have established just how common dural pain is in either acute or chronic low back pain.

EPIDURAL PLEXUS

The epidural veins are innervated by the lumbar sinuvertebral nerves[103,180] and are therefore a possible source of pain. Presumably, pain could occur if these veins became distended when flow through them was obstructed by lesions such as massive disc herniation or spinal stenosis. However, circumstantial evidence of this concept has been provided in only one published study[181] and the concept has not otherwise been further explored.

LIGAMENTS

Many patients presenting with low back pain provide a history and clinical features that are analogous to those of patients with ligamentous injuries of the appendicular skeleton. This similarity invites the generic diagnosis of 'ligament strain' of the lumbar spine, but this diagnosis raises the question 'Which ligament?'.

The intertransverse ligament is actually a membrane and does not constitute a ligament in any true sense. Moreover, because it is buried between the erector spinae and quadratus lumborum, it is highly unlikely that any diagnostic test could distinguish lesions of the intertransverse membranes from lesions in the surrounding muscles.

The ligamentum flavum is poorly innervated[104,125,126,182,183] and is therefore unlikely to be a source of pain. Furthermore, there are no known lesions that affect the ligamentum flavum that could render it painful, and because the ligament is elastic, it is not susceptible to sprain. It has a distensibility far in excess of that of the posterior longitudinal ligament and other collagenous ligaments of the lumbar spine.[184]

The so-called supraspinous ligament has been shown to consist of collagen fibres derived from the thoracolumbar fascia, the erector spinae aponeurosis and the tendons of multifidus.[185,186] Technically, it is therefore a raphe rather than a ligament, but the most decisive evidence against the supraspinous ligament being a source of back pain at L4 and L5 (the most common location of low back pain) is that the ligament is totally lacking. It is consistently absent at L5, frequently so at L4, and even at L3 it is poorly developed and irregularly present.[186]

The posterior longitudinal ligament is innervated by the sinuvertebral nerves, and the anterior longitudinal ligament by fibres from the lumbar sympathetic trunk and grey rami communicantes.[103,180,187] Reports that probing the back of a lumbar disc at operation under local anaesthetic reproduces the patient's back pain,[188,189] engender the belief that the pain naturally stems from the overlying posterior longitudinal ligaments. However, the posterior longitudinal ligament blends intimately with the anulus fibrosus of the intervertebral disc at each segmental level. Anatomically the longitudinal ligaments are not separable from the anulus fibrosus other than at a microscopic level. It is therefore not legitimate to consider disorders of the ligaments separately from those of the anulus fibrosus (see below).

Otherwise, it is only with respect to two substantive ligaments of the lumbar spine – the interspinous and iliolumbar ligaments – that recordable data exist about their being sources of back pain.

Interspinous ligaments

The interspinous ligaments receive an innervation from the medial branches of the lumbar dorsal rami,[44,105,124–127] and experimental stimulation of the interspinous ligament produces low back pain and referred pain in the lower limbs.[190–192] This renders the interspinous ligament as an attractive source of low back pain.

Post-mortem studies have shown that the interspinous ligaments are frequently 'degenerated' in their central portions,[186] but it is not known whether or not such lesions are painful. Otherwise, it is conceivable that interspinous ligaments might be subject to strain following excessive flexion of lumbar motion segments, but evidence of this is currently still lacking, even by way of comparing clinical history with the presence of midline interspinous tenderness and relief of pain following infiltration with local anaesthetic.

Clinical studies of the prevalence of interspinous ligament sprain are sobering. Steindler and Luck[193] reported that in a heterogeneous population of 145 patients, 13 obtained complete relief of their pain following anaesthetisation of interspinous ligaments, suggesting a prevalence of less than 10%. A more recent audit of the experience of a musculoskeletal general practice found only 10 patients in a series of 230 whose pain could be relieved by anaesthetising an interspinous ligament.[194] Since these injections were not controlled, the observed prevalence of 4% must be construed as a best-case estimate.

Iliolumbar ligament

The iliolumbar ligament has not explicitly been shown to have an innervation but presumably it is innervated by the dorsal rami or ventral rami of the L4 and L5 spinal nerves. Biomechanically, the iliolumbar ligament serves to resist flexion, rotation and lateral bending of the L5 vertebra,[195–197] and could therefore be liable to strain during such movements. However, the evidence implicating the iliolumbar ligament as a source of back pain is inconclusive.

Some investigators have regarded tenderness over the posterior superior iliac spine as a sign of iliolumbar ligament sprain[198] but this is hard to credit, for the ligament lies anterior to the ilium and is buried by the mass of the erector spinae and multifidus. Consequently, tenderness in this region cannot be explicitly ascribed to the iliolumbar ligament. Some have claimed to have relieved back pain by infiltrating the iliolumbar ligament,[199] but because of the deep location of this structure, there can be no guarantee that, without radiological confirmation, the ligament was accurately or selectively infiltrated.

Other investigators have been more circumspect in interpreting tenderness near the posterior superior iliac spine, and question whether the pain stems from the iliolumbar ligament, the lumbosacral joint or the back muscles.[200–202] Indeed, radiographic studies of injections made into the tender area reveal spread, not into the iliolumbar ligament but extensively along the iliac crest.[198] Accordingly, the rubric – iliac crest syndrome – has been adopted to describe this entity.[200,201] Others have referred to it simply as lumbosacral strain.[202]

What all investigators have overlooked is that the site of tenderness in iliac crest syndrome happens to overlie the site of attachment of the lumbar intermuscular aponeurosis (LIA), which constitutes a common tendon for the lumbar fibres of longissimus thoracis.[203,204] The LIA attaches to the iliac crest rostromedial to the posterior superior iliac spine and exhibits a morphology not unlike that of the common extensor origin of the elbow. Thus, a basis for pain and tenderness in this region could be a tendonopathy of the LIA. On the other hand, it could be no more specific than tenderness in the posterior back muscles, which has been recognised for many years under different rubrics.[202,205,206]

Regardless of its underlying pathology, the putative advantage of recognising an iliac crest syndrome is that perhaps specific therapy might be applied. In this regard, if iliac crest syndrome is defined simply as tenderness over the medial part of the iliac crest, the kappa score for its diagnosis is 0.57.[207] If the criteria are extended to include reproduction of typical pain, the kappa score rises to 0.66.[207] These scores indicate that the syndrome can be identified. Its prevalence seems to be about 30–50%.[200] However, as long as the syndrome amounts to no more than tenderness, it is not evident whether it is a unique disorder or a feature that could occur in association with other sources and causes of back pain.

Recognising the syndrome, however, has little impact on treatment. Injecting the area with local anaesthetic is significantly more effective than injecting it with normal saline, but only some 50% of patients benefit and only 30% obtain more than 80% improvement.[200]

SACROILIAC JOINT

The sacroiliac joint is reported to have an innervation. Branches of the L4–L5 and S1–S2 dorsal rami are directed to the posterior sacroiliac and interosseous sacroiliac ligaments,[208] but it is not known whether these nerves actually reach the sacroiliac joint itself which lies substantially ventral of these ligaments. Anteriorly, the sacroiliac joint is said to receive branches from the obturator nerve, the lumbosacral trunk and the superior gluteal nerve,[209] but the original sources for this claim are obscure. Modern studies provide conflicting results, with some reporting an innervation from both the front and the back,[210] while others report an exclusively posterior innervation.[211]

In normal volunteers, stressing the sacroiliac joint with injections of contrast medium produces somatic pain focused over the joint, and a variable referral pattern into the lower limb.[212] Thus, the joint is quite capable of being a source of back pain.

In orthodox medical circles, recognised disorders of the sacroiliac joint include ankylosing spondylitis, other spondylarthropathies, various infectious and metabolic diseases,[213] and an idiopathic sacroiliitis that typically befalls women,[214] but controversy surrounds alleged mechanical disorders of the joint. Manual therapists claim that such disorders can be diagnosed on the basis of palpable hypomobility of the joint and abnormal relations between the sacrum and ilium.[215-220] However, biomechanical and radiographic studies reveal only a very small range of movement in the sacroiliac joint, even in patients diagnosed as having hypermobility.[221-223] Nor does manipulation of the joint alter its position.[224] These data provide grounds for scepticism as to whether pathological disturbances of movement can be palpated in a joint that has only 1° of movement.

However, formal studies have shown that sacroiliac joint pain can be diagnosed using intra-articular injections of local anaesthetic. In patients with chronic low back pain, the prevalence of sacroiliac joint pain is about 15%.[225,226] The pathology of this pain is not known, although ventral capsular tears seem to underlie some cases.[226]

Although it can be diagnosed using intra-articular injections of local anaesthetic, sacroiliac joint pain cannot be diagnosed using orthodox clinical examination.[226] Furthermore, it cannot be diagnosed using osteopathic or chiropractic techniques. Although these latter procedures have good reliability, they have no validity; they cannot distinguish patients who respond to diagnostic blocks from those who do not.[227] Thus, although sacroiliac joint pain is common in patients with chronic low back pain, it can only be diagnosed using diagnostic local anaesthetic blocks.

ZYGAPOPHYSIAL JOINTS

The lumbar zygapophysial joints are well innervated by the medial branches of the lumbar dorsal rami.[103-105,124,228] Their capacity to produce low back pain has been established in normal volunteers. Stimulation of the joints with injections of hypertonic saline or with injections of contrast medium produces back pain and somatic referred pain identical to that commonly seen in patients.[229,230] Conversely, certain patients can have their pain relieved by anaesthetising one or more of the lumbar zygapophysial joints.[230-234]

Referred pain from the lumbar zygapophysial joints occurs predominantly in the buttock and thigh but does not follow any clinically reliable segmental pattern.[229]

Radiation of referred pain below the knee can occur, even as far as the foot,[230,231] but typically the pain involves the more proximal segments of the lower limb. There is some evidence that the distance of radiation is proportional to the intensity of the pain generated in the back.[230]

Belief in lumbar zygapophysial joint pain dates back to 1933 when Ghormley[235] coined the term 'facet syndrome'. The entity has enjoyed a resurgence of interest over the last 20 years and, for reference, the history of this interest is recorded in detail elsewhere.[236,237] However, much of the literature on the prevalence of zygapophysial joint pain has been made redundant.

Prevalence

In the past, the criterion standard for diagnosing lumbar zygapophysial joint pain was complete relief of pain following anaesthetisation of one or more of these joints.[236-238] However, it has now been shown that such blocks are not valid because they are associated with an unacceptable false-positive rate.[237,239] Only one in three patients who respond to a first diagnostic block respond to subsequent repeat blocks.[233] Moreover, the placebo response rate to diagnostic blocks is 32%.[234] This means that previous data, based on uncontrolled diagnostic blocks, overestimate the prevalence of this condition.

To be valid, diagnostic blocks must be controlled in some way, in each and every patient. Unless such precautions are taken, for every three apparently positive cases, two will be false-positive.[234]

Using controlled diagnostic blocks, several studies have tried to estimate the prevalence of lumbar zygapophysial joint pain. Variously they have reported the prevalence to be 15% in a sample of injured workers in the USA,[232] 40% in an Australian population of elderly patients in a rheumatology practice[234] and 45% among patients of various ages attending a pain clinic in the USA.[240]

Collectively, these studies suggest that lumbar zygapophysial joint pain is quite common. However, in all of these studies the criterion for a positive response to blocks was not complete relief of pain but only at least 50% relief of pain. This is a somewhat contentious criterion, for it does not explain the remnant pain. Although the investigators presumed that incomplete relief of pain indicates another, concurrent source of pain, this has never been verified. The only studies that have addressed this question found that multiple sources of pain, in the one patient, were uncommon. Patients tend to have discogenic pain, sacroiliac joint pain, or lumbar zygapophysial joint pain, in isolation. Fewer than 5% have zygapophysial joint pain as well as discogenic pain,[241] or lumbar zygapophysial joint pain as well as sacroiliac joint pain.[226] The alternative interpretation – that back pain was imperfectly relieved by the blocks – has not been excluded. If the latter applies, the cited prevalence rates may be an overestimate.

When complete relief of pain, following lumbar zygapophysial joint blocks, has been used as the criterion for zygapophysial joint pain, studies have reported a much lower prevalence: substantially less than 10%.[242,243] In a general population, therefore, lumbar zygapophysial joint pain may not be as common as previously believed. Nevertheless, one study, which used 90% relief of pain as the criterion, did find the prevalence of lumbar zygapophysial joint pain to be 32% in an elderly population.[234]

Overall, it would seem that amongst younger workers with a history of injury to their lumbar spine, lumbar zygapophysial joint pain is uncommon, accounting for 10% or less of these patients. Amongst older patients, with no history of injury, the prevalence is greater, and may exceed 30%.

Clinical features

Despite beliefs to the contrary,[244,245] controlled studies have shown that lumbar zygapophysial joint pain cannot be diagnosed clinically.[232,234,246] Controlled diagnostic blocks are the only means available to date of establishing a diagnosis of lumbar zygapophysial joint pain.

Pathology

Although the prevalence of zygapophysial joint pain is known, what remains elusive is its pathology. The lumbar zygapophysial joints can be affected by rheumatoid arthritis,[247-249] ankylosing spondylitis[250] or un-united epiphyses of the inferior articular processes,[251-253] and there have been case reports of rare conditions such as pigmented villonodular synovitis[254,255] and suppurative arthritis.[256-259] However, these conditions have not been identified as the cardinal causes of pain in patients responding to diagnostic zygapophysial joint blocks.

Post-mortem studies[131,260,261] and radiological surveys[262,263] have shown that the lumbar zygapophysial joints are frequently affected by osteoarthrosis, and studies of joints excised at operation revealed changes akin to chondromalacia patellae.[264] Although it is asserted that zygapophysial arthritis is usually secondary to disc degeneration or spondylosis,[131] in about 20% of cases it can be a totally independent disease.[260]

The prevalence of zygapophysial osteoarthrosis attracts the belief that this condition is the underlying cause in patients with zygapophysial joint pain.[244,264-266] However, on plain radiographs zygapophysial osteoarthrosis appears as commonly in asymptomatic individuals as in patients with back pain.[262,263] Features indicative of osteoarthritis on CT scans were once held to be indicative of zygapophysial joint pain[264,265,267] but controlled studies have shown that CT is of no diagnostic value for lumbar zygapophysial joint pain.[268] These data preclude making the diagnosis of painful zygapophysial arthropathy on the basis of plain radiography. They also indicate either that osteoarthrosis is not a cause of zygapophysial joint pain or that, when it is, the pain is due to some factor other than the simple radiological presence of this condition.

Injuries

Biomechanics studies have shown that the lumbar zygapophysial joints can be injured in a variety of ways and to various extents.

Extension of the lumbar spine may be limited by impaction of an inferior articular process on the lamina below (see Ch. 8). Under these conditions, continued application of an extension force results in rotation of the affected segment around the impacted articular process, which draws the inferior articular process of the contralateral zygapophysial joint backwards (Fig. 15.1). As a result, the capsule of that joint is disrupted.[269]

Rotation of a lumbar intervertebral joint normally occurs around an axis located in the posterior third of the vertebral bodies and intervertebral disc (see Ch. 8). Rotation is limited by impaction of the zygapophysial joint opposite the direction of movement but if torque continues to be applied rotation can continue around a new axis located in the impacted joint. As a result, the contralateral inferior articular process is drawn backwards and medially and the joint capsule on that side is disrupted (Fig. 15.2). The lesions that occur in biomechanics experiments include tears of the capsule, avulsion of the capsule or fracture-avulsion of the capsule.[270] The impacted joint may sustain fractures of its subchondral bone or articular processes, or the pars interarticularis may fail.[271-276]

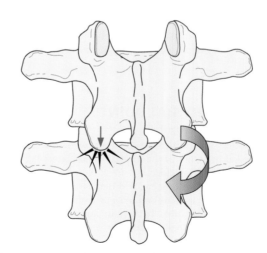

Figure 15.1 Extension injury to a lumbar zygapophysial joint. When extension is arrested by impaction of an inferior articular process on the lamina, the contralateral inferior articular process is forced backwards into rotation, resulting in capsular disruption.

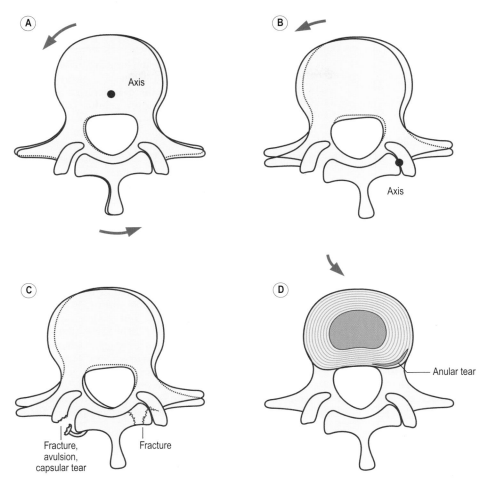

Figure 15.2 Torsion injuries to a lumbar intervertebral joint. (A) Rotation initially occurs about an axis through the posterior third of the intervertebral disc but is limited by impaction of a zygapophysial joint. (B) Further rotation occurs about a new axis through the impacted joint; the opposite joint rotates backwards while the disc undergoes lateral shear. (C) The impacted joint may suffer fractures of its articular processes, its subchondral bone or the pars interarticularis; the opposite joint may suffer capsular injuries. (D) Subjected to torsion and lateral shear, the anulus fibrosus suffers circumferential tears.

Capsular tears, capsular avulsion, subchondral fractures, intra-articular haemorrhage and fractures of the articular processes, such as those produced in biomechanics studies, have all been found in post-mortem studies.[277,278] However, in no case were any of these lesions evident on plain radiographs.

Fractures of the zygapophysial joints have occasionally been recorded in the past in the radiology literature[251,279–281] but by and large, these fractures cannot be detected on plain radiographs.[277,278] Fractures should be visible on CT scans although fractures have not been reported in the CT scans of patients with proven painful lumbar zygapophysial joints.[268] Thus, fractures are either not the basis for most cases of zygapophysial joint pain, or they are too small or subtle to be detected by conventional use of lumbar CT.

Lesions such as capsular tears cannot be detected by radiography, CT or MRI. It may be that these lesions underlie zygapophysial joint pain, or it may be that the mechanism of pain is due to some process that is both radiologically invisible and still to be determined.

Meniscus extrapment

A relatively common clinical syndrome is 'acute locked back'. In this condition, the patient, having bent forward, is unable to straighten because of severe focal pain on attempted extension. Because this condition does not lend itself to high resolution investigations like CT scanning and MRI, its cause remains speculative. However, theories have been advanced involving the concept of meniscus extrapment.

Normal lumbar zygapophysial joints are endowed with fibroadipose meniscoids (see Ch. 3),[282,283] and following trauma, segments of articular cartilage still attached to joint capsules may be avulsed from the articular surface to form an acquired cartilaginous meniscoid.[284] These meniscoid structures could feasibly act as loose bodies within the joint or be trapped in the subcapsular pockets of the joints.

Upon flexion, one of the fibroadipose meniscoids is drawn out of the joint but upon attempted extension it fails to re-enter the joint cavity (Fig. 15.3). Instead, it impacts against the edge of the articular cartilage, and in this location it buckles and acts like a space-occupying lesion under the capsule, causing pain by distending the capsule.[285] Maintaining flexion is comfortable for the patient because that movement disengages the meniscoid. Treatment by manipulation becomes logical. Passive flexion of the segment reduces the impaction, and rotation gaps the joint, encouraging the meniscoid to re-enter the joint cavity (see Fig. 15.3).[285]

This condition of meniscoid entrapment is only theoretical, for it is difficult, if not impossible, to visualise meniscoids radiologically. However, it reigns as one of the plausible explanations for some cases of acute locked back, particularly those amenable to manipulative therapy.[285]

DISCOGENIC PAIN

The concept that the lumbar intervertebral discs might be a source of pain is not new. As long ago as 1947, it was recognised that the discs received a nerve supply and so could be intrinsically painful.[286] However, this concept remained suppressed by erroneous declarations that the discs were not innervated and so could not be painful.[287]

There is now no doubt that the lumbar discs are innervated.[103–105,187,287–292] Consequently, there can be no objection on anatomical grounds that they *could* be sources of back pain.

Disc stimulation

Despite its chequered and controversial history, disc stimulation (formerly known as discography) remains the only means of determining whether or not a disc is painful.[293–295] The procedure involves introducing a needle into the nucleus pulposus of the target disc and using it to distend the disc with an injection of normal saline or contrast medium.[295] The test is positive if upon stimulating a disc the patient's pain is reproduced *provided that stimulation of adjacent discs does not reproduce their pain.*[1,295,296] Moreover, modern guidelines insist that the pressure of injection is critical.[295] Discs are considered symptomatic only if pain is reproduced at pressures of injection less than 50 psi and preferably less than 15 psi.

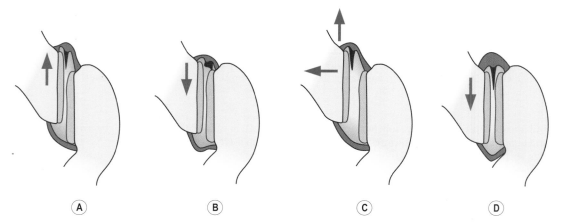

Figure 15.3 Meniscus extrapment. (A) Upon flexion, the inferior articular process of a zygapophysial joint moves upwards, taking a meniscoid with it. (B) Upon attempted extension, the inferior articular process returns towards its neutral position but the meniscoid, instead of re-entering the joint cavity, impacts against the edge of the articular cartilage, and buckles, forming a space-occupying 'lesion' under the capsule. Pain occurs as a result of capsular tension, and extension is inhibited. (C) Manipulation of the joint, involving flexion and gapping, reduces the impaction and opens the joint to encourage re-entry of the meniscoid into the joint space (D).

At low pressures of injection, disc stimulation does not cause pain in normal volunteers. In a normal disc the innervated outer third of the anulus fibrosus is buffered by the dense inner two-thirds of the anulus fibrosus from mechanical and chemical stimuli directed to the central nucleus pulposus. The anulus fibrosus is designed to withstand immense pressures within the nucleus pulposus, and therefore one should not expect disc stimulation to be able to cause pain in a normal disc. Only at high pressures of injection, over the order of 80 psi or more, are some discs painful in normal individuals.

Previous studies that reported painful stimulation of discs in normal volunteers[297] have been refuted on methodological grounds,[298] and a stringent study found no painful discs in asymptomatic individuals.[299] A more recent study found painful discs in only 10% of normal volunteers.[300] Another study showed that discs are not painful in normal volunteers if they are stimulated at pressures less than 40 psi.[301] A systematic review found that disc stimulation has a false-positive rate of less than 10%.[302] Disc stimulation, therefore, is specific for painful discs, and a positive response implies an abnormality that has rendered the disc painful.

This experience with stimulation of lumbar discs by injection has been complemented by another approach. Discs can be stimulated thermally, by heating a wire electrode inserted into the anulus of the disc.[303] Heating the disc evokes pain, which is initially perceived in the back, but which can be referred in different patterns into the lower limb. The referred pain may be perceived in the buttock, or posterior thigh, and even in the leg (i.e. below the knee). Since the noxious stimulus is restricted to the disc, and does not affect the nerve roots, thermal heating provides evidence not only that lumbar discs can be painful, but also that they can be responsible for somatic referred pain in the thigh and leg.

Pathology

At present, data on the pathology of disc pain are incomplete and are largely circumstantial but there are sufficient data to enable three entities to be described: discitis; torsion injuries; and internal disc disruption.[304]

Discitis

Iatrogenic discitis is the archetypical lesion that renders a disc painful.[305,306] In this condition, the disc is infected by bacteria introduced by needles used for discography. The process is restricted to the disc and is evident on bone scans and MRI. The condition is intensely painful and there is no evidence that the pain arises from sources other than the infected disc.

Fortunately iatrogenic discitis is rare but as an example it serves to establish the principle that discs, affected internally by a known and demonstrable lesion, can be painful.

Torsion injury

When an intervertebral joint is forcibly rotated, injuries can occur to the disc as well as the posterior elements (see Fig. 15.2). Rotation about the normal axis of rotation pre-stresses the anulus, but once further rotation ensues around the secondary axis through the impacted zygapophysial joint (see Fig. 15.2B), the disc is subjected to an additional lateral shear. The combination of torsion and lateral shear results in circumferential tears in the outer anulus (see Fig. 15.2D).[270,307,308] The risk of injury is greater if rotation is undertaken in flexion, for then the flexion pre-stresses the anulus to a near maximal extent, and the added rotation takes the collagen fibres of the anulus beyond their normal strain limit.[309]

In discs with concave posterior surfaces, circumferential tears occur in the posterolateral corner of the anulus fibrosus; in discs with convex posterior surfaces the tears occur posteriorly. The reason for these locations lies in the stress distribution across a disc subjected to torque.[273,308] These are locations where the lamellae of the anulus fibrosus exhibit the greatest relative curvature and where torsional strains are maximal. Consequently, they are sites where collagen fibres are most likely initially to fail under torsion.

Torsion injuries, however, are only a theoretical diagnosis. The condition can be suspected on clinical grounds given the appropriate mechanical history of a flexion–rotation strain. Neurological examination is normal because the lesion is restricted to the anulus fibrosus and does not involve nerve root compression. For the same reason, CT scanning, myelography and MRI are normal, and discography will be normal since the nucleus pulposus is not involved in the lesion. The condition is essentially a ligament sprain and behaves as such. Theoretically, the pain should be aggravated by any movements that stress the anulus fibrosus, but in particular flexion and rotation in the same direction that produced the lesion.[310] However, these clinical features are not enough to prove the diagnosis.

Circumferential tears of the anulus are not visible on any contemporary imaging technique, including MRI,[311] but it is possible to identify the lesion by other means.[312,313] Contrast medium and local anaesthetic can be injected into the putatively painful tear in the anulus fibrosus. If the tear is painful, the local anaesthetic relieves the pain, and the contrast medium outlines the tear, which can then be seen on a post-procedural CT scan as a crescent in the outer anulus fibrosus (Fig. 15.4).

This procedure, however, is still experimental, and no studies have reported the prevalence of torsion injuries diagnosed in vivo. Consequently, torsion injury remains a

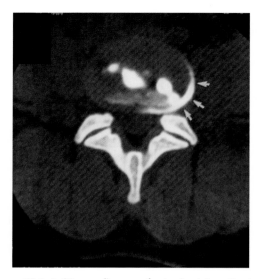

Figure 15.4 A CT scan diagram of a torsion injury. Contrast medium and local anaesthetic were injected into a putatively painful circumferential tear in the anulus fibrosus. The contrast medium shows that the injectate was deposited in a crescent fashion in the anulus. The local anaesthetic abolished the patient's pain. The nucleus is outlined because of an earlier discogram, which was painless. *(Courtesy of Hunter Valley X-Ray, Newcastle, Australia.)*

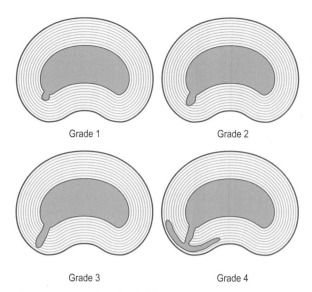

Figure 15.5 Grades of radial fissures in internal disc disruption. Grade 1: disruption extends into the inner third of the anulus fibrosus. Grade 2: disruption extends as far as the inner two-thirds of the anulus. Grade 3: disruption extends into the outer third of the anulus fibrosus. Grade 4: a grade 3 fissure spreads circumferentially between the lamellae of the outer anulus.

theoretical diagnosis but one that may assume greater prominence in the future.

Internal disc disruption

Internal disc disruption (IDD) has emerged as the most extensively studied, and best understood, causes of chronic low back pain. For no other condition are there such strong correlations between the morphology of the condition, its biophysics and pain.

Morphologically, IDD is characterised by degradation of the nuclear matrix and the presence of radial fissures, extending from the nucleus into the anulus fibrosus. For descriptive purposes, the fissures can be graded according to the extent to which they penetrate the anulus (Fig. 15.5):[314]

- Grade 1 fissures reach only the inner third of the anulus.
- Grade 2 fissures reach the second, or middle, third.
- Grade 3 fissures extend into the outer third of the anulus.
- Some investigators recognise a fourth grade, which is a grade 3 fissure that expands circumferentially around the outer anulus.[315]

IDD is not disc degeneration, as commonly understood. It is not a diffuse process affecting the entire disc. Rather, it is a focal disorder, affecting a single sector of the anulus

fibrosus. The remainder of the anulus remains intact and normal.

Also, IDD is not equivalent to disc herniation. Although the radial fissures contain nuclear material, that material has not herniated. It remains contained within the disc. The external perimeter of the anulus remains intact. The disc may exhibit a diffuse bulge, but there is no focal protrusion of nuclear material beyond the normal perimeter of the anulus.

The extent to which the anulus is penetrated by radial fissures correlates strongly with the affected disc being painful on disc stimulation.[316,317] Grade 1 fissures are typically not painful. Grade 2 fissures may or may not be painful but some 70% of grade 3 fissures are associated with pain, and some 70% of painful discs exhibit a grade 3 fissure.[316].

This pattern correlates with the density of innervation of the disc. The inner third of the anulus lacks an innervation and so grade 1 fissures do not have access to a nerve supply. The middle third of the anulus may or may not have an innervation. So, grade 2 fissures may or may not have access to a nerve supply. The outer third of the anulus is consistently innervated. So, grade 3 fissures consistently have access to the nerve supply of the disc.

Studies using multivariate analysis have shown that IDD is independent of degenerative changes.[317] Degenerative changes increase with age but do not correlate with the

Table 15.2 The correlation between anular disruption and reproduction of pain by disc stimulation. The numbers refer to the number of patients exhibiting the features tabulated. $\chi^2 = 148$; $P < 0.001$. (Based on Moneta et al. 1994.[317])

Pain reproduction	Anular disruption			
	Grade 3	Grade 2	Grade 1	Grade 0
Exact	43	29	6	4
Similar	32	36	21	8
Dissimilar	9	11	6	2
None	16	24	67	86

Stress

2MPa

Normal

Posterior

Anterior

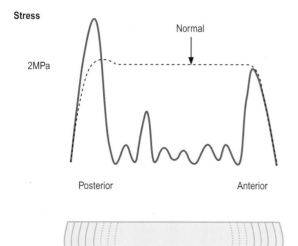

Table 15.3 The correlation between disc stimulation and changes in stress profile of the disc (Based on McNally et al. 1996.[318])

Anular stress	Pain	No pain	Fisher's exact test
Stressed	17	2	
Normal	1	11	$P = 0.001$
Nuclear stress			
Depressurised	11	0	
Normal	7	13	$P = 0.017$

Figure 15.6 The stress profile of a disc with internal disc disruption. The graph shows the irregular and reduced stress profile across the nucleus pulposus and a raised stress in the posterior anulus. The dotted line indicates the normal stress profile. *(Based on McNally et al. 1996.[318])*

disc being painful. Radial fissures occur at an early age and their prevalence does not increase with age. Yet fissures are strongly correlated with pain, independently of age changes (Table 15.2).[317]

Discs affected by IDD exhibit abnormal stress profiles (see Ch. 8). Nuclear stresses are reduced, irregular or absent (Fig. 15.6).[318] Meanwhile, stresses in the posterior anulus are increased greatly above normal. These features indicate that the degraded nuclear matrix is no longer able to retain water and does not contribute to sustaining compression loads on the disc. Instead, the compression load is transferred to the posterior anulus.

Each of these changes in the biophysical properties of the disc correlate with the disc becoming painful. Decreased nuclear stresses and increased stresses in the

posterior anulus each correlate with reproduction of pain by disc stimulation (Table 15.3).[318]

Collectively, these data constitute evidence of convergent validity. Different, and independent, techniques point to the same conclusion. IDD has a distinctive morphology that correlates strongly with pain and IDD has biophysical properties that correlate strongly with pain. For no other cause of low back pain have such multiple and strong correlations been demonstrated.

For many years, the aetiology of IDD remained elusive. It was addressed only by theoretical arguments. The reasons for this were that it was ethically impossible to induce IDD in normal volunteers, and it was not possible to study the evolution of the disorder in individuals affected by it because there is no marker of its onset.

Early proponents argued that IDD was the result of compression injuries to the disc. This proposition was based on intuition and studies of the mechanism of failure of discs subjected to compression.[273,308,319,320] This is consonant with the available biomechanical evidence.

Despite traditional wisdom in this regard, when compressed, intervertebral discs do not fail by prolapsing. In biomechanical experiments, it is exceedingly difficult to induce disc failure by prolapse. Even if a channel is cut

189

into the anulus fibrosus, the nucleus fails to herniate.[321-323] A normal nucleus is intrinsically cohesive and resists herniation. Even in specimens with partially herniated discs, completion of the prolapse rarely occurs even after repeated flexion and compression.[324]

When compressed, intervertebral discs typically fail by fracture of a vertebral endplate.[323,325-330] The forces required are usually quite large,[327,331] of the order of 10 000 N, but can be as low as 3000 N.[332] Although seemingly large, these forces are of a magnitude such as might be encountered in a sudden fall, landing on the buttocks or as a result of forceful muscle activity.[333] In a heavy lift, the back muscles can exert a longitudinal force of some 4000 N.[334] It transpires, therefore, that certain individuals could be susceptible to compression injury of their vertebral endplates if their vertebral bodies were weaker than the maximum strength of their muscles.

In such individuals, fracture of the vertebral endplate could occur during unaccustomed inordinate heavy lifting, or if they maximally exerted their back muscles in activities such as pulling on a stubborn tree root while gardening. In these situations the individual voluntarily exerts their back muscles to a severe degree, but the muscles act on a vertebral column that is unaccustomed to bearing the large loads involved. Training and physical exercise appear to condition vertebral bodies, rendering them stronger and better able to withstand the longitudinal stresses imposed upon them by severe efforts of the back muscles,[331,335] but the risk of endplate fracture prevails if athletes, workers and other individuals with relatively weak vertebral endplates are not conditioned to their task, and take on lifting activities for which their back muscles might be capable but their vertebrae are not.

These considerations presuppose sudden static loading. However, modern research has shown that endplate failure can occur at loads substantially less than ultimate failure strength of the endplate, if the endplate is fatigued (see Ch. 8).

If a normal disc is repetitively loaded, in compression or in compression with flexion, at loads between 37 and 50% of its ultimate failure strength, it can resist 1000 or 2000 repetitions without failing.[336,337] However, if it is loaded to between 50% and 80% of its ultimate strength, the endplate can fail, by fracturing, after as few as 100 repetitions.[336]

These latter figures are within the ranges encountered during normal working activities. Loads of between 50% and 80% of ultimate compression strength of the disc are not atypical of those encountered in heavy lifting or bending, and 100 repetitions are not atypical of a normal course of work. Thus, instead of sudden compression loads, endplate fractures can occur as a result of fatigue failure after repeated, submaximal compression loading.

An endplate fracture is of itself not symptomatic and may pass unnoticed. Furthermore, an endplate fracture may heal and cause no further problems (Fig. 15.7).

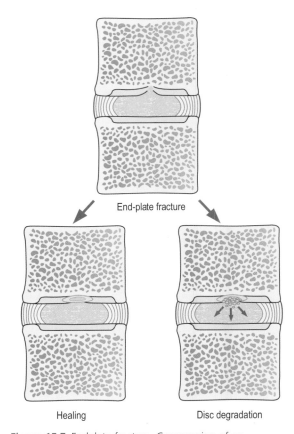

End-plate fracture

Healing

Disc degradation

Figure 15.7 Endplate fracture. Compression of an intervertebral disc results in fracture of a vertebral endplate. The fracture may heal or may trigger degradation of the intervertebral disc.

However, it is possible for an endplate fracture to set in train a series of sequelae that manifest as pain and a variety of endstages.

Early proponents of internal disc disruption argued that an endplate fracture simply elicited an unbridled, inflammatory repair response[273,274,308,319] that failed to heal the fracture but proceeded to degrade the matrix of the underlying nucleus pulposus.

Others subsequently ventured a bolder interpretation, suggesting that through the fracture, the proteins of the nuclear matrix are exposed to the circulation in the vertebral spongiosa, and elicit an autoimmune inflammatory response.[304,338,339] This proposal was based on evidence that showed that disc material was antigenic[55-59,340] and was consistent with observations that acute intraosseous disc herniation was associated with inflammation of the spongiosa.[341] The model invited an analogy with the condition of sympathetic ophthalmia in which release of lens proteins after an injury to an eye causes an autoimmune reaction that, in due course, threatens the integrity of the healthy eye. What lens proteins and disc proteins have in common is that neither has ever been exposed to the body's immune system, because the two tissues are avascular. Their proteins, therefore, are not recognised as self.

A more conservative interpretation could be that an endplate fracture interferes with the delicate homeostasis of the nuclear matrix. The matrix contains degradative enzymes whose activity is normally limited by tissue inhibitors of metalloproteinases.[60,61,342-345] Furthermore, the balance between synthesis and degradation of the matrix is very sensitive to changes in pH.[344,346] This invites the conjecture that an injury, such as an endplate fracture, might disturb the metabolism of the nucleus, perhaps by lowering the pH, and precipitate degradation of the matrix without an explicit inflammatory reaction. Indeed, recent biochemical studies suggest that increased activation of disc proteinases occurs progressively from the endplate into the nucleus, and that these proteinases either may be activated by blood in the vertebral body or may even stem from cells in the bone marrow.[347]

Regardless of its actual mechanism, the endplate theory supposes that fractures result in progressive degradation of the nuclear matrix. Nuclear 'degradation' may appear synonymous with disc 'degeneration' and, indeed, other authors have implicated the same biochemical processes described above as the explanation for disc degeneration.[348] However, they view this as an idiopathic phenomenon, and do not relate it to endplate fracture. In the present context, nuclear 'degradation' is not intended to mean 'degeneration'. 'Degeneration' is an emotive term, conjuring images of inevitable decay and destruction, yet many of the pathological changes said to characterise disc degeneration are little more than normal age changes (see Ch. 13). In contrast, nuclear degradation is a process, initiated by an endplate fracture, that progressively destroys the nucleus pulposus. It is an active consequence of trauma not a passive consequence of age.

When degradation is restricted to the nucleus pulposus, proteolysis and deaggregation of the nuclear matrix result in a progressive loss of water-binding capacity and a deterioration of nuclear function. Less able to bind water, the nucleus is less able to sustain pressures, and greater loads must be borne by the anulus fibrosus. In time, the anulus buckles under this load and the disc loses height, which compromises the functions of all joints in the affected segment (Fig. 15.8). As a result, reactive changes occur in the form of osteophyte formation in the zygapophysial joints and anulus fibrosus. This state, characterised by osteophytes and disc narrowing, has been recognised clinically and described as 'isolated disc resorption',[348,349] which becomes symptomatic if nerve roots are compromised by canal stenosis or foraminal stenosis.

In Chapter 13, it was explained that disc narrowing is not a consequence of age: discs retain their height with age.[350] A different explanation is required for disc narrowing, especially if it occurs at only one in five lumbar segments. The explanation lies in disc narrowing being a consequence of nuclear degradation following endplate fracture. However, disc narrowing and isolated disc resorption comprise only one possible endstage of disc degradation. This occurs when the anulus fibrosus remains intact circumferentially but when nuclear degradation and dehydration are severe.

In contrast, the water-binding capacity of the nucleus may not be so severely affected by nuclear degradation, whereupon the disc relatively retains its height. However, in time, nuclear degradation extends peripherally to erode the anulus fibrosus, typically along radial fissures, to establish the definitive features of internal disc disruption (see Fig. 15.8).

Ultimately, it is possible for internal disc disruption to progress to disc herniation (see Fig. 15.8). This occurs if the inflammatory degradation extends along a radial fissure for the entire thickness of the anulus. The conditions for disc herniation are thereby set – a defect has been produced in the anulus fibrosus and the nucleus pulposus has been denatured into a form that is expressible. In such a disc, compression loading during normal flexion may be sufficient to herniate the nucleus.

However, disc herniation is only one possible endstage of internal disc disruption, hence its relative rarity. In the meantime, the condition that prevails and renders the disc painful, without rupturing, is internal disc disruption.

Further evidence. Two lines of evidence have recently corroborated the importance of compression injury and endplate fracture in the aetiology of IDD. Both come from laboratory studies.

When cadaveric discs are repeatedly loading in compression, the onset of fatigue failure of the endplate can be detected by the sudden change in mechanical behaviour.[333] Harvesting the specimen at this time reveals the endplate fracture (Fig. 15.9). When stress profiles in the disc have been monitored during loading, another correlate has appeared. At the time of failure, the disc exhibits the onset of the biophysical changes of IDD. Nuclear stresses reduce and posterior anulus stress rises sharply (Fig. 15.10).

In laboratory animals, experimental induction of an endplate fracture precipitates the biochemical, morphological and biophysical changes of IDD.[351] The water content of the nucleus decreases, and proteoglycans decrease, the inner anulus delaminates and nuclear pressure falls.

Both of these experiments addressed only the immediate effects of endplate fracture. Neither examined what the long-term effects might be. Therefore, the experiments did not produce the full effects of what might be called 'full-blown' IDD. Nevertheless, both showed the onset of the features of IDD. Together they provide strong

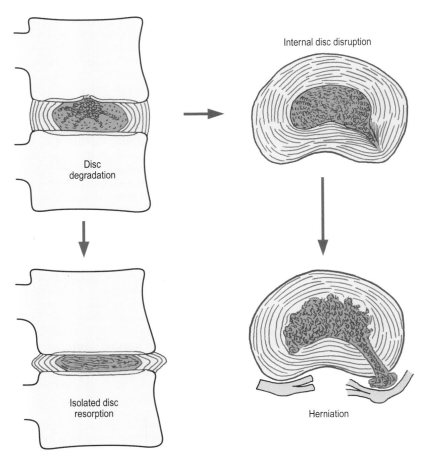

Internal disc disruption

Disc
degradation

Isolated disc
resorption

Herniation

Figure 15.8 Disc degradation. If restricted to the nucleus pulposus, disc degradation may lead to isolated disc resorption. Otherwise, it results in internal disc disruption, which is characterised by degradation of the nucleus pulposus and radial fissuring of the anulus fibrosus. If fissures reach the periphery of the anulus fibrosus, the degraded nucleus may herniate if the disc is subjected to compression.

circumstantial evidence that endplate fracture is the critical, initiating factor for the development of IDD.

Symptoms. The mechanism by which IDD becomes painful has not been explicitly demonstrated but two explanations apply. In the first instance, chemicals from the degraded nuclear matrix that enter the radial fissure might irritate nerve endings in the outer third of the anulus. This becomes the basis for chemical nociception from the disc. To this effect, there is evidence that inflammatory cells penetrate the anulus fibrosus of disrupted discs,[352] whereupon inflammatory chemical mediators may trigger nociceptive nerve endings.

Secondly, the disruption of the anulus provides a basis for mechanical nociception. In an intact anulus, mechanical loads would be borne uniformly across all the laminae of the anulus in any given sector. However, when a radial fissure penetrates the anulus, two-thirds or more of the

laminae are disrupted and cannot contribute to resisting mechanical loads. Consequently, the load is thrust onto the remaining intact laminae, which, therefore, are required to bear three times their normal load.

Chemical and mechanical processes may act simultaneously. Chemicals may sensitise the nerve endings in the outer anulus and amplify their response to mechanical stimulation.

These models predict the clinical features of IDD. The chemical nociception would produce a background of constant, dull, aching pain that is difficult to localise but which is felt deeply in the back. Mechanical nociception would be manifest as aggravation of that pain by any movements that strain the outer anulus. Movements that strain the anulus most would be the cardinal aggravating factors. Meanwhile, movements that strain the anulus less would be less aggravating.

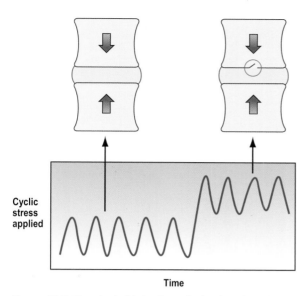

Figure 15.9 The physical behaviour of a lumbar disc when subjected to cyclic compression loading. During early cycles the disc remains intact. Failure is indicated by a sudden loss of resistance. This coincides with the onset of an endplate fracture.

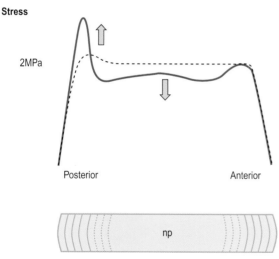

Figure 15.10 The stress profile of a disc at the time of failure when subjected to cyclic compression loading. There is a sudden decrease in nuclear stress and an increase in stress in the posterior anulus. *(Based on Adams et al. 1993.[333])*

There would be no other specific clinical features. In particular, since there is no herniation of disc material, radicular pain or radiculopathy would be absent. The features are no more specific than constant pain aggravated by movements. These are the features exhibited by patients in whom IDD is detected.

Diagnosis. There are no means by which IDD can be diagnosed clinically. The diagnosis requires reproduction of the patient's pain by disc stimulation, and the demonstration by postdiscography CT of a radial fissure (Fig. 15.11).

In some patients, the condition can be detected by MRI. In these patients, internal disc disruption is manifest by a signal of high intensity in the posterior anulus (Fig. 15.12). This signal is discontinuous with that of the nucleus and is somewhat brighter. Empirically, the presence of this high-intensity zone correlates strongly both with the disc being painful and with the presence of a grade 4 radial fissure.[315,353] Morphologically, the high-intensity zone seems to have the appearance, in sagittal section, of nuclear material running circumferentially in the posterior anulus.[315] Its relative brightness distinguishes it from asymptomatic transverse fissures and suggests that symptomatic fissures are ones that somehow have become 'activated', perhaps by inflammation of the tissue contained in the fissure.

A high-intensity zone is not exhibited by all patients who have IDD but it is evident in about 30% of patients with chronic back pain. When evident, it strongly implicates the affected disc as the source of pain.

Prevalence. IDD is the single most common detectable cause of chronic low back pain. Under the strictest of diagnostic criteria, and using worst-case analysis, its prevalence has been measured as 39%.[296] Under more liberal criteria, and allowing for multilevel disease, its prevalence may be considerable higher than this.

SUMMARY

This review of the possible sources and causes of back pain generates an interesting matrix of data. For each putative source of pain, one can check which of the postulates are satisfied and to what extent (see Table 15.4). In turn, this indicates the depth and quality of evidence to substantiate belief in any particular source or cause.

Structures such as muscle are innervated and have been shown to be sources of pain in normal volunteers. However, there are no data on underlying pathology that justify the belief that muscles can be a source of chronic low back pain. Nor are there any reliable data to indicate how often muscles are a source of chronic back pain, if indeed they ever are.

The interspinous ligaments are innervated and can be painful in normal volunteers. Presumably, they might become painful if sprained. Moreover, ligament pain can be diagnosed by anaesthetising the affected ligament. However, clinical data indicate that, at best, interspinous ligament pain is an uncommon basis for chronic low back pain.

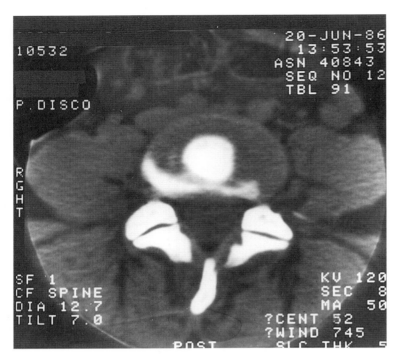

Figure 15.11 A CT discogram showing internal disc disruption. Contrast medium has been injected into the nucleus but outlines a radial fissure that spreads circumferentially around the anulus. The perimeter of the disc is intact; there is no herniation or disc bulge. This disc was symptomatic. *(Courtesy of Dr Charles Aprill, New Orleans, USA.)*

Table 15.4 The extent to which various proposed sources and causes of back pain satisfy the postulates for a structure to be a source of back pain. Muscle sprain, muscle spasm, trigger points and iliac crest syndrome are presumed to have been produced in normal volunteers in as much as pain from muscles, in general, has been so produced

Structure or cause	Postulates					
	Innervated	Pain in normal volunteers	Pathology known	Identified in patients	Prevalence	
					Acute back pain	*Chronic back pain*
Vertebral bodies	Yes	No	Yes	Yes	Rare	Rare
Kissing spines	Yes	No	Presumed	Yes	Unknown	Unknown
Lamina impaction	Yes	No	Presumed	No	Unknown	Unknown
Spondylolysis	Yes	No	Yes	Yes	<6%	<6%
Muscle sprain	Yes	Yes	Yes	Anecdotal	Unknown	Unknown
Muscle spasm	Yes	Yes	No	No	Unknown	Unknown
Muscle imbalance	Yes	No	No	Uncontrolled	Unknown	Unknown
Trigger points	Yes	Yes	No	Unreliable	Unknown	Unknown
Iliac crest syndrome	Yes	Yes	No	Yes	Unknown	30–50%
Compartment syndrome	Yes	No	No	Yes	Unknown	Unknown
Fat herniation	Yes	No	Yes	Yes	Unknown	Unknown
Dural pain	Yes	Yes	Presumed	Yes	Unknown	Unknown

Table 15.4 The extent to which various proposed sources and causes of back pain satisfy the postulates for a structure to be a source of back pain. Muscle sprain, muscle spasm, trigger points and iliac crest syndrome are presumed to have been produced in normal volunteers in as much as pain from muscles, in general, has been so produced—cont'd

Structure or cause	Postulates					
	Innervated	Pain in normal volunteers	Pathology known	Identified in patients	Prevalence	
					Acute back pain	*Chronic back pain*
Epidural plexus	Yes	No	No	No	Unknown	Unknown
Interspinous ligament	Yes	Yes	Presumed	Uncontrolled	Unknown	<10%
Iliolumbar ligament	Probably	No	No	No	Unknown	Unknown
Sacroiliac joint pain	Yes	Yes	No	Controlled studies	Unknown	13% (±7%)
Zygapophysial joint pain	Yes	Yes	No	Controlled studies	Unknown	<10% 32% (elderly)
Internal disc disruption	Yes	No	Yes	Controlled studies	Unknown	39% (±10%)

Figure 15.12 A magnetic resonance image of a lumbar spine showing a high-intensity zone lesion in the posterior anulus of the L4–L5 intervertebral disc.

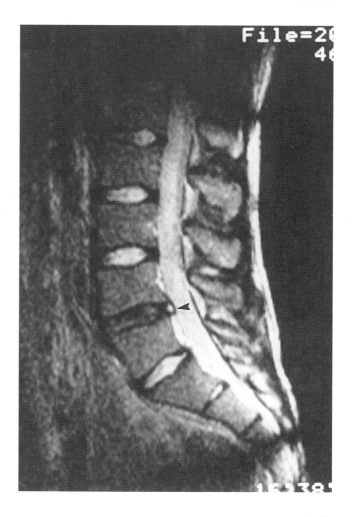

The causative pathology of lumbar zygapophysial joint pain is unknown. So too is the cause of sacroiliac joint pain. However, in both instances, the joint is innervated and has been shown to be capable of producing low back pain and referred pain in normal volunteers. Furthermore, controlled studies have established the prevalence of these conditions in patients with chronic low back pain.

For anatomical reasons, it is impossible to produce pain from an intervertebral disc in normal volunteers, but the discs are innervated and so have the appropriate apparatus to become sources of pain. The pathology of a painful disc is evident in internal disc disruption, and controlled studies have shown this condition to be a common cause of chronic low back pain.

Fascinatingly, there is a perverse correlation evident in this matrix (see Table 15.3). It emerges that those conditions that have attracted the greatest popularity in clinical practice – muscle pain, ligament pain, trigger points – are associated with the smallest amount of scientific evidence. Data on the mechanism of pain in these conditions and its prevalence are simply lacking. Also, no reliable means of diagnosis have been established. When subjected to scientific scrutiny, clinical examination for the diagnosis of these conditions has failed.

In contrast, the less popular diagnoses – zygapophysial joint pain, sacroiliac joint pain, IDD – are the ones that have the greatest amount of scientific data. No other conditions have survived as much scientific scrutiny as these. Diagnostic techniques are available and can be controlled if required. Prevalence data indicate that these conditions are common and, indeed, collectively account for over 60% of patients with chronic low back pain.

A second correlation that emerges is that the scientifically valid entities are all ones that require sophisticated techniques and specialised radiological facilities for their diagnoses. In contrast, the hitherto popular diagnoses are ones that are easy to make, and do not require sophisticated techniques or facilities: they are 'office' diagnoses and their treatments are 'office' procedures. Yet it is these diagnoses and treatments that are least supported by scientific evidence.

Perhaps this says more about the state of practitioners in spine medicine than the state of the art of spine science. If it is easy and simple, it will be believed in and adopted even though the evidence and science are lacking.

REFERENCES

1. Merskey H, Bogduk N, eds. *Classification of Chronic Pain. Descriptions of chronic pain syndromes and definitions of pain terms*, 2nd ed. Seattle: IASP Press; 1994.

2. Bogduk N. On the definitions and physiology of back pain, referred, pain and radicular pain. *Pain*. 2009;147:17–19.

3. Hadley LA. Apophyseal subluxation. Disturbances in and about the intervertebral foramen causing back pain. *J Bone Joint Surg*. 1936;18:428–433.

4. Hadley LA. Intervertebral joint subluxation, bony impingement and foramen encroachment with nerve root changes. *Am J Roentgenol*. 1951;65:377–102.

5. Arnoldi CC, Brodsky AE, Cauchoix J. Lumbar spinal stenosis. *Clin Orthop*. 1976;115: 4–5.

6. Ehni G. Significance of the small lumbar spinal canal: cauda equina compression syndromes due to spondylosis. *J Neurosurg*. 1962; 31:490–494.

7. Epstein JA, Epstein BS, Levine L. Nerve root compression associated with narrowing of the lumbar spinal canal. *J Neurol Neurosurg Psychiatry*. 1962;25:165–176.

8. Kirkaldy-Willis WH, Wedge JH, Yong-Hing K, et al. Pathology and pathogenesis of lumbar spondylosis and stenosis. *Spine*. 1978;3:319–328.

9. Verbiest H. A radicular syndrome from developmental narrowing of the lumbar vertebral canal. *J Bone Joint Surg*. 1954;36B: 230–237.

10. Verbiest H. Fallacies of the present definition, nomenclature and classification of the stenoses of the lumbar vertebral canal. *Spine*. 1976;1:217–225.

11. Cophignon J, Fischer G, Fuentes JM, et al. Les sciatiques chirurgicales non discales. *Neurochirurgie*. 1978;24:283–336.

12. Epstein BS. *The Spine. A radiological text and atlas*, 4th ed. Philadelphia: Lea & Febiger; 1976.

13. Epstein JA, Epstein BS, Levine LS, et al. Lumbar nerve root compression at the intervertebral foramina caused by arthritis of the posterior facets. *J Neurosurg*. 1973;39:362–369.

14. Naffziger HC, Inman V, Saunders JB. Lesions of the intervertebral disc and ligamenta flava. *Surg Gynecol Obstet*. 1938;66:288–299.

15. Haase J. Extradural cyst of ligamentum flavum L4 – a case. *Acta Orthop Scand*. 1972;43:32–38.

16. Pou-Serradell A, Casademont M. Syndrome de la queue de cheval et présence d'appendices apophysaires vertébraux, ou apophyses articulaires accessoires, dans la région lombaire. *Rev Neurol*. 1972;126:435–440.

17. Feldman R, McCulloch J. Juxta facet cysts of the lumbar spine. *Neuro-Orthopedics*. 1987;4:31–35.

18. Gritzka TL, Taylor TKF. A ganglion arising from a lumbar articular facet associated with low back pain and sciatica. Report of a case. *J Bone Joint Surg*. 1970;52B: 528–531.

19. Jackson DE, Atlas SW, Mani JR, et al. Intraspinal synovial cysts:

MR imaging. *Radiology*. 1989;170: 527–530.

20. Kao CC, Uihein A, Bichel WH, et al. Lumbar intraspinal extradural ganglion. *J Neurosurg*. 1968;29:168–172.

21. Reust P, Wendling D, Lagier R, et al. Degenerative spondylolisthesis, synovial cyst of the zygapophyseal joints, and sciatic syndrome: report of two cases and review of the literature. *Arthritis Rheum*. 1988;31:288–294.

22. Galibert P, Estefan G, Le Gars D, et al. Conflits mécaniques sciatalgiques par synovialome bénin des articulations rachidiennes. A propos de quatre cas. *Neurochirurgie*. 1983;29: 377–380.

23. Hadjipavlou AG, Lander PH. Paget's disease. In: White AH, ed. *Spine Care*, Vol. 2. St Louis: Mosby; 1995:1720–1737.

24. Dietmann JL, Bonneville JF, Runge M, et al. Computed tomography of lumbar apophyseal joint lipoma: report of three cases. *Neuroradiology*. 1989;31:60–62.

25. Husson JL, Chales G, Lancien G, et al. True intra-articular lipoma of the lumbar spine. *Spine*. 1987;12: 820–822.

26. Cloward RB. Congenital spinal extradural cysts. *Ann Surg*. 1968;168:851–864.

27. Fortuna A, La Torre E, Ciappetta P. Arachnoid diverticula: a unitary approach to spinal cysts communicating with the subarachnoid space. *Acta Neurochir*. 1977;39:259–268.

28. Glasauer FE. Lumbar extradural cysts. *J Neurosurg*. 1966;25: 567–570.

29. Tarlov IM. Spinal perineurial and meningeal cysts. *J Neurol Neurosurg Psychiatry*. 1970;33:833–843.

30. Varughese G. Lumbosacral intradural periradicular ossification. *J Neurosurg*. 1978;49:132–137.

31. Naftulin S, Fast A, Thomas M. Diabetic lumbar radiculopathy: sciatica without disc herniation. *Spine*. 1993;18:2419–2422.

32. Howe JF. A neurophysiological basis for the radicular pain of nerve root compression. In: Bonica JJ, Liebeskind JC, Albe-Fessard DG, eds. *Advances in Pain Research and Therapy*, Vol. 3. New York: Raven Press; 1979: 647–657.

33. Howe JF, Loeser JD, Calvin WH. Mechanosensitivity of dorsal root ganglia and chronically injured axons: a physiological basis for the radicular pain of nerve root compression. *Pain*. 1977;3:25–41.

34. MacNab I. The mechanism of spondylogenic pain. In: Hirsch C, Zotterman Y, eds. *Cervical Pain*. Oxford: Pergamon; 1972:89–95.

35. Smyth MJ, Wright V. Sciatica and the intervertebral disc. An experimental study. *J Bone Joint Surg*. 1959;40A:1401–1418.

36. Norlen G. On the value of the neurological symptoms in sciatica for the localization of a lumbar disc herniation. *Acta Chir Scand*. 1944;95(Suppl.):1–96.

37. McCulloch JA, Waddell G. Variation of the lumbosacral myotomes with bony segmental anomalies. *J Bone Joint Surg*. 1980;62B:475–480.

38. Friberg S. Lumbar disc degeneration in the problem of lumbago sciatica. *Bull Hosp Joint Dis*. 1954;15:1–20.

39. Horal J. The clinical appearance of low back disorders in the city of Gothenburg, Sweden. *Acta Orthop Scand*. 1969;1(Suppl.):118.

40. Mooney V. Where is the pain coming from? *Spine*. 1987;12: 754–759.

41. Deyo RA, Tsui-Wu YJ. Descriptive epidemiology of low-back pain and its related medical care in the United States. *Spine*. 1987;12: 264–268.

42. Boden SD, Davis DO, Dina TS, et al. Abnormal magnetic-resonance scans of the lumbar spine in asymptomatic subjects. *J Bone Joint Surg*. 1990;72A: 403–408.

43. Hitselberger WE, Witten RM. Abnormal myelograms in asymptomatic patients. *J Neurosurg*. 1968;28:204–206.

44. Jensen MC, Brant-Zawadzki MN, Obuchowski N, et al. Magnetic resonance imaging of the lumbar spine in people without back pain. *New Engl J Med*. 1994;331:69–73.

45. Wiesel SW, Tsourmas N, Feffer HL, et al. A study of computer-assisted tomography. 1. The incidence of positive CAT scans in an asymptomatic group of patients. *Spine*. 1984;9:549–551.

46. Delauche-Cavalier MC, Budet C, Laredo JD, et al. Lumbar disc herniation. Computed tomography scan changes after conservative treatment of nerve root compression. *Spine*. 1992;17:927–933.

47. Maigne JY, Rime B, Delinger B. Computed tomographic follow-up study of forty-eight cases of non-operatively treated lumbar intervertebral disc herniation. *Spine*. 1992;17:1071–1074.

48. Greenbarg PE, Brown MD, Pallares VS, et al. Epidural anesthesia for lumbar spine surgery. *J Spinal Disord*. 1988;1:139–143.

49. Murphy RW. Nerve roots and spinal nerves in degenerative disk disease. *Clin Orthop*. 1977;129: 46–60.

50. Irsigler FJ. Mikroskopische Befunde in den Ruckenlarkswurzeln beim lumbalen un lumbalsakralen (dorsolateral) Diskusprolaps. *Acta Neurochir*. 1951;1:478–516.

51. Lindahl O, Rexed B. Histologic changes in spinal nerve roots of operated cases of sciatica. *Acta Orthop Scand*. 1951;20:215–225.

52. Lindblom K, Rexed B. Spinal nerve injury in dorsolateral protrusions of lumbar disks. *J Neurosurg*. 1949;5:413–432.

53. Marshal LL, Trethewie ER. Chemical irritation of nerve-root in disc prolapse. *Lancet*. 1973;2: 320.

54. Marshall LL, Trethewie ER, Curtain CC. Chemical radiculitis. A clinical, physiological and immunological study. *Clin Orthop*. 1977;129:61–67.

55. McCarron RF, Wimpee MW, Hudkins PG, et al. The inflammatory effect of nucleus pulposus: a possible element in the pathogenesis of low-back pain. *Spine*. 1987;12:760–764.

56. Bobechko WT, Hirsch C. Autoimmune response to nucleus pulposus in the rabbit. *J Bone Joint Surg*. 1965;47B:574–580.

57. Gertzbein SD. Degenerative disk disease of the lumbar spine:

immunological implications. *Clin Orthop*. 1977;129:68–71.

58. Gertzbein SD, Tait JH, Devlin SR. The stimulation of lymphocytes by nucleus pulposus in patients with degenerative disk disease of the lumbar spine. *Clin Orthop*. 1977;123:149–154.

59. Gertzbein SD, Tile M, Gross A, et al. Autoimmunity in degenerative disc disease of the lumbar spine. *Orthop Clin North Am*. 1975;6:67–73.

60. Naylor A. The biochemical changes in the human intervertebral disc in degeneration and nuclear prolapse. *Orthop Clin North Am*. 1971;2:343–358.

61. Naylor A. Intervertebral disc prolapse and degeneration. The biochemical and biophysical approach. *Spine*. 1976;1:108–114.

62. Naylor A, Happey F, Turner RL, et al. Enzymic and immunological activity in the intervertebral disc. *Orthop Clin North Am*. 1975;6:51–58.

63. De Silva M, Hazleman BL, Ward M, et al. Autoimmunity and the prolapsed intervertebral disc syndrome. *Rheumatology*. 1981;1:35–38.

64. Olmarker K, Rydevik B, Holm S. Edema formation in spinal nerve roots induced by experimental, graded compression. *Spine*. 1989;14:569–573.

65. Rydevik BL, Myers R, Powell HC. Pressure increase in the dorsal root ganglion following mechanical compression. Closed compartment syndrome in nerve roots. *Spine*. 1989;14:574–576.

66. McCarron RF, Wimpee MW, Hudkins PG, et al. The inflammatory effect of nucleus pulposus: a possible element in the pathogenesis of low-back pain. *Spine*. 1987;12:760–764.

67. Olmarker K, Rydevik B, Nordborg C. Autologous nucleus pulposus induces neurophysiologic and histologic changes in porcine cauda equina nerve roots. *Spine*. 1993;18:1425–1432.

68. Olmarker K, Blomquist J, Stromberg J, et al. Inflammatogenic properties of nucleus pulposus. *Spine*. 1995;20:665–669.

69. Yabuki S, Kikuchi S, Olmarker K, et al. Acute effects of nucleus pulposus on blood flow and endoneural fluid pressure in rat dorsal root ganglia. *Spine*. 1998;23:2517–2523.

70. Olmarker K, Byrod G, Cornefjord M, et al. Effects of methylprednisolone on nucleus pulposus-induced nerve root injury. *Spine*. 1994;19:1803–1808.

71. Olmarker K, Nordborg C, Larsson K, et al. Ultrastructural changes in spinal nerve roots induced by autologous nucleus pulposus. *Spine*. 1996;21:411–414.

72. Olmarker K, Myers RR. Pathogenesis of sciatic pain: role of herniated nucleus pulposus and deformation of spinal nerve root and dorsal root ganglion. *Pain*. 1998;78:99–105.

73. Kayama S, Olmarker K, Larsson K, et al. Cultured, autologous nucleus pulposus cells induce functional changes in spinal nerve roots. *Spine*. 1998;23:2155–2158.

74. Kawakami M, Tamaki T, Weinstein JN, et al. Pathomechanism of pain-related behavior produced by allografts of intervertebral disc in the rat. *Spine*. 1996;21:2101–2107.

75. Kawakami M, Tamaki T, Hashizume H, et al. The role of phospholipase A2 and nitric oxide in pain-related behavior produced by an allograft of intervertebral disc material to the sciatic nerve of the rat. *Spine*. 1997;22:1074–1079.

76. Kawakami M, Tamaki T, Hayashi N, et al. Possible mechanism of painful radiculopathy in lumbar disc herniation. *Clin Orthop*. 1998;351:241–251.

77. Olmarker K, Larson K. Tumor necrosis factor α and nucleus pulposus-induced nerve root injury. *Spine*. 1998;23:2538–2544.

78. Olmarker K, Rydevik B. Selective inhibition of tumor necrosis factor α prevents nucleus pulposus-induced thrombus formation, intraneural edema, and reduction of nerve conduction velocity. Possible implications for future pharmacologic treatment strategies of sciatica. *Spine*. 2001;26:863–869.

79. Chen C, Cavanaugh JM, Ozaktay AC, et al. Effects of phospholipase A2 on lumbar nerve roots structure and function. *Spine*. 1997;22:1057–1064.

80. Hashizume K, Kawakami M, Nishi H, et al. Histochemical demonstration of nitric oxide in herniated lumbar discs: a clinical and animal model study. *Spine*. 1997;22:1080–1084.

81. Kawakami M, Matsumoto T, Kuribayashi K, et al. mRNA expression of interleukins, phospholipase A2, and nitric oxide synthetase in the nerve root and dorsal root ganglion induced by autologous nucleus pulposus in the rat. *J Orthop Res*. 1999;17:941–946.

82. Igarashi T, Kikuchi S, Shubayev V, et al. Exogenous TNF-α mimics nucleus pulposus-induced neuropathology: molecular, histologic, and behavioural comparisons in rats. *Spine*. 2000;25:2975–2980.

83. Gronblad M, Virri J, Tolonen J, et al. A controlled immunohistochemical study of inflammatory cells in disc herniation tissue. *Spine*. 1994;19:2744–2751.

84. Doita M, Kanatani T, Harada T, et al. Immunohistologic study of rupture intervertebral disc of lumbar spine. *Spine*. 1996;21:235–241.

85. Haro H, Shinomiya K, Komori H, et al. Upregulated expression of chemokines in herniated nucleus pulposus resorption. *Spine*. 1996;21:1647–1652.

86. Habtemariam A, Gronblad M, Virri J, et al. Immunohistochemical localization of immunoglobulins in disc herniation. *Spine*. 1996;21:1864–1869.

87. Ito T, Yamada M, Ikuta F, et al. Histologic evidence of absorption of sequestration-type herniated disc. *Spine*. 1996;21:230–234.

88. Habtemariam A, Gronblad M, Virri J, et al. A comparative immunohistochemical study of inflammatory cells in acute-stage and chronic-stage disc herniations. *Spine*. 1998;23:2159–2165.

89. Park JB, Chang H, Kim YS. The pattern of interleukin-12 and T-helper types 1 and 2 cytokine

expression in herniated lumbar disc tissue. *Spine*. 2002;27: 2125–2128.

90. Takahashi H, Sugaro T, Okazima Y, et al. Inflammatory cytokines in the herniated disc of the lumbar spine. *Spine*. 1996;21:218–224.

91. Saal JS, Franson RC, Dobrow R, et al. High levels of inflammatory phospholipase A2 activity in lumbar disc herniations. *Spine*. 1990;15:674–678.

92. Franson RC, Saal JS, Saal JA. Human disc phospholipase A2 is inflammatory. *Spine*. 1992;17: S129–S132.

93. Kang JD, Georgescu HI, Larkin L, et al. Herniated lumbar interverte-bral discs spontaneously produce matrix metalloproteinases, nitric oxide, interleukin-6 and prostaglandin E2. *Spine*. 1996;21: 271–277.

94. Kang JD, Stefanovic-Racic M, McIntyre LA, et al. Toward a biochemical understanding of human intervertebral disc degeneration and herniation: contributions of nitric oxide, interleukins, prostaglandin E2 and matrix metalloproteinases. *Spine*. 1997;22:1065–1073.

95. Nygaard OP, Mellgren SI, Osterud B. The inflammatory properties of contained and noncontained lumbar disc herniation. *Spine*. 1997;22:2484–2488.

96. Ahn SH, Cho YW, Ahn MW, et al. mRNA expression of cytokines in herniated lumbar intervertebral discs. *Spine*. 2002;27:911–917.

97. Brisby H, Olmarker K, Larsson K, et al. Proinflammatory cytokines in cerebrospinal fluid and serum in patients with disc herniation and sciatica. *Eur Spine J*. 2002;11: 62–66.

98. Spiliopoulou II, Korovessis P, Konstantinou D, et al. IgG and IgM concentration in the prolapsed human intervertebral disc and sciatica etiology. *Spine*. 1994;19:1320–1323.

99. Brisby H, Balague F, Schafer D, et al. Glycosphingolipid antibodies in serum in patients with sciatica. *Spine*. 2002;27:380–386.

100. Suguwara O, Atsuta Y, Iwahara T, et al. The effects of mechanical compression and hypoxia on nerve root and dorsal root ganglia. *Spine*. 1996;21:2089–2094.

101. Cavanaugh JM. Neural mechanisms of lumbar spinal pain. *Spine*. 1995;16:1804–1809.

102. Cavanaugh JM, Ozaktay AC, Yamashita T, et al. Mechanisms of low back pain: a neurophysiologic and neuroanatomic study. *Clin Orthop*. 1997;335:166–180.

103. Groen G, Baljet B, Drukker J. The nerves and nerve plexuses of the human vertebral column. *Am J Anat*. 1990;188:282–296.

104. Hirsch C, Ingelmark BE, Miller M. The anatomical basis for low back pain. *Acta Orthop Scand*. 1963;33:1–17.

105. Jackson HC, Winkelmann RK, Bickel WH. Nerve endings in the human lumbar spinal column and related structures. *J Bone Joint Surg*. 1966;48A:1272–1281.

106. Inman VT, Saunders JB. Referred pain from skeletal structures. *J Nerv Ment Dis*. 1944;99:660–667.

107. Hadjipavlou AG, Lander PH. Paget's disease. In: White AH, ed. *Spine Care*, Vol. 2. St Louis: Mosby; 1995:1720–1737.

108. Parfitt AM, Duncan H. Metabolic bone disease affecting the spine. In: Rothman RH, Simeone FA, eds. *The Spine*, Vol. II. Philadelphia: Saunders; 1975:599–720.

109. Francis KC. Tumors of the spine. In: Rothman RH, Simeone FA, eds. *The Spine*, Vol. II. Philadelphia: Saunders; 1975:811–822.

110. Nugent PJ. Surgical treatment of spinal tumours. In: White AH, ed. *Spine Care*, Vol. 2. St Louis: Mosby; 1995:1457–1484.

111. Gornet MF. Spinal infection. In: White AH, ed. *Spine Care*, Vol. 2. St Louis: Mosby; 1995:1543–1551.

112. Hodgson AR. Infectious disease of the spine. In: Rothman RH, Simeone FA, eds. *The Spine*, Vol. II. Philadelphia: Saunders; 1975:567–598.

113. Gershon-Cohen J. Asymptomatic fractures in osteoporotic spine of the aged. *JAMA*. 1953;153: 625–627.

114. Nathanson L, Lewitan A. Deformities and fractures of vertebrae as a result of senile and presenile osteoporosis. *Am J Roentgenol*. 1941;46:197–202.

115. Wyke B. The neurology of low-back pain. In: Jayson MIV, ed. *The Lumbar Spine and Back Pain*. Edinburgh: Churchill Livingstone; 1987:56–99.

116. Niv D, Gofeld M, Devor M. Cause of pain in degenerative bone and joint disease: a lesson from vertebroplasty. *Pain*. 2003;105: 387–392.

117. Buonocore M, Aloisi AM, Barbieri M, et al. Vertebral body innervation: implications for pain. *J Cell Physiol*. 2010;222:488–491.

118. Bogduk N, MacVicar K, Borowczyk J. The pain of vertebral compression fractures can arise in the posterior elements. *Pain Med*. 2010;11:1666–1673.

119. Arnoldi CC. Intravertebral pressures in patients with lumbar pain. *Acta Orthop Scand*. 1972;43: 109–117.

120. Arnoldi CC. Intraosseous hypertension: a possible cause of low-back pain? *Clin Orthop*. 1976;115:30–34.

121. Deyo RA, Diehl AK. Lumbar spine films in primary care: current use and effects of selective ordering criteria. *J Gen Int Med*. 1986;1: 20–25.

122. Baastrup CI. Proc. Spin. vert. Lumb. und einige zwischen diesen leigende Gelenkbildungen mit pathologischen Prozessen in dieser Region. *Fortschritee auf den Gebiete der Rontgenstrahlen*. 1933;48: 430–435.

123. Epstein BS. *The Spine. A radiological text and atlas*, 4th ed. Philadelphia: Lea & Febiger; 1976.

124. Bogduk N, Wilson AS, Tynan W. The human lumbar dorsal rami. *J Anat*. 1982;134:383–397.

125. Rhalmi S, Yahia L, Newman N, et al. Immunohistochemical study of nerves in lumbar spine ligaments. *Spine*. 1993;18:264–267.

126. Yahia LH, Newman NA. A light and electron microscopic study of spinal ligament innervation. *Z mikroskop anat Forsch Leipzig*. 1989;103:664–674.

127. Yahia LH, Newman N, Rivard CH. Neurohistology of lumbar spine ligaments. *Acta Orthop Scand*. 1988;59:508–512.

128. Beks JWF. Kissing spines: fact or fancy? *Acta Neurochir.* 1989;100: 134–135.

129. Hadley LA. Subluxation of the apophyseal articulations with bony impingement as a cause of back pain. *Am J Roentgenol.* 1935;33:209–213.

130. Harris RI, MacNab I. Structural changes in the lumbar intervertebral discs. Their relationship to low back pain and sciatica. *J Bone Joint Surg.* 1954;36B:304–322.

131. Vernon-Roberts B, Pirie CJ. Degenerative changes in the intervertebral discs of the lumbar spine and their sequelae. *Rheumatol Rehab.* 1977;16:13–21.

132. Cyron BM, Hutton WC. The fatigue strength of the lumbar neural arch in spondylolysis. *J Bone Joint Surg.* 1978;60B: 234–238.

133. O'Neill DB, Micheli LJ. Postoperative radiographic evidence for fatigue fracture as the etiology in spondylolysis. *Spine.* 1989;14:1342–1355.

134. Wiltse LL, Widell EH, Jackson DW. Fatigue fracture: the basic lesion in isthmic spondylolisthesis. *J Bone Joint Surg.* 1975;57A:17–22.

135. Eisenstein SM, Ashton IK, Roberts S, et al. Innervation of the spondylolysis 'ligament'. *Spine.* 1994;19:912–916.

136. Schneiderman GA, McLain RF, Hambly MF, et al. The pars defect as a pain source: a histological study. *Spine.* 1995;20:1761–1764.

137. Moreton R. Spondylolysis. *JAMA.* 1966;5:671–674.

138. Libson E, Bloom RA, Dinari G. Symptomatic and asymptomatic spondylolysis and spondylolisthesis in young adults. *Int Orthop.* 1982;6:259–261.

139. Fredrickson BE, Baker D, McHolick WJ, et al. The natural history of spondylosis and spondylolisthesis. *J Bone Joint Surg.* 1984;66A:699–707.

140. Su PB, Esses SI, Kostuik JP. Repair of a pars interarticularis defect – the prognostic value of pars infiltration. *Spine.* 1991;16(Suppl. 8):S445–S448.

141. Bogduk N, McGuirk B. Imaging. In: Bogduk N, McGuirk B, eds. *Medical Management of Acute and Chronic Low Back Pain. An Evidence-Based Approach.* Amsterdam: Elsevier; 2002:49–63.

142. Williams PL, ed. *Gray's Anatomy*, 38th ed. Edinburgh: Churchill Livingstone; 1995.

143. Cave AJE. The innervation and morphology of the cervical intertransverse muscles. *J Anat.* 1937;71:497–515.

144. Bogduk N. Lumbar dorsal ramus syndrome. *Med J Aust.* 1980;2: 537–541.

145. Kellgren JH. Observations on referred pain arising from muscle. *Clin Sci.* 1938;3:175–190.

146. Garrett WE, Nikoloau PK, Ribbeck BM, et al. The effect of muscle architecture on the biomechanical failure properties of skeletal muscle under passive tension. *Am J Sports Med.* 1988;16:7–12.

147. Garrett WE, Saffrean MR, Seaber AV, et al. Biomechanical comparison of stimulated and non-stimulated skeletal muscle pulled to failure. *Am J Sports Med.* 1987;15:448–454.

148. Nikoloau PK, MacDonald BL, Glisson RR, et al. Biomechanical and histological evaluation of muscle after controlled strain injury. *Am J Sports Med.* 1987; 15:9–14.

149. Garrett W, Bradley W, Byrd S, et al. Muscle: basic science perspectives. In: Frymoyer JW, Gordon SL, eds. *New Perspectives on Low Back Pain.* Park Ridge: American Academy of Orthopedic Surgeons; 1989: 335–372.

150. Garrett W, Anderson G, Richardson W. Muscle: future directions. In: Frymoyer JW, Gordon SL, eds. *New Perspectives on Low Back Pain.* Park Ridge: American Academy of Orthopedic Surgeons; 1989:373–379.

151. Roland MO. A critical review of the evidence for a pain–spasm–pain cycle in spinal disorders. *Clin Biomech.* 1986;1:102–109.

152. Jull GA, Janda V. Muscles and motor control in low back pain: assessment and management. In: Twomey LT, Taylor JR, eds. *Physical Therapy of the Low Back.* New York: Churchill Livingstone; 1987: 253–278.

153. Simons DG. Myofascial pain syndromes: where are we? Where are we going? *Arch Phys Med Rehab.* 1988;69:207–212.

154. Simons DG. Myofascial trigger points: a need for understanding. *Arch Phys Med Rehab.* 1981;62: 97–99.

155. Simons DG, Travell J. Myofascial trigger points, a possible explanation. (letter). *Pain.* 1981;10:106–109.

156. Travell J, Rinzler SH. The myofascial genesis of pain. *Postgrad Med.* 1952;11:425–434.

157. Sola AE, Kuitert JH. Quadratus lumborum myofasciitis. *Northwest Med.* 1954;53:1003–1005.

158. Nice DA, Riddle DL, Lamb RL, et al. Intertester reliability of judgments of the presence of trigger points in patients with low back pain. *Arch Phys Med Rehab.* 1992;73:893–898.

159. Njoo KH, van der Does E. The occurrence and interrater reliability of myofascial trigger points in the quadratus lumborum and gluteus medius: a prospective study in non-specific low back pain patients and controls in general practice. *Pain.* 1994; 58:317–323.

160. Yahia LH, Rhalmi S, Isler M. Sensory innervation of human thoracolumbar fascia: an immunohistochemical study. *Acta Orthop Scand.* 1992;63:195–197.

161. Stillwell DL. Regional variations in the innervation of deep fasciae and aponeuroses. *Anat Rec.* 1957;127:635–653.

162. Carr D, Gilbertson L, Frymoyer J, et al. Lumbar paraspinal compartment syndrome: a case report with physiologic and anatomic studies. *Spine.* 1985;10:816–820.

163. Peck D, Nicholls PJ, Beard C, et al. Are there compartment syndromes in some patients with idiopathic back pain? *Spine.* 1986;11: 468–475.

164. Styf J, Lysell E. Chronic compartment syndrome in the erector spinae muscle. *Spine.* 1987;12:680–682.

165. Konno S, Kikuchi S, Nagaosa Y. The relationship between intramuscular pressure of the

paraspinal muscles and low back pain. *Spine*. 1994;19:2186–2189.

166. Bonner CD, Kasdon SC. Herniation of fat through lumbo-dorsal fascia as a cause of low-back pain. *New Engl J Med*. 1954;251:1101–1104.

167. Copeman WSC, Ackerman WL. 'Fibrositis' of the back. *Quart J Med*. 1944;13:37–52.

168. Copeman WSC, Ackerman WL. Edema or herniations of fat lobules as a cause of lumbar and gluteal 'fibrositis'. *Arch Int Med*. 1947;79:22–35.

169. Faille RJ. Low back pain and lumbar fat herniation. *Am Surg*. 1978;44:359–361.

170. Herz R. Herniation of fascial fat as a cause of low-back pain. *JAMA*. 1945;128:921–925.

171. Hucherson DC, Gandy JR. Herniation of fascial fat: a cause of low-back pain. *Am J Surg*. 1948;76:605–609.

172. Singewald ML. Sacroiliac lipomata – an often unrecognised cause of low back pain. *Bull Johns Hopkins Hosp*. 1966;118:492–498.

173. Woollgast GF, Afeman CE. Sacroiliac (episacral) lipomas. *Arch Surg*. 1961;83:925–927.

174. Edgar MA, Nundy S. Innervation of the spinal dura mater. *J Neurol Neurosurg Psychiatry*. 1964;29:530–534.

175. El Mahdi MA, Latif FYA, Janko M. The spinal nerve root innervation, and a new concept of the clinicopathological interrelations in back pain and sciatica. *Neurochirurgia*. 1981;24:137–141.

176. Walton JN, ed. *Brain's Diseases of the Nervous System*, 8th ed. Oxford: OUP; 1977:407–408.

177. Spencer DL, Irwin GS, Miller JAA. Anatomy and significance of fixation of the lumbosacral nerve roots in sciatica. *Spine*. 1983;8:672–679.

178. Cuatico W, Parker JC, Pappert E, et al. An anatomical and clinical investigation of spinal meningeal nerves. *Acta Neurochir*. 1988;90:139–143.

179. Cuatico W, Parker JC. Further observations on spinal meningeal nerves and their role in pain production. *Acta Neurochir*. 1989;101:126–128.

180. Pedersen HE, Blunck CFJ, Gardner E. The anatomy of lumbosacral posterior rami and meningeal branches of spinal nerves (sinu-vertebral nerves): with an experimental study of their function. *J Bone Joint Surg*. 1956;38A:377–391.

181. Boas RA. Post-surgical low back pain. In: Peck C, Wallace M, eds. *Problems in Pain*. Sydney: Pergamon; 1980:188–191.

182. Ramsey RH. The anatomy of the ligamenta flava. *Clin Orthop*. 1966;44:129–140.

183. Yong-Hing K, Reilly J, Kirkaldy-Willis WH. The ligamentum flavum. *Spine*. 1976;1:226–234.

184. Kirby MC, Sikoryn TA, Hukins DWL, et al. Structure and mechanical properties of the longitudinal ligaments and ligamentum flavum of the spine. *J Biomed Eng*. 1989;11:192–196.

185. Heylings DJA. Supraspinous and interspinous ligaments of the human spine. *J Anat*. 1978;125:127–131.

186. Rissanen PM. The surgical anatomy and pathology of the supraspinous and interspinous ligaments of the lumbar spine with special reference to ligament ruptures. *Acta Orthop Scand*. 1960;46(Suppl.):1–100.

187. Bogduk N, Tynan W, Wilson AS. The nerve supply to the human lumbar intervertebral discs. *J Anat*. 1981;132:39–56.

188. Falconer MA, McGeorge M, Begg AC. Observations on the cause and mechanism of symptom-production in sciatica and low-back pain. *J Neurol Neurosurg Psychiatry*. 1948;11:13–26.

189. Wiberg G. Back pain in relation to the nerve supply of the intervertebral disc. *Acta Orthop Scand*. 1947;19:211–221.

190. Feinstein B, Langton JNK, Jameson RM, et al. Experiments on pain referred from deep structures. *J Bone Joint Surg*. 1954;36A:981–997.

191. Hockaday JM, Whitty CWM. Patterns of referred pain in the normal subject. *Brain*. 1967;90:481–496.

192. Kellgren JH. On the distribution of pain arising from deep somatic structures with charts of segmental pain areas. *Clin Sci*. 1939;4:35–46.

193. Steindler A, Luck JV. Differential diagnosis of pain low in the back: allocation of the source of pain by the procain hydrochloride method. *JAMA*. 1938;110:106–112.

194. Wilk V. Pain arising from the interspinous and supraspinous ligaments. *Australas Musculoskeletal Med*. 1995;1:21–31.

195. Chow DHK, Luk KDK, Leong JCY, et al. Torsional stability of the lumbosacral junction: significance of the iliolumbar ligament. *Spine*. 1989;14:611–615.

196. Leong JCY, Luk KDK, Chow DHK, et al. The biomechanical functions of the iliolumbar ligament in maintaining stability of the lumbosacral junction. *Spine*. 1987;12:669–674.

197. Yamamoto I, Panjabi MM, Oxland TR, et al. The role of the iliolumbar ligament in the lumbosacral junction. *Spine*. 1990;15:1138–1141.

198. Hirschberg GG, Froetscher L, Naeim F. Iliolumbar syndrome as a common cause of low-back pain: diagnosis and prognosis. *Arch Phys Med Rehab*. 1979;60:415–419.

199. Hackett GS. Referred pain from low back ligament disability. *AMAArch Surg*. 1956;73:878–883.

200. Collee G, Dijkmans AC, Vandenbroucke JP, et al. Iliac crest pain syndrome in low back pain: frequency and features. *J Rheumatol*. 1991;18:1064–1067.

201. Fairbank JCT, O'Brien JP. The iliac crest syndrome: a treatable cause of low-back pain. *Spine*. 1983;8:220–224.

202. Ingpen ML, Burry HC. A lumbo-sacral strain syndrome. *Ann Phys Med*. 1970;10:270–274.

203. Bogduk N. A reappraisal of the anatomy of the human lumbar erector spinae. *J Anat*. 1980;131:525–540.

204. Macintosh JE, Bogduk N. The morphology of the lumbar erector spinae. *Spine*. 1986;12:658–668.

205. Bauwens P, Coyer AB. The 'multifidus triangle' syndrome as a cause of recurrent low-back pain. *BMJ*. 1955;2:1306–1307.

206. Livingstone WK. Back disabilities due to strain of the multifidus

muscle. *West J Surg*. 1941;49: 259–263.

207. Njoo KH, van der Does E, Stam HJ. Interobserver agreement on iliac crest pain syndrome in general practice. *J Rheumatol*. 1995;22:1532–1535.

208. Paris SV. Anatomy as related to function and pain. *Orthop Clin North Am*. 1983;14:475–489.

209. Pitkin HC, Pheasant HC. Sacrarthogenetic telalgia I. A study of referred pain. *J Bone Joint Surg*. 1936;18:111–133.

210. Ikeda R. Innervation of the sacroiliac joint: macroscopical and histological studies. *Nippon Ika Daigaku Zasshi*. 1991;58:587–596.

211. Grob KR, Neuhuber WL, Kissling RO. Innervation of the human sacroiliac joint. *Z Rheumatol*. 1995;54:117–122.

212. Fortin JD, Dwyer AP, West S, et al. Sacroiliac joint: pain referral maps upon applying a new injection/ arthrography technique. Part I. Asymptomatic volunteers. *Spine*. 1994;19:1475–1482.

213. Bellamy N, Park W, Rooney PJ. What do we know about the sacroiliac joint? *Semin Arthritis Rheum*. 1983;12:282–313.

214. Davis P, Lentle BC. Evidence for sacroiliac disease as a common cause of low backache in women. *Lancet*. 1978;2:496–497.

215. Aitken GS. Syndromes of lumbo-pelvic dysfunction. In: Grieve GP, ed. *Modern Manual Therapy of the Vertebral Column*. Edinburgh: Churchill Livingstone; 1986:473–478.

216. Lee D. *The Pelvic Girdle*. Edinburgh: Churchill Livingstone; 1989.

217. Lewit K. The diagnosis of sacroiliac movement restriction in ankylosing spondylitis. *Man Med*. 1987;3:67–68.

218. Rantanen P, Airaksinen O. Poor agreement between so-called sacroiliacal joint tests in ankylosing spondylitis patients. *J Man Med*. 1989;4:62–64.

219. Schmid HJA. Sacroiliac diagnosis and treatment. *Man Med*. 1984;1: 33–38.

220. Wells PE. The examination of the pelvic joints. In: Grieve GP, ed. *Modern Manual Therapy of the Vertebral Column*. Edinburgh: Churchill Livingstone; 1986: 473–478.

221. Egund N, Olsson TH, Schmid H, et al. Movements in the sacroiliac joints demonstrated with roentgen stereophotogrammetry. *Acta Radiol*. 1978;19:833–846.

222. Sturesson B, Selvik G, Uden A. Movements of the sacroiliac joints: a roentgen stereophotogrammetric analysis. *Spine*. 1989;14:162–165.

223. Sturesson B, Uden A, Vlemming A. A radiostereometric analysis of movements of the sacroiliac joints during the standing hip flexion test. *Spine*. 2000;25:364–366.

224. Tulberg T, Blomberg S, Branth B, et al. Manipulation does not alter the position of the sacroiliac joint. A Roentgen stereophoto-grammetric analysis. *Spine*. 1998;23:1124–1129.

225. Maigne JY, Aivaliklis A, Pfeffer F. Results of sacroiliac joint double block and value of sacroiliac pain provocation tests in 54 patients with low back pain. *Spine*. 1996;21:1889–1892.

226. Schwarzer AC, Aprill CN, Bogduk N. The sacroiliac joint in chronic low back pain. *Spine*. 1995;20: 31–37.

227. Dreyfuss P, Michaelsen M, Pauza K, et al. The value of history and physical examination in diagnosing sacroiliac joint pain. *Spine*. 1996;21:2594–2602.

228. Bogduk N. The innervation of the lumbar spine. *Spine*. 1983;8:286–293.

229. McCall IW, Park WM, O'Brien JP. Induced pain referral from posterior lumbar elements in normal subjects. *Spine*. 1979;4:441–446.

230. Mooney V, Robertson J. The facet syndrome. *Clin Orthop*. 1976;115: 149–156.

231. Fairbank JCT, Park WM, McCall IW, et al. Apophyseal injections of local anaesthetic as a diagnostic aid in primary low-back pain syndromes. *Spine*. 1981;6: 598–605.

232. Schwarzer AC, Aprill CN, Derby R, et al. Clinical features of patients with pain stemming from the lumbar zygapophysial joints. Is the lumbar facet syndrome a clinical entity? *Spine*. 1994;19:1132–1137.

233. Schwarzer AC, Aprill CN, Derby R, et al. The false-positive rate of uncontrolled diagnostic blocks of the lumbar zygapophysial joints. *Pain*. 1994;58:195–200.

234. Schwarzer AC, Wang S, Bogduk N, et al. Prevalence and clinical features of lumbar zygapophysial joint pain: a study in an Australian population with chronic low back pain. *Ann Rheum Dis*. 1995;54:100–106.

235. Ghormley RK. Low back pain with special reference to the articular facets, with presentation of an operative procedure. *JAMA*. 1933;101:1773–1777.

236. Bogduk N, Aprill C, Derby R. Diagnostic blocks of synovial joints. In: White AH, ed. *Spine Care, Vol. 1. Diagnosis and conservative treatment*. St Louis: Mosby; 1995:298–321.

237. Bogduk N. Evidence-informed management of chronic back pain with facet injections and radiofrequency neurotomy. *Spine J*. 2008;8:56–64.

238. Bogduk N, Aprill C, Derby R. Lumbar zygapophysial joint pain: diagnostic blocks and therapy. In: Wilson DJ, ed. *Interventional Radiology of the Musculoskeletal System*. London: Edward Arnold; 1995:73–86.

239. Bogduk N. On the rational use of diagnostic blocks for spinal pain. *Neurosurg Q*. 2009;19:88–100.

240. Manchikanti L, Pampati V, Fellows B, et al. Prevalence of lumbar facet joint pain in chronic low back pain. *Pain Physician*. 1999;2:59–64.

241. Schwarzer AC, Aprill CN, Derby R, et al. The relative contributions of the disc and zygapophyseal joint in chronic low back pain. *Spine*. 1994;19:801–806.

242. Jackson RP, Jacobs RR, Montesano PX. Facet joint injection in low-back pain. *Spine*. 1988;13: 966–971.

243. Carette S, Marcoux S, Truchon R, et al. A controlled trial of corticosteroid injections into facet joints for chronic low back pain. *New Engl J Med*. 1991;325: 1002–1007.

244. Eisenstein SM, Parry CR. The lumbar facet arthrosis syndrome. *J Bone Joint Surg.* 1987;69B:3–7.

245. Lippit AB. The facet joint and its role in spine pain. *Spine.* 1984;9:746–750.

246. Schwarzer AC, Derby R, Aprill CN, et al. Pain from the lumbar zygapophysial joints: a test of two models. *J Spinal Disord.* 1994;7:331–336.

247. Jayson MIV. Degenerative disease of the spine and back pain. *Clin Rheum Dis.* 1976;2:557–584.

248. Lawrence JS, Sharpe J, Ball J, et al. Rheumatoid arthritis of the lumbar spine. *Ann Rheum Dis.* 1964;23:205–217.

249. Sims-Williams H, Jason MIV, Baddeley H. Rheumatoid involvement of the lumbar spine. *Ann Rheum Dis.* 1977;36:524–531.

250. Ball J. Enthesopathy of rheumatoid and ankylosing spondylitis. *Ann Rheum Dis.* 1971;30:213–223.

251. Bailey W. Anomalies and fractures of the vertebral articular processes. *JAMA.* 1937;108:266–270.

252. Fulton WS, Kalbfleisch WK. Accessory articular processes of the lumbar vertebrae. *Arch Surg.* 1934;29:42–48.

253. King AB. Back pain due to loose facets of the lower lumbar vertebrae. *Bull Johns Hopkins Hosp.* 1955;97:271–283.

254. Campbell AJ, Wells IP. Pigmented villonodular synovitis of a lumbar vertebral facet joint. *J Bone Joint Surg.* 1982;64A:145–146.

255. Titelbaum DS, Rhodes CH, Brooks JS, et al. Pigmented villonodular synovitis of a lumbar facet joint. *Am J Neuroradiol.* 1992;13:164–166.

256. Chevalier X, Marty M, Larget-Piet B. *Klebsiella pneumoniae* septic arthritis of a lumbar facet joint. *J Rheumatol.* 1992;19:1817–1819.

257. Halpin DS, Gibson RD. Septic arthritis of the lumbar facet joint. *J Bone Joint Surg.* 1987;69B:457–459.

258. Rousselin B, Gires F, Vallee C, et al. Case report 627. *Skeletal Radiol.* 1990;19:453–455.

259. Rush J, Griffiths J. Suppurative arthritis of a lumbar facet joint.

J Bone Joint Surg. 1989;71B:161–162.

260. Lewin T. Osteoarthritis in lumbar synovial joints. *Acta Orthop Scand.* 1964;Suppl. 19;73:1–112.

261. Shore LR. On osteoarthritis in the dorsal intervertebral joints: a study in morbid anatomy. *Br J Surg.* 1935;22:833–849.

262. Lawrence JS, Bremner JM, Bier F. Osteoarthrosis: prevalence in the population and relationship between symptoms and X-ray changes. *Ann Rheum Dis.* 1966;25:1–24.

263. Magora A, Schwartz A. Relation between the low back pain syndrome and X-ray findings. 1. Degenerative osteoarthritis. *Scand J Rehab Med.* 1976;8:115–125.

264. Abel MS. The radiology of low back pain associated with posterior element lesions of the lumbar spine. *Crit Rev Diagn Imaging.* 1984;20:311–352.

265. Carrera GF, Williams AL. Current concepts in evaluation of the lumbar facet joints. *Crit Rev Diagn Imaging.* 1984;21:85–104.

266. Lynch MC, Taylor JF. Facet joint injection for low back pain. *J Bone Joint Surg.* 1986;68B:138–141.

267. Hermanus N, De Becker D, Baleriaus D, et al. The use of CT scanning for the study of posterior lumbar intervertebral articulations. *Neuroradiology.* 1983;24:159–161.

268. Schwarzer AC, Wang S, O'Driscoll D, et al. The ability of computed tomography to identify a painful zygapophysial joint in patients with chronic low back pain. *Spine.* 1995;20:907–912.

269. Yang KH, King AI. Mechanism of facet load transmission as a hypothesis for low-back pain. *Spine.* 1984;9:557–565.

270. Farfan HF, Cossette JW, Robertson GH, et al. The effects of torsion on the lumbar intervertebral joints: the role of torsion in the production of disc degeneration. *J Bone Joint Surg.* 1970;52A:468–497.

271. Adams MA, Hutton WC. The relevance of torsion to the mechanical derangement of the lumbar spine. *Spine.* 1981;6:241–248.

272. Farfan HF. *Mechanical Disorders of the Low Back.* Philadelphia: Lea & Febiger; 1973.

273. Farfan HF. A reorientation in the surgical approach to degenerative lumbar intervertebral joint disease. *Orthop Clin.* 1977;8:9–21.

274. Farfan HF, Kirkaldy-Willis WH. The present status of spinal fusion in the treatment of lumbar intervertebral joint disorders. *Clin Orthop.* 1981;158:198–214.

275. Lamy C, Kraus H, Farfan HF. The strength of the neural arch and the etiology of spondylosis. *Orthop Clin North Am.* 1975;6:215–231.

276. Sullivan JD, Farfan HF. The crumpled neural arch. *Orthop Clin North Am.* 1975;6:199–213.

277. Taylor JR, Twomey LT, Corker M. Bone and soft tissue injuries in post-mortem lumbar spines. *Paraplegia.* 1990;28:119–129.

278. Twomey LT, Taylor JR, Taylor MM. Unsuspected damage to lumbar zygapophyseal (facet) joints after motor-vehicle accidents. *Med J Aust.* 1989;151:210–217.

279. Jacoby RK, Sims-Williams H, Jayson MIV, et al. Radiographic stereoplotting: a new technique and its application to the study of the spine. *Ann Rheum Dis.* 1976;35:168–170.

280. Mitchell CL. Isolated fractures of the articular processes of the lumbar vertebrae. *J Bone Joint Surg.* 1933;15:608–614.

281. Sims-Williams H, Jayson MIV, Baddeley H. Small spinal fractures in back pain patients. *Ann Rheum Dis.* 1978;37:262–265.

282. Bogduk N, Engel R. The menisci of the lumbar zygapophyseal joints. A review of their anatomy and clinical significance. *Spine.* 1984;9:454–460.

283. Engel R, Bogduk N. The menisci of the lumbar zygapophyseal joints. *J Anat.* 1982;135:795–809.

284. Taylor JR, Twomey LT. Age changes in lumbar zygapophyseal joints. *Spine.* 1986;11:739–745.

285. Bogduk N, Jull G. The theoretical pathology of acute locked back: a basis for manipulative therapy. *Man Med.* 1985;1:78–82.

286. Inman VT, Saunders JB, de CM. Anatomicophysiological aspects of injuries to the intervertebral disc.

J Bone Joint Surg. 1947;29:461–475, 534.

287. Bogduk N. The innervation of intervertebral discs. In: Ghosh P, ed. *The Biology of the Intervertebral Disc*, Vol. I. Boca Raton: CRC Press; 1988:135–149.

288. Ehrenhaft JC. Development of the vertebral column as related to certain congenital and pathological changes. *Surg Gynecol Obst*. 1943;76:282–292.

289. Malinsky J. The ontogenetic development of nerve terminations in the intervertebral discs of man. *Acta Anat*. 1959;38:96–113.

290. Rabischong P, Louis R, Vignaud J, et al. The intervertebral disc. *Anat Clin*. 1978;1:55–64.

291. Roofe PG. Innervation of annulus fibrosus and posterior longitudinal ligament. *Arch Neurol Psychiatry*. 1940;44:100–103.

292. Yoshizawa H, O'Brien JP, Thomas-Smith W, et al. The neuropathology of intervertebral discs removed for low-back pain. *J Path*. 1980;132:95–104.

293. Bogduk N. Diskography. *Am Pain Soc J*. 1994;3:149–154.

294. Bogduk N, Aprill C, Derby R. Discography. In: White AH, ed. *Spine Care*, Vol. 1. *Diagnosis and conservative treatment*. St Louis: Mosby; 1995:219–238.

295. International Spinal Injection Society. Lumbar disc stimulation. In: Bogduk N, ed. *Practice Guidelines for Spinal Diagnostic and Treatment Procedures*. San Francisco: International Spinal Injection Society; 2004.

296. Schwarzer AC, Aprill CN, Derby R, et al. The prevalence and clinical features of internal disc disruption in patients with chronic low back pain. *Spine*. 1995;20:1878–1883.

297. Holt EP. The question of lumbar discography. *J Bone Joint Surg*. 1968;50A:720–726.

298. Simmons JW, Aprill CN, Dwyer AP, et al. A reassessment of Holt's data on 'the question of lumbar discography'. *Clin Orthop*. 1988;237:120–124.

299. Walsh TR, Weinstein JN, Spratt KF, et al. Lumbar discography in normal subjects. *J Bone Joint Surg*. 1990;72A:1081–1088.

300. Carragee EJ, Tanner CM, Khurana S, et al. The rates of false-positive lumbar discography in select patients without low back symptoms. *Spine*. 2000;25:1373–1381.

301. Derby R, Lee SH, Kim BJ, et al. Pressure-controlled lumbar discography in volunteers without low back symptoms. *Pain Med*. 2005;6:213–221.

302. Wolfer LR, Derby R, Lee JE, et al. Systematic review of lumbar provocation discography in asymptomatic subjects with a meta-analysis of false positive rates. *Pain Physician*. 2008;11:513–538.

303. O'Neill CW, Kurgansky ME, Derby R, et al. Disc stimulation and patterns of referred pain. *Spine*. 2002;27:2776–2781.

304. Bogduk N. The lumbar disc and low back pain. *Neurosurg Clin North Am*. 1991;2:791–806.

305. Fraser RD, Osti OL, Vernon-Roberts B. Discitis after discography. *J Bone Joint Surg*. 1987;69B:26–35.

306. Guyer RD, Collier R, Stith WJ, et al. Discitis after discography. *Spine*. 1988;13:1352–1354.

307. Farfan HF, Gracovetsky S. The nature of instability. *Spine*. 1984;9:714–719.

308. Farfan HF, Huberdeau RM, Dubow HI. Lumbar intervertebral disc degeneration. The influence of geometrical features on the pattern of disc degeneration – a post-mortem study. *J Bone Joint Surg*. 1972;54A:492–510.

309. Pearcy MJ. Inferred strains in the intervertebral discs during physiological movements. *J Man Med*. 1990;5:68–71.

310. Farfan HF. The use of mechanical etiology to determine the efficacy of active intervention in single joint intervertebral joint problems. *Spine*. 1985;10:350–358.

311. Yu S, Sether LA, Ho PSP, et al. Tears of the anulus fibrosus: correlation between MR and pathologic findings in cadavers. *Am J Neuroradiol*. 1988;9:367–370.

312. Finch PM, Khangure MS. Analgesic discography and magnetic resonance imaging (MRI). *Pain*. 1990;5(Suppl.):S285.

313. Finch P. Analgesic discography in the diagnosis of spinal pain. Paper presented at 'Spinal Pain': precision diagnosis and treatment. Official Satellite Meeting of the VIth World Congress on Pain, Perth, April 8–10, 1990. Meeting Abstracts: 8.

314. Sachs BL, Vanharanta H, Spivey MA, et al. Dallas discogram description: a new classification of CT/discography in low-back disorders. *Spine*. 1987;12:287–294.

315. Aprill C, Bogduk N. High intensity zone: a pathognomonic sign of painful lumbar disc on MRI. *Br J Radiol*. 1992;65:361–369.

316. Vanharanta H, Sachs BL, Spivey MA, et al. The relationship of pain provocation to lumbar disc deterioration as seen by CT/discography. *Spine*. 1987;12:295–298.

317. Moneta GB, Videman T, Kaivanto K, et al. Reported pain during lumbar discography as a function of anular ruptures and disc degeneration. A re-analysis of 833 discograms. *Spine*. 1994;17:1968–1974.

318. McNally DS, Shackleford IM, Goodship AE, et al. In vivo stress measurement can predict pain on discography. *Spine*. 1996;21:2500–2587.

319. Farfan HF. *Mechanical Disorders of the Low Back*. Philadelphia: Lea & Febiger; 1973.

320. Farfan HF, Kirkaldy-Willis WH. The present status of spinal fusion in the treatment of lumbar intervertebral joint disorders. *Clin Orthop*. 1981;158:198–214.

321. Brinckmann P. Injury of the annulus fibrosus and disc protrusions: an in vitro investigation on human lumbar discs. *Spine*. 1986;11:149–153.

322. Markolf KL, Morris JM. The structural components of the intervertebral disc. *J Bone Joint Surg*. 1974;56A:675–687.

323. Virgin WJ. Experimental investigations into the physical properties of the intervertebral disc. *J Bone Joint Surg*. 1951;33B:607–611.

324. Adams MA, Hutton WC. Gradual disc prolapse. *Spine*. 1985;10:524–531.

325. Adams MA, Hutton WC. Prolapsed intervertebral disc. A hyperflexion injury. *Spine.* 1982;7:184–191.

326. Brown T, Hansen RJ, Yorra AJ. Some mechanical tests on the lumbosacral spine with particular reference to the intervertebral discs. *J Bone Joint Surg.* 1957; 39A:1135–1164.

327. Hutton WC, Adams MA. Can the lumbar spine be crushed in heavy lifting? *Spine.* 1982;7:586–590.

328. Jayson MIV, Herbert CM, Barks JS. Intervertebral discs: nuclear morphology and bursting pressures. *Ann Rheum Dis.* 1973;32:308–315.

329. Perey O. Fracture of the vertebral end-plate in the lumbar spine. *Acta Orthop Scand.* 1957; 25(Suppl.):1–101.

330. Rolander SD, Blair WE. Deformation and fracture of the lumbar vertebral end plate. *Orthop Clin North Am.* 1975;6:75–81.

331. Porter RW, Adams MA, Hutton WC. Physical activity and the strength of the lumbar spine. *Spine.* 1989;14:201–203.

332. Brinckmann P, Frobin W, Hierholzer E, et al. Deformation of the vertebral end-plate under axial loading of the spine. *Spine.* 1983;8:851–856.

333. Adams MA, McNally DS, Wagstaff J, et al. Abnormal stress concentrations in lumbar intervertebral discs following damage to the vertebral bodies: a cause of disc failure? *Eur Spine J.* 1993;1:214–221.

334. McNeill T, Warwick D, Andersson G, et al. Trunk strengths in attempted flexion, extension, and lateral bending in healthy subjects and patients with low-back disorders. *Spine.* 1980;5:529–538.

335. Granhed H, Johnson R, Hansson T. The loads on the lumbar spine during extreme weight lifting. *Spine.* 1987;12:146–149.

336. Hansson TH, Keller TS, Spengler DM. Mechanical behaviour of the human lumbar spine. II. Fatigue strength during dynamic compressive loading. *J Orthop Res.* 1987;5:479–487.

337. Liu YK, Njus G, Buckwalter J, et al. Fatigue response of lumbar intervertebral joints under axial cyclic loading. *Spine.* 1983;8:857–865.

338. Bogduk N. Sources of low back pain. In: Jayson MIV, ed. *The Lumbar Spine and Back Pain.* Edinburgh: Churchill Livingstone; 1992:61–88, Ch. 4.

339. Bogduk N, Twomey L. *Clinical Anatomy of the Lumbar Spine,* 2nd ed. Melbourne: Churchill Livingstone; 1991.

340. Elves MW, Bucknill T, Sullivan MF. In vitro inhibition of leukocyte migration in patients with intervertebral disk lesions. *Orthop Clin North Am.* 1975;6:59–65.

341. McCall IW, Park WM, O'Brien JP, et al. Acute traumatic intraosseous disc herniation. *Spine.* 1985;10:134–137.

342. Kalebo P, Kadziolka R, Sward L. Compression–traction radiography of lumbar segmental instability. *Spine.* 1990;15:351–355.

343. Maroudas A. Nutrition and metabolism of the intervertebral disc. In: Ghosh P, ed. *The Biology of the Intervertebral Disc,* Vol. II. Boca Raton: CRC Press; 1988:1–37, Ch. 9.

344. Melrose J, Ghosh P. The noncollagenous proteins of the intervertebral disc. In: Ghosh P, ed. *The Biology of the Intervertebral Disc,* Vol. I. Boca Raton: CRC Press; 1988:189–237, Ch. 8.

345. Sedowfia KA, Tomlinson IW, Weiss JB, et al. Collagenolytic enzyme systems in human intervertebral disc. *Spine.* 1982;7:213–222.

346. Ohshima H, Urban JPG. The effect of lactate and pH on proteoglycan and protein synthesis rates in the intervertebral disc. *Spine.* 1992;17:1079–1082.

347. Fujita K, Nakagawa T, Hirabayashi K, et al. Neutral proteinases in human intervertebral disc: role in degeneration and probable origin. *Spine.* 1993;18:1766–1773.

348. Crock HV. A reappraisal of intervertebral disc lesions. *Med J Aust.* 1970;1:983–989 (and supplementary pages i–ii).

349. Venner RM, Crock HV. Clinical studies of isolated disc resorption in the lumbar spine. *J Bone Joint Surg.* 1981;63B:491–494.

350. Twomey L, Taylor J. Age changes in lumbar intervertebral discs. *Acta Orthop Scand.* 1985;56:496–499.

351. Holm S, Kaigle-Holm A, Ekstrom L, et al. Experimental disc degeneration due to endplate injury. *J Spinal Disord Tech.* 2004;17:64–71.

352. Jaffray D, O'Brien JP. Isolated intervertebral disc resorption: a source of mechanical and inflammatory back pain? *Spine.* 1986;11:397–401.

353. Schellhas KP, Pollei SR, Gundry CR, et al. Lumbar disc high-intensity zone: correlation of magnetic resonance imaging and discography. *Spine.* 1996;21:79–86.

Chapter | 16 |

Instability

The term 'instability' has crept into the literature on low back pain as a diagnostic entity. The implication is that the patient has something wrong biomechanically in their back, and that this is somehow the cause of their pain. Furthermore, since the cause of pain is biomechanical in nature, its treatment should be mechanical. The notion of lumbar instability, however, has become very controversial, as is evident in several reviews[1,2] and symposia.[3-5] Physicians have abused the term and have applied it clinically without discipline and without due regard to available biomechanical definitions and diagnostic techniques.

BIOMECHANICS

Instability has been defined as a condition of a system in which the application of a small load causes an inordinately large, perhaps catastrophic, displacement.[6] This definition conveys the more colloquial sense of something that is about to fall apart or could easily fall apart. Bioengineers have insisted that instability is a mechanical entity and should be treated as such,[7] but how biomechanists have portrayed the definition graphically in mathematical terms has evolved over recent years, as more and more embellishments and alternatives have been added.

Stiffness

An early definition simply maintained that instability was loss of stiffness.[7] A later elaboration introduced a clinical dimension, to the effect that instability is a

> *loss of spinal motion segment stiffness such that force application to the structure produces a greater displacement(s) than would be seen in a normal structure, resulting in a painful condition, the potential for progressive deformity, and that places neurologic structures at risk.*[8]

Other engineers have disagreed, insisting that any definition of instability should include the sense of sudden, unpredictable behaviour; that a small load causes a large, perhaps catastrophic, displacement.[6] They argue that loss of stiffness may simply describe loose or hypermobile segments that are not at risk of catastrophic collapse.

Indeed, any definition expressed simply in terms of stiffness is inadequate and inappropriate. It is inadequate because it raises the question 'How much less stiff should a segment become before it is considered unstable?'. It is inappropriate because it does not convey the sense of impending failure. In that regard the definition that includes the terms 'catastrophic displacement' is more appropriate but there is still the question 'What constitutes a "catastrophic displacement"?'.

There may well be conditions of the lumbar spine that involve loss of stiffness and the production of symptoms, but these do not necessarily constitute instability in the full sense of the word, and perhaps an alternative term should be applied, such as 'segmental looseness' or simply 'hypermobility'.

Neutral zone

A refreshing new definition that has emerged is one that essentially defines instability as an increased neutral zone. Explicitly, the definition is

> *a significant decrease in the capacity of the stabilising system of the spine to maintain the intervertebral neutral zones within the physiological limits so that there is no neurological dysfunction, no major deformity, and no incapacitating pain.*[9]

The neutral zone is that part of the range of physiological intervertebral motion, measured from the neutral position, within which the spinal motion is produced with a minimal internal resistance.[9] In essence, although not exactly the same mathematically, it is similar to the length of the toe phase of the stress–strain curve that describes the behaviour of the segment (Fig. 16.1).

This definition describes joints that are loose but early in range. Their ultimate strength may be normal but early in range they exhibit excessive displacement (Fig. 16.2). This definition captures the sense of excessive displacement; it captures the sense of excessive displacement under minor load but it defies the engineering sense of impending catastrophic failure. However, it does so deliberately and not totally without regard to catastrophe.

The neutral zone concept directs attention away from the terminal behaviour of a joint to its earlier behaviour. This allows the definition to be applied to circumstances more common than those associated with impending failure of the spine; it is applicable to the conditions otherwise described as 'looseness'. The sense of catastrophe, and hence instability, is nonetheless retained in a modified form.

As a joint moves through an extended neutral zone it is undergoing an inordinate displacement. If extrapolated, this behaviour predicts that the joint will eventually fall apart. Hence the sense of impending catastrophe applies. It transpires, however, that eventually the inordinate motion of the joint is arrested and catastrophe does not ensue. Nevertheless, during the neutral zone, the movement looks and feels inordinate and threatening.

Instability factor

The engineering definitions of instability describe what might be called terminal instability: the behaviour of a system at its endpoint. It is there that the sense of impending failure arises. Another interpretation addresses instability during movement rather than at its endpoint. It focuses on the quality of movement during range, not on terminal behaviour.

Flexion–extension of the lumbar spine is not a singular movement; it involves a combination of rotation and translation (see Ch. 8). Notwithstanding the range of

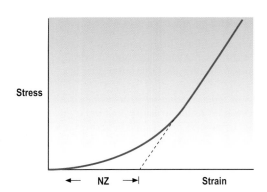

Figure 16.1 An archetypical stress–strain curve showing the location of the neutral zone (NZ).

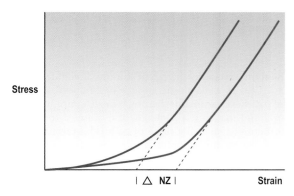

Figure 16.2 The stress–strain curve of a lumbar segment that exhibits instability in terms of an increased neutral zone (ΔNZ) compared to a normal curve.

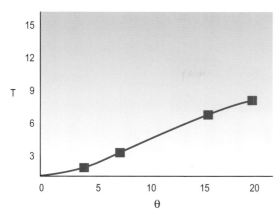

Figure 16.3 A normal movement pattern of a lumbar segment in terms of the ratio between translation and rotation. *(Based on Weiler et al. 1990.[10])*

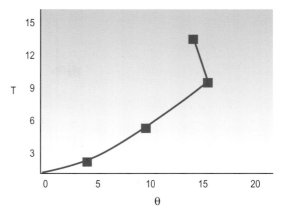

Figure 16.4 A movement pattern of a lumbar segment showing an aberrant ratio between translation and rotation, and an abnormally high instability factor. *(Based on Weiler et al. 1990.[10])*

motion, the quality of motion may be defined in terms of the ratio between the amplitude of translation and the amplitude of rotation. For each phase of movement there should be a certain amount of translation accompanied by an appropriate degree of rotation. If this ratio is disturbed, the motion becomes abnormal and the sense of instability may arise. In this regard, the instability would be defined as an inordinate amount of translation for the degree of rotation undergone, or vice versa.

Normal lumbar segments exhibit an essentially uniform ratio of translation to rotation during flexion–extension.[10] The overall pattern of movement looks smooth; translation progresses regularly, as does rotation (Fig. 16.3). The ratio between translation and rotation at any phase of movement is the same as the ratio between total translation and total rotation.

It may be defined that instability occurs when, at any time in the movement, there is an aberration to this ratio. The segment suddenly exhibits an inordinate translation for the degree of rotation undergone, or may translate without any rotation (Fig. 16.4).

This definition conveys the sense of inordinate displacement but places it during the normal range of motion instead of at its endpoint. The segment may be terminally stable but expresses instability during range. The sense of catastrophe does not obtain in the conventional sense, in that the segment will not fall apart, but it is present qualitatively. For that brief moment when the unexpected inordinate movement suddenly occurs, the sensation will be the same as that of impending failure. The fact that the joint is ultimately stable is not sufficiently reassuring, for during the unstable phase the movement is alarming and qualitatively the same as if the spine were about to fall apart.

Special techniques are required to detect this form of instability. They involve taking serial radiographs of the motion, at least five exposures for the entire range of motion, and determining the ratios of translation to rotation for each phase. From these ratios, an instability factor (IF) can be computed, namely.

$$IF = \Sigma \, (\Delta T)_i / \Sigma \, (\Delta \theta)_i$$

where $(\Delta T)_i$ is the range of translation for each phase of motion (i) and $(\Delta \theta)_i$ is the range of rotation for each phase.[10] In normal spines, the instability factor has a mean value of 25 (mm radian^{-1}) and a standard deviation of 8.7. Values beyond the upper two SD range nominally qualify for instability.

ANATOMY

Although biomechanical definitions for instability are available, for them to be meaningful clinically they require translation into anatomy. For treatment to be rational and targeted, the structure must be specified which is responsible for the decreased stiffness, the increased neutral zone or the excessive translation versus rotation.

In principle, a spectrum of possibilities arises (Fig. 16.5). Instability may be related to the extent of injury to a segment and the factors that remain trying to stabilise it. At one extreme lies complete dislocation, where no factors maintain the integrity of the segment. At the opposite extreme lies an intact segment that is absolutely stable. Between lies a hierarchy of possibilities.

In a totally disrupted segment, instability will be overt. Gravity may be the only factor keeping it together. As long as the patient remains upright, the compressive loads between vertebrae keep them in place. However, if the patient leans forwards, the affected segment can simply

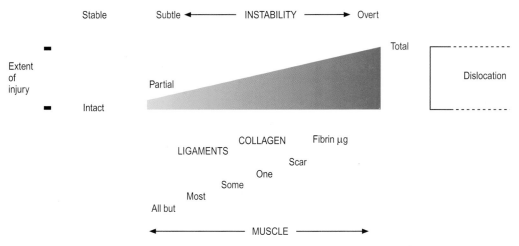

Figure 16.5 The relationship between instability, extent of injury and the factors maintaining stability.

slip forwards under gravity. Friction, fibrin deposits or scar tissue may offer token resistance to displacement but are insufficient practically to stabilise the segment.

For any degree of stability, the segment requires its stabilising elements: its facets and ligaments (see Chs 3 and 4). The fewer of these that are intact, the more liable the segment is to catastrophic failure; the more that are intact, the more stable the segment becomes.

Numerous studies have been conducted that demonstrate how progressively removing each of the restraining elements progressively disables a lumbar motion segment. Transecting the posterior longitudinal ligament and posterior anulus fibrosus produces hypermobility, even when other elements remain intact.[11] Progressively transecting the supraspinous and interspinous ligaments, ligamentum flavum, joint capsules, facets, the posterior longitudinal ligament and the posterior anulus fibrosus leads to progressively greater displacements when a segment is loaded in flexion, with the greatest increase in displacement occurring after transection of the posterior disc.[12] Short of transecting the disc, the zygapophysial joints appear to be the major stabilising elements in flexion.[13,14]

Superimposed on the facets and ligaments are muscles. These contribute to stability in two ways. The lesser mechanism is to pull directly against threatened displacements. In this regard, however, the back muscles are not well oriented to resist anterior or posterior shear or torsion; they run longitudinally and can only resist sagittal rotation (see Ch. 9). However, whenever the muscles act they exert compressive loads on the lumbar spine. This achieves a stabilising effect. By compressing joints, the muscles make it harder for the joints to move, and a variety of studies have now documented the stabilising effect of muscles on the lumbar spine.[15,16] Specifically, muscle contraction decreases the range of motion and decreases the

neutral zone of lumbar spinal segments, with the multifidus contributing the strongest influence.[16]

Notwithstanding the range of possible explanations for instability, across the spectrum of possibilities a transition occurs from concerns about terminal failure to interest in looseness, or instability within range. Overall, a segment may have most of its restraining elements intact and not be at risk of terminal failure, but the absence of a single restraining element may allow the segment to exhibit a partial inordinate movement within range. For clinical practice, two challenges obtain:

- Overt failure or impending failure is readily recognised radiographically in conditions such as fracture-dislocation when a vertebra exhibits malposition or an excessive motion apparent to the unaided eye. In such circumstances, instability is beyond doubt because the evident motion could not possibly have occurred unless the restraining elements were totally disrupted. However, the challenge obtains to determine the threshold for instability when the abnormal motion is not readily apparent.
- For instability within range, the challenge is to demonstrate its presence and to be certain that the abnormal motion is responsible for the patient's symptoms.

HYPOTHETICAL MODELS

The concepts offered by biomechanists can be collated and summarised graphically using a unifying device: a force and displacement graph (Fig. 16.6). For any lumbar movement there will be a force that induces displacement.

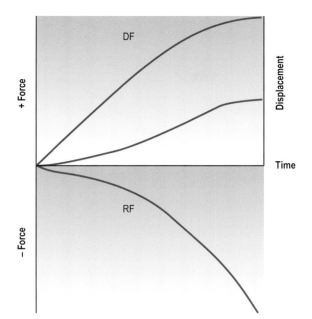

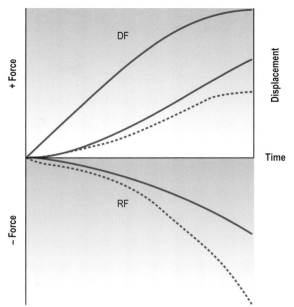

Figure 16.6 A force and displacement diagram. The difference between displacing forces (DF) and restraining forces (RF) results in displacement of a motion segment. The slope of the displacement curve is the velocity of movement. In a normal coordinated movement, the velocity curve is smooth and regular. Towards the end of range, the velocity slows to zero as movement is arrested.

Figure 16.7 A force and displacement diagram of a motion segment with decreased stiffness. Throughout the range, the restraining forces (RF) are considerably less than the displacing forces (DF) and the segment develops a higher than normal velocity towards end of range. For comparison, the normal curves for restraining forces and displacement (see Fig. 16.6) are shown as dotted lines.

Acting against this force will be restraining forces that stem from the facets, ligaments and muscles of the segment. These restraining forces act to prevent uncontrolled acceleration of the segment, under gravity for example. Given an appropriate combination of displacing forces and restraining forces, motion occurs; displacement progresses with time, and a velocity of motion emerges. The graph (see Fig. 16.6) shows the two opposing sets of forces and the change of displacement. The slope of this latter curve will be the velocity of movement. Under normal conditions, as displacing forces build up, the segment accelerates. As long as displacing forces exceed the restraining forces, movement continues. Towards the end of range, restraining forces exceed the displacing forces and movement decelerates, eventually stopping at end of range.

If a segment suffers a loss of stiffness, the restraining forces that resist forward flexion are reduced, but the gravitational forces that produce forward bending are unaltered and displacing forces remain the same (Fig. 16.7). As a result, the acceleration and eventual velocity of the resultant movement must, prima facie, be greater. Instability ensues if the balance between the displacing and restraining forces is insufficient to prevent inordinate dis-

placement or the threat of failure of the segment. Such instability obtains both throughout range and at terminal range.

If a segment suffers a loss of restraints that operate early in range but no loss of terminal restraints, the restraining forces will exhibit an increased neutral zone, but the displacing forces are unchanged (Fig. 16.8). As a result, the motion segment exhibits an essentially normal early velocity but as the difference between displacing and restraining forces increases, it accelerates and eventually exhibits a higher than normal velocity. The sense of instability arises because the terminal velocity is excessive and unexpected. Instead of the accustomed pattern of motion, there is an unfamiliar acceleration, which is alarming because it predicts (albeit inappropriately) that, at this rate of displacement, the segment threatens to fall apart.

If a segment suffers a loss of restraints that operate in mid-range or late in range, initial movements may be normal but the loss of restraints results in an acceleration late in range (Fig. 16.9). This acceleration is alarming because it feels as if the segment is about to shoot out of control.

These models convert the concept from one of abnormal range or abnormal displacement to one of excessive

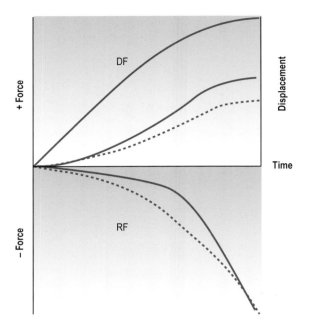

Figure 16.8 A force and displacement diagram of a motion segment with an increased neutral zone. The displacing forces (DF) and restraining forces (RF) are imbalanced early in range, and the segment accelerates towards end of range and develops a higher than normal terminal velocity. For comparison, the normal curves for restraining forces and displacement (see Fig. 16.6) are shown as dotted lines.

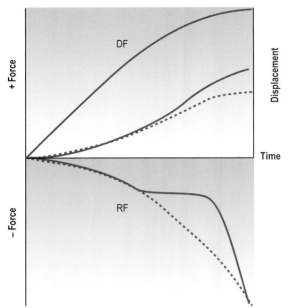

Figure 16.9 A force and displacement diagram of a motion segment exhibiting instability in mid-range. Early in range the balance between displacing forces (DF) and restraining forces (RF) is normal, and a normal velocity of movement occurs. When suddenly a restraining component fails to engage, the movement accelerates, reaching a higher than normal terminal velocity. For comparison, the normal curves for restraining forces and displacement (see Fig. 16.6) are shown as dotted lines.

acceleration. It is the degree of acceleration that corresponds to the degree of instability. The models also implicitly invoke a neurophysiological dimension. Instability arises when there is a mismatch between the expected and actual velocity of motion.

In neurophysiological terms, the mismatch is between the proprioceptive feedback and the motor programme for the movement. For a given movement, the individual will be accustomed to a particular pattern of motion, and therefore to a particular pattern of proprioceptive feedback. Habitually, they will have used a correspondingly appropriate pattern of activity of their back muscles. When, however, the pattern of motion changes, the proprioceptive feedback will be different, but if the individual uses their habitual motor pattern it will be inappropriate for the velocity of movement occurring. In essence, at a time when the individual is accustomed to expecting 'n' units of velocity and 'm' units of motor control, they actually suffer 'n + x' units of velocity, for which 'm' units of motor control are insufficient. As a result, the segment will feel as if it is 'getting away' or 'falling apart'. Hence the sensation of instability.

There is no guarantee that the nervous system can adapt to changes in the behaviour of mechanical constraints,

other than in a crude way. The changes in motion occur too quickly for the proprioceptive feedback to correct the motor activity by reflex. Instead, warned of the unaccustomed acceleration, the nervous system recruits a sudden muscle contraction, as if to deal with an 'emergency'. Clinically, this would manifest as a jerk or a 'catch'. Otherwise, in a very unstable segment, muscles may be persistently active to guard the affected segment against any movement that risks accelerating the segment.

In terms of these models, how instability relates to pain is a vexatious issue. Notionally, a hypermobile segment, or one with loss of stiffness, should not be painful. Pain might occur only at end of range when restraints were being excessively strained. If the loss of stiffness is due to injury, pain may arise from the injured structures, but in this regard the pain is independent of the instability; the pain may be aggravated by the movement, not because of instability but simply because the injured part is being irritated.

Segments with an increased neutral zone or with mid-range loss of restraints exhibit a marked terminal acceleration. A model that might explain pain under these circumstances invokes what might be referred to as abnormal 'attack'. Normally, terminal restraints in a segment would be engaged at a normal, accustomed velocity. However, in an unstable segment, these restraints will be engaged, or 'attacked', at a greater than normal velocity. Perhaps the more forceful attack on these restraints stimulates nociceptors in them.

However, notwithstanding these speculations, it may well be that there is no need to explain the pain of instability because there is no direct relationship. Pain may arise from a segment simply because it is injured. Instability may be present but in parallel. Movement is painful as in any painful segment. But if the movement is suddenly jerked or arrested, the sudden compression load exerted by the back muscles might be the aggravating factor for the pain, rather than a painful engagement of restraints.

CLINICAL INSTABILITY

Almost antithetical to the biomechanists' notion of instability is the concept of 'clinical instability'. Two uses of this latter term obtain.

One use is explicitly clinical and temporal; it bears no relationship to biomechanics. It maintains that clinical instability is a condition in which the clinical status of a patient with back problems steps, with the least provocation, from the mildly symptomatic to the severe episode.[17] Philosophically and semantically this does amount to instability in the sense that a trivial force causes a major displacement, but the displacement is not of a mechanical entity; it is a displacement of the patient's *symptoms* or of their clinical course. This use of the term is akin to speaking of an individual's mood or emotions being 'unstable'. This use of the term should not be confused or equated with the biomechanical use. More seriously, because it lacks any relationship to biomechanics, a diagnosis of clinical instability does not suggest, let alone indicate, mechanical therapy. There is a risk that, because 'clinical instability' and 'biomechanical instability' sound alike, they are equivalent. They are not.

A second definition of clinical instability has a more evident and legitimate relationship to biomechanics. It refers to biomechanical instability that reaches clinical significance, in that it produces symptoms. In this regard, the clinical features are immaterial to the basic definition; the definition rests on biomechanical abnormalities. The addition of the adjective 'clinical' simply promotes the biomechanical instability to one of ostensible clinical relevance. However, and most particularly, it does not imply that the instability is clinical evident; it implies only that the instability is clinically relevant.

The diagnosis of instability still hinges on biomechanical tests.

DIAGNOSIS

Instability is readily abused as a diagnostic rubric. It is easy to say a patient has instability; it is much harder to satisfy any criteria that justify the use of this term.

Most irresponsible in this regard is the fashion to label as instability any spinal pain that is aggravated by movement. This is patently flawed. Conditions can occur which are painful and which are aggravated by movement but which involve no instability of the spine. The movements of the affected segment are normal in quality and in range; they are not excessive. Indeed, the range of movement may be restricted rather than excessive. For example, a septic arthritis is very painful, and any movement may aggravate the pain, but the joint and its segment are essentially intact and there is no risk of them falling apart. Osteoarthritis may be painful and aggravated by movements, and if anything, the joint is stiffer and more stable than normal.

If an anatomic or pathological diagnosis is available, it should be used, but 'instability' is not an arbitrary alternative that can be applied when no other diagnosis is apparent. Instability is clearly a biomechanical term and if it is to be applied, a biomechanical criterion must be satisfied. Pain on movement is not that criterion.

Criteria

Various authorities have issued guidelines for the legitimate use of the term instability.[8,18] The major categories are shown in Table 16.1. Categories I, II and III are beyond controversy. Each involves a condition that threatens the integrity of the spine and which can be objectively diagnosed by medical imaging, perhaps supplemented by biopsy.

Spondylolisthesis is a controversial category. Traditionally, the appearance of this condition has been interpreted as threatening. Even under normal circumstances, the L5 vertebra appears to be precariously perched on the sloping upper surface of the sacrum. Defects in the posterior elements, notably pars interarticularis fractures, threaten to allow the L5 vertebra to slip progressively across the

Table 16.1 Lumbar segmental instabilities

Category	Causes
I	Fractures and fracture-dislocations
II	Infections of the anterior elements
III	Neoplasms
IV	Spondylolisthesis
V	Degenerative

sacrum. However, the available data mitigate against this fear.

Spondylolisthesis rarely progresses in adults[19] or teenagers,[20] and therefore it appears inherently stable, despite its threatening appearance. Indeed, biplanar radiography studies of moving patients have shown that, if anything, grade 1 and grade 2 spondylolisthesis are associated with reduced range of motion rather than instability.[21] However, some patients with spondylolisthesis may exhibit forward slipping upon standing from a lying position,[22] but it is not clear whether the extent of slip in such cases is abnormal. Studies, using implanted tantalum balls in order to establish landmarks accurately, have found no evidence of instability.[23] In some patients, movement abnormalities may be revealed using special radiographic techniques, which include having the patient stand loaded with a 20 kg pack and hanging by their hands from an overhead bar.[24,25] These extreme measures, however, have been criticised as unrealistic and cumbersome.[6]

It is with respect to degenerative instability that the greatest difficulties arise. A classification system of this category of lumbar instability has been proposed (Box 16.1).[8,18] The secondary instabilities are easy to accept and understand. They involve surgical destruction of one or more of the restraining elements of the spine, and are thereby readily diagnosed on the basis of prior surgery and subsequent excessive or abnormal motion. It is the primary instabilities that pose the greatest difficulties.

Rotational instability has been described as a hypothetical entity.[26] Based on clinical intuition, certain qualitative radiographic signs have been described[17] but their normal limits have not been defined, nor has their reliability or validity been determined. Consequently, rotational instability remains only a hypothetical entity.

Translational instability is perhaps the most classic of all putative instabilities. It is characterised by excessive anterior translation of a vertebra during flexion of the lumbar spine. However, anterior translation is a normal component of flexion (see Ch. 8). The difficulty that arises is setting an upper limit of normal translation. Posner et al.[12] prescribed a limit of 2.3 mm or 8% of the length of the vertebral endplate for the L1–L4 vertebrae, and 1.6 mm or 6% for the L5 vertebra. Boden and Wiesel[27] however, demonstrated that many asymptomatic individuals exhibited static slips of such magnitude, and emphasised that, in the first instance, any slip should be dynamic before instability could be considered. A dynamic slip is one that is evident in full flexion but not in extension, or vice versa. Furthermore, even dynamic slips of up to 3 mm can occur in asymptomatic individuals; only 5% of an asymptomatic population exhibited slips greater than 3 mm. Accordingly, Boden and Wiesel[27] have advocated that 3 mm should be the threshold limit for diagnosing anterior translational instability. Hayes et al.,[28] however, found that 4 mm of translation occurred in 20% of their asymptomatic patients. Accordingly, 4 mm might be a better threshold limit.

Belief in retrolisthetic instability dates to the work of Knutsson.[29] He maintained that degenerative discs exhibited instability in the form of abnormal motions, notably retrolisthesis upon extension of the lumbar spine. This contention, however, was subsequently disproved when it was shown that similar appearances occurred in asymptomatic individuals.[28,30] As a result, there are no operational criteria for instability due to retrolisthesis, other than the guidelines of Boden and Wiesel[27] or Hayes et al.,[28] which state that up to 3 mm or 4 mm of translation can be normal.

Scoliotic instability amounts to no more than rotational instability or translational instability, alone or in combination, in a patient who happens to have scoliosis. Adding the adjective 'scoliotic' in no way changes the difficulties in defining and satisfying the diagnostic criteria for these putative instabilities.

There is no evidence, to date, that internal disc disruption is associated with instability. Radiographic biomechanical studies simply have not been conducted on patients with proven internal disc disruption.

Although positive correlations are lacking between disc degeneration and retrolisthetic rotational and translational instability, there are associations between disc degeneration and a raised instability factor.[10] Patients with disc degeneration exhibit a greater mean value of instability factor that is statistically significant (Fig. 16.10). However, because the technique for determining the instability factor is very demanding and time consuming, this method of studying instability has not been pursued further, to date.

Clinical diagnosis

Various clinical criteria have been proclaimed as indicative or diagnostic of lumbar instability.[17,31,32] At best, these constitute fancy. To be valid, clinical signs have to be validated

---

Box 16.1 Degenerative lumbar instabilities

Primary

- axial rotational
- translational
- retrolisthetic
- scoliotic
- internal disc disruption

Secondary

- post-disc excision
- post-laminectomy
- post-fusion

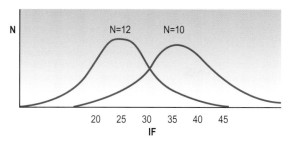

Figure 16.10 The distribution of values of instability factor (IF) in a normal population (left curve) and a population of patients with degenerative disc disease (right curve). *(Based on Weiler et al. 1990.[10])*

against a criterion standard. The only available criterion standard for instability is offered by radiographic signs, but the radiographic signs of instability are themselves beset with difficulties. Consequently, no studies have yet validated any of the proclaimed clinical signs of instability.

SUMMARY

Instability is a biomechanical term. Biomechanists have offered three distinct definitions of instability. One invokes decreased resistance to movement; the second invokes an increased neutral zone; and the third invokes altered ratios between translation and rotation. The first pertains to terminal instability while the latter two refer to instability within a normal range of motion.

The anatomical substrate for instability is damage to one or more of the restraining elements of the lumbar spine. For major types of instability, substantial damage to these elements is usually obvious radiographically. However, the anatomical basis for more subtle forms of instability remains elusive, as is the case for increased neutral zone or increased instability factor.

The diagnosis of major types of instability is relatively straightforward and relies on overt radiographic features. What remains contentious is whether or not so-called degenerative spinal disorders are associated with instability, and whether this type of instability can be diagnosed. There are no operational criteria for rotational and retrolisthetic instability. Operational criteria are available only for translational instability. The criteria for instability factor have been tested in only one study. There are no validated clinical signs by which instability might be diagnosed.

It is perhaps lamentable that for an entity that has attracted so much clinical attention, there is so little basis for its valid diagnosis. Nevertheless, the concepts of increased neutral zone and instability factor provide a likely explanation of what clinicians believe they have been diagnosing in patients who seem to suffer instability but who lack signs of overt instability. The challenge remains to correlate clinical wisdom with demonstrable radiographic biomechanical signs.

REFERENCES

1. Nachemson AL. Instability of the lumbar spine: pathology, treatment, and clinical evaluation. *Neurosurg Clin North Am.* 1991;2:785–790.

2. Pope MH, Frymoyer JW, Krag MH. Diagnosing instability. *Clin Orthop.* 1992;279:60–67.

3. Kirkaldy-Willis WH. Presidential symposium on instability of the lumbar spine: introduction. *Spine.* 1985;10:254.

4. Nachemson A. Lumbar spine instability: a critical update and symposium summary. *Spine.* 1985;10:290–291.

5. Wiesel S. Editor's corner. *Semin Spine Surg.* 1991;3:91.

6. Ashton-Miller JA, Schultz AB. Spine instability and segmental hypermobility biomechanics: a call for the definition and standard use of terms. *Semin Spine Surg.* 1991;3:136–148.

7. Pope MH, Panjabi M. Biomechanical definitions of spinal instability. *Spine.* 1985;10:255–256.

8. Frymoyer JW, Pope MH. Segmental instability. *Semin Spine Surg.* 1991;3:109–118.

9. Panjabi MM. The stabilizing system of the spine. Part II. Neutral zone and instability hypothesis. *J Spinal Disord.* 1992;5:390–397.

10. Weiler PJ, King GJ, Gertzbein SD. Analysis of sagittal plane instability of the lumbar spine in vivo. *Spine.* 1990;15:1300–1306.

11. Akkerveeken PF, O'Brien JP, Parl WM. Experimentally induced hypermobility in the lumbar spine: a pathologic and radiologic study of the posterior ligament and annulus fibrosus. *Spine.* 1979;4:236–241.

12. Posner I, White AA, Edwards WT, et al. A biomechanical analysis of the clinical stability of the lumbar and lumbosacral spine. *Spine.* 1982;:374–389.

13. Abumi K, Panjabi MM, Kramer KM, et al. Biomechanical evaluation of lumbar spinal stability after graded facetectomies. *Spine.* 1990;15:1142–1147.

14. Pintar FA, Cusick JF, Yoganandan N, et al. The biomechanics of lumbar facetectomy under compression–flexion. *Spine.* 1992;17:804–810.

15. Panjabi M, Abumi K, Duranceau J, et al. Spinal stability and intersegmental muscle forces: a biomechanical model. *Spine.* 1989;14:194–200.

16. Wilke HJ, Wolf S, Claes LE, et al. Stability increase of the lumbar spine with different muscle groups: a biomechanical in vitro study. *Spine*. 1995;20:192–198.

17. Kirkaldy-Willis WH, Farfan HF. Instability of the lumbar spine. *Clin Orthop*. 1982;165:110–123.

18. Hazlett JW, Kinnard P. Lumbar apophyseal process excision and spinal instability. *Spine*. 1982;7:171–176.

19. Fredrickson BE, Baker D, McHolick WJ, et al. The natural history of spondylosis and spondylolisthesis. *J Bone Joint Surg*. 1984;66A:699–707.

20. Danielson BI, Frennered AK, Irstam LKH. Radiologic progression of isthmic lumbar spondylolisthesis in young patients. *Spine*. 1991;16:422–425.

21. Pearcy M, Shepherd J. Is there instability in spondylolisthesis? *Spine*. 1985;10:175–177.

22. Lowe RW, Hayes TD, Kaye J, et al. Standing roentgenograms in spondylolisthesis. *Clin Orthop*. 1976;117:80–84.

23. Axelsson P, Johnsson R, Stromqvist B. Is there increased intervertebral mobility in isthmic adult spondylolisthesis? A matched comparative study using roentgen stereophotogrammetry. *Spine*. 2000;25:1701–1703.

24. Friberg O. Lumbar instability: a dynamic approach by traction-compression radiography. *Spine*. 1987;12:119–129.

25. Kalebo P, Kadziolka R, Sward L. Compression–traction radiography of lumbar segmental instability. *Spine*. 1990;15:351–355.

26. Farfan HF, Gracovetsky S. The nature of instability. *Spine*. 1984;9:714–719.

27. Boden SD, Wiesel SW. Lumbosacral segmental motion in normal individuals. Have we been measuring instability properly? *Spine*. 1990;15:571–576.

28. Hayes MA, Howard TC, Gruel CR, et al. Roentgenographic evaluation of lumbar spine flexion–extension in asymptomatic individuals. *Spine*. 1989;14:327–331.

29. Knutsson F. The instability associated with disk degeneration in the lumbar spine. *Acta Radiol*. 1944;25:593–609.

30. La Rocca H, MacNab I. Value of pre-employment radiographic assessment of the lumbar spine. *Ind Med Surg*. 1970;39:31–36.

31. Grieve GP. Lumbar instability. In: Grieve G, ed. *Modern Manual Therapy of the Vertebral Column*. Edinburgh: Churchill Livingstone; 1986;416–441.

32. Paris SV. Physical signs of instability. *Spine*. 1985;10:277–279.

Chapter | **17** |

Reconstructive anatomy

Anatomy is often perceived by students as a subject devoted to listing the names of parts of the body. Names are important, for they are the vocabulary that health professionals use to communicate with one another; but anatomy does not stop there.

Advanced anatomy is sometimes perceived as the study and knowledge of details, e.g. the so-called minutiae of structure. Although burdensome and overwhelming to beginners, such detail has the habit, sooner or later, of assuming clinical relevance.

The preceding chapters of this book have, to various extents, addressed these two domains of anatomy. They provide the names of bones, joints, muscles, blood vessels and nerves and they provide various details about these structures.

There is, however, another objective of anatomy education. It is to provide students with a global, comprehensive appreciation of a structure or a region. Such an appreciation is fundamental to competent clinical practice. For someone examining the lumbar spine, it should be more than an anonymous, mysterious structure buried under the skin of the back. For someone reading radiographs or magnetic resonance images, it should be more than a bewildering array of black, white and grey masses. Whatever the medium that they use, clinical practitioners should have a comfortable understanding of the lumbar spine in its entirety. They should be able to move from bones to joints to muscles, vessels and nerves in a seamless fashion. Yet this may be difficult to do, for someone armed with just a litany of names, through which they scramble desperately, in an effort to make sense of the global structure.

There is a device by which students can become comfortable with the anatomy of regions. It is the discipline of reconstructive anatomy. Instead of scrambling through jumbled memories of names and the shape of structures, students can use a step-wise approach to organise the recall of facts. This chapter outlines such an approach, and it predicates the next chapter (Ch. 18) on radiographic anatomy.

PRINCIPLES

The principles of reconstructive anatomy are to start with the bones; arrange them into their normal configuration, and thereby establish their joints. Then, progressively add additional structures in some form of logical order; for example, add the ligaments (because these are next most intimately associated with the bones) followed by the muscles and fasciae (because these are next most intimately associated). Thereafter, thread the vessels and nerves around the bones and into the muscles.

For the purposes of recall, all that is required is to remember the order in which the region was reconstructed. If and once students can remember that, they will forever be equipped to reproduce the process. Then, in clinical practice, if confronted by the need to recall the entire region, they can quickly use the principles to reconstruct the region, and use the various steps to precipitate recall of necessary detail.

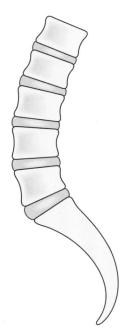

Figure 17.1 The appearance of the five lumbar vertebral bodies and their discs, as seen in a lateral view, forming a column resting on the sacrum.

This will not happen automatically, or by magic. Some degree of rehearsal and practice is required. The first iteration of that practice is what follows.

THE LUMBAR SPINE

The starting point is to recall that the lumbar spine consists of five vertebrae. The quintessential elements of those vertebrae are the **vertebral bodies**. These are stacked into a column, standing on the sacrum. The vertebral bodies are separated by the **intervertebral discs**.

It is the lateral view of this column that introduces the next level of detail. The vertebrae are stacked in a curved fashion, forming the lumbar **lordosis** (Fig. 17.1) A feature of reference in this column is that, most often, the third lumbar vertebra is the most horizontal. Higher vertebrae tilt forwards and upwards; lower vertebrae tilt forwards and downwards. Students able to invoke detail will recall that the average L1–S1 **lordosis angle** is about 70°, which dictates how curved the lordosis should be.

In an anterior view, there is nothing remarkable about this column. The vertebral bodies appear as rectangles, separated by their discs (Fig. 17.2A). Similarly, in a posterior view the column of vertebral bodies is unremarkable. The one new feature is that the posterior surfaces of the

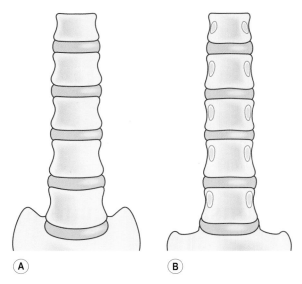

Figure 17.2 The appearance of the five lumbar vertebral bodies and their discs, forming a column resting on the sacrum. (A) Anterior view. (B) Posterior view.

vertebral bodies are marked by the origin of the **pedicles** (Fig. 17.2B).

The next layer of reconstruction, in the anterior view, introduces the **anterior longitudinal ligament** (Fig. 17.3A). Correspondingly, in the posterior view, the **posterior longitudinal ligament** is introduced (Fig. 17.3B).

For the time being, the reconstruction focuses on what lies behind the vertebral bodies. This introduces the **dural sac**, lying in the vertebral canal, and containing the caudal end of the **spinal cord**, which terminates opposite the L1–2 level (Fig. 17.4A). Hanging from the spinal cord are the nerve roots forming the **cauda equina** and the **lumbar nerve roots** passing around the pedicles to their intervertebral foramina (Fig. 17.4B). Eventually, these are enclosed by the posterior half of the dural sac (Fig. 17.4C).

The vertebral canal is then covered by the **posterior elements** of the lumbar vertebral column (Fig. 17.5A). They consist of the **laminae** and **zygapophysial joints**, the **transverse processes** and the **spinous processes**. The laminae are joined by the **ligamentum flavum**, while the spinous processes are joined by the **interspinous ligaments**. At this stage of the reconstruction, the anterior view has changed little. The transverse processes are the only posterior elements evident in an anterior view. They are seen projecting laterally behind the vertebral bodies (Fig. 17.5B).

A lateral view of this stage of reconstruction shows the posterior elements projecting behind the vertebral bodies, and enclosing the dural sac; the lumbar **spinal nerves** lie below the pedicles in their **intervertebral foramina** (Fig. 17.6). In a lateral view, the superior articular processes cover the inferior articular processes of the vertebra above. So, the inferior articular processes are not evident. At typical lumbar levels, the transverse processes project towards the viewer, from the posterior end of the pedicles; but the transverse process of L5 has a large root, which

expands across the lateral surface of the L5 pedicle and onto the L5 vertebral body. The boundaries of the intervertebral foramina are the pedicles above and below, the vertebral body and intervertebral disc anteriorly, and the ligamentum flavum and zygapophysial joints posteriorly.

Around the waists of the vertebral bodies run the **lumbar arteries** and **lumbar veins**. In an anterior view, their origins and terminals await connection to the aorta and inferior vena cava; but their trunks disappear posteriorly around the vertebral bodies (Fig. 17.7A). In a lateral view, these vessels cross the vertebral body, heading towards the intervertebral foramina and posterior elements (Fig. 17.7B).

These vessels are covered by the muscles that flank the vertebral bodies, and lie anterior to the plane of the transverse processes. In an anterior view, the **quadratus lumborum** covers the outer ends of the transverse processes; and the **psoas major** covers the roots of the transverse processes and the lateral surfaces of the vertebral bodies and intervertebral discs (Fig. 17.8A). The quadratus lumborum is broad but flat and thin. The psoas major is narrow in the upper lumbar spine but broadens progressively caudally, as more fibres are added to it, and becomes relatively massive at lower lumbar levels. As the psoas enlarges, it bulges over the quadratus lumborum. In a lateral view, the psoas major covers the vertebral bodies and intervertebral discs, while the quadratus lumborum is seen in profile, as a narrow flat plane of muscle covering the tips of the transverse processes (Fig. 17.8B).

The final stage of reconstruction of the anterior region of the lumbar spine involves placing the great vessels. In

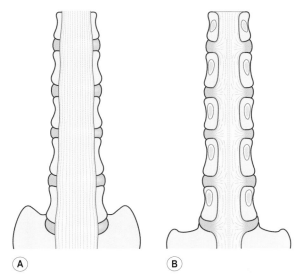

Figure 17.3 The lumbar vertebral bodies and their discs, onto which the longitudinal ligaments have been added (*cf.* Fig. 17.2). (A) Anterior longitudinal ligament. (B) Posterior longitudinal ligament.

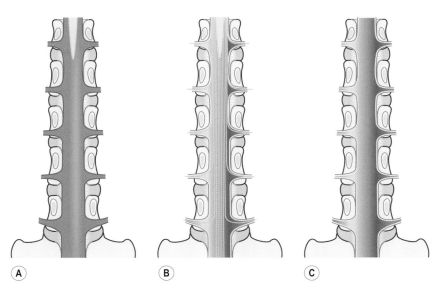

Figure 17.4 The contents of the vertebral canal. (A) The anterior half of the dural sac, and the spinal cord terminating at L1–2. (B) The lumbar nerve roots and roots of the cauda equina. (C) The posterior half of the dural sac enclosing the cauda equina.

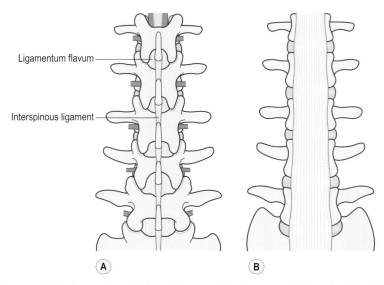

Figure 17.5 The lumbar vertebral column after addition of the posterior elements. (A) Posterior view. (B) Anterior view. lf, ligamentum flavum; isl, interspinous ligament.

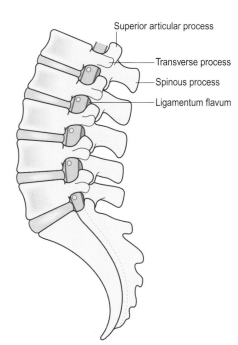

Figure 17.6 A lateral view of the lumbar vertebral column, showing the posterior elements and the intervertebral foramina containing the lumbar spinal nerves. tp, transverse process; sap, superior articular process; sp, spinous process; lf, ligamentum flavum.

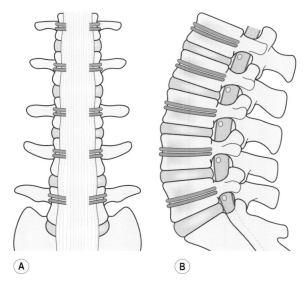

Figure 17.7 The lumbar spine, to which the lumbar arteries and veins have been added. (A) Anterior view. (B) Lateral view. (*cf.* Figs 17.5B and 17.6.)

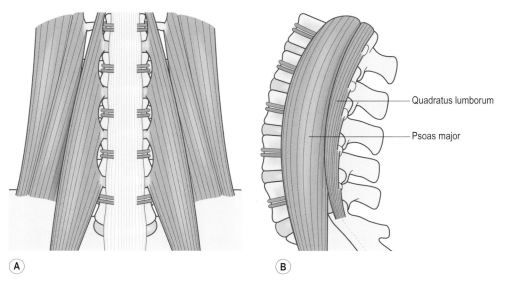

Figure 17.8 The lumbar spine, to which the quadratus lumborum and psoas major have been added (*cf.* Fig. 17.7). (A) anterior view. (B) lateral view.

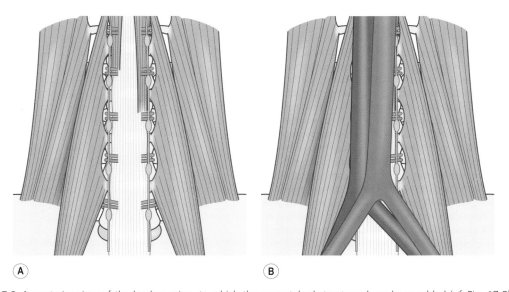

Figure 17.9 An anterior view of the lumbar spine, to which the prevertebral structures have been added (*cf.* Fig. 17.8). (A) The left crus and right crus have been added, together with the left and right lumbar sympathetic trunks and their ganglia. (B) The inferior vena cava and abdominal aorta have been added.

the upper lumbar region, the aorta and inferior vena cava are related to the crura of the diaphragm. The **left crus** attaches to the vertebral column, in a tapering fashion, as far down as the L3 vertebra. The **right crus** is shorter, reaching only as far as L2 (Fig. 17.9A). With the crura placed, it is a convenient time to introduce the **lumbar**

sympathetic trunks. These issue from the crura and run caudally along the medial border of the psoas major (Fig. 17.9A).

The **inferior vena cava** is formed by the convergence of the common iliac veins in front of the L5 vertebra (Fig. 17.9B). It then ascends across the right-hand side of the

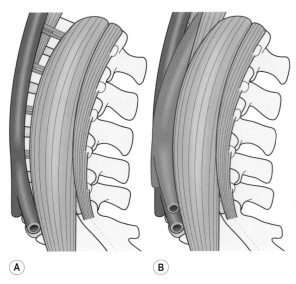

(A)   (B)

Figure 17.10 A lateral view of the lumbar spine (viewed from the left), to which (A) the right crus and the inferior vena cava have been added, and (B) the aorta and left crus have been added.

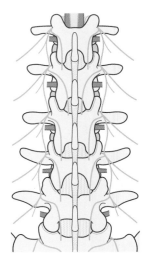

Figure 17.11 A posterior view of the lumbar spine showing the branches of the lumbar dorsal rami.

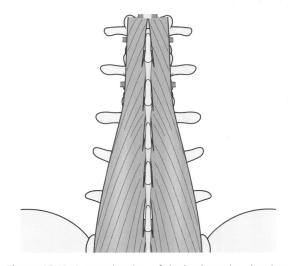

Figure 17.12 A posterior view of the lumbar spine showing the multifidus muscle.

lumbar vertebral column. At the L1 level, it is pushed forwards by the right crus, so that it can penetrate the central tendon of the diaphragm to reach the heart (Fig. 17.10A). The abdominal aorta starts between the left and right crura, and descends across the left-hand side of the lumbar vertebral column (Fig. 17.9B). It terminates in front of the L4 vertebra by dividing into the common iliac arteries (Figs 17.9B, 17.10B). As a result of this arrangement, the vascular relations of the lumbar vertebrae differ. At L1, both the inferior vena cava and aorta are present, but the inferior vena cava is being pushed forwards by the right crus. At L2, both great vessels are present, but the inferior vena cava is closer to the vertebral column as the right crus tapers. At L3, the crura have both dissipated, and the two great vessels lie directly in front of the vertebral column. At L4, the inferior vena cava persists, but the aorta divides. Therefore, three vessels lie in front of L4: the inferior vena cava and the two common iliac arteries. At L5, the inferior vena cava is formed. Therefore, four vessels lie in front of L5: the two common iliac arteries and the two common iliac veins.

The remaining phase of the reconstruction is to complete the posterior compartment. This contains several nerves and three large muscles.

The branches of the **lumbar dorsal rami** lie in the deepest layer of the posterior compartment (Fig. 17.11), and enter their respective muscles through their deep aspects. The **medial branches** enter the multifidus, the **intermediate branches** enter longissimus thoracis pars

lumborum and the **lateral branches** enter iliocostalis lumborum.

In the upper lumbar region, the **multifidus** is restricted to the region behind the laminae, but from L3 caudally the muscle expands to assume its insertions into the posterior surface of the sacrum (Fig. 17.12). As a result, it is virtually the only muscle present in the lumbosacral region.

The **longissimus thoracis pars lumborum** flanks the multifidus. It arises from the lumbar intermuscular aponeurosis, which is anchored to the medial aspect of the posterior segment of the ilium. The muscle fibres insert into the region around the accessory processes of the lumbar transverse processes (Fig. 17.13).

The **iliocostalis lumborum pars lumborum** completes the three major posterior lumbar back muscles. Rising from the iliac crest, it inserts into the distal ends of the upper four lumbar transverse processes (Fig. 17.14).

When the three posterior back muscles are viewed from a lateral perspective, certain features become apparent. The multifidus is the most medial of the three muscles. It lies behind the depth of the articular processes and lamina. Its fibres largely run dorsally and cephalad, and are evident throughout the lumbar region (Fig. 17.15A).

The lumbar fibres of the longissimus thoracic run ventrally and cephalad, i.e. contrary to the direction of the fibres of the multifidus muscle (Fig. 17.15B). Furthermore, these fibres fill only the ventral-caudal half of the posterior lumbar region, leaving a space vacant in the

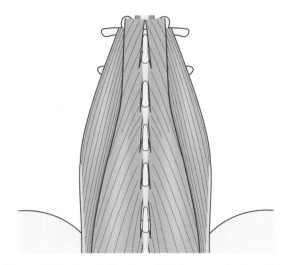

Figure 17.13 A posterior view of the lumbar spine to which the longissimus thoracis pars lumborum and the lumbar intermuscular aponeurosis have been added (*cf.* Fig. 17.12).

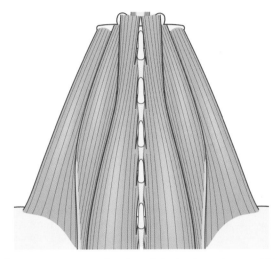

Figure 17.14 A posterior view of the lumbar spine to which the iliocostalis lumborum pars lumborum has been added (*cf.* Fig. 17.13).

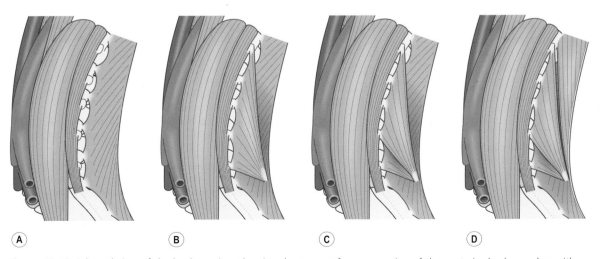

(A) (B) (C) (D)

Figure 17.15 A lateral view of the lumbar spine, showing the stages of reconstruction of the posterior back muscles, with individual muscles being progressively added. (A) Multifidus. (B) Longissimus thoracis pars lumborum. (C) Iliocostalis lumborum pars lumborum. (D) The lower thoracic fibres of erector spinae.

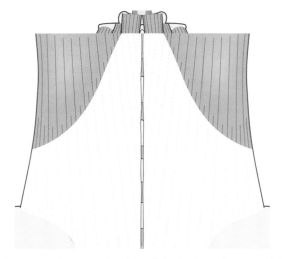

Figure 17.16 A posterior view of the lumbar spine, to which the erector spinae aponeurosis and lower thoracic fibres of iliocostalis lumborum and longissimus thoracic have been added (*cf.* Fig. 17.14).

dorsal-cephalad half. A similar appearance arises upon the addition of the lumbar fibres of iliocostalis lumborum (Fig. 17.15C). Its fibres, too, run ventrally and cephalad, filling the ventral-caudal half of the region, and leaving vacant the dorsal-cephalad half.

The vacant dorsal-cephalad corner is filled by the lower, thoracic fibres of longissimus thoracis and iliocostalis lumborum (Fig. 17.15D). These fibres arise from the ventral surface of the erector spinae aponeurosis and so, complete the posterior lumbar region when that aponeurosis is finally added to the region. In posterior view, the erector spinae aponeurosis covers all the foregoing muscles, and completes the posterior surface of the lumbar region (Fig. 17.16).

SYNOPSIS

The method of reconstructive anatomy involves taking a starting point and systematically applying, in order, the structures that are encountered in various directions from the starting point. For purposes of recall, all that is required is to remember the short lists of structures in each direction.

Thus, starting with the column of vertebral bodies and intervertebral discs:

- Anteriorly, we expect to encounter: the **anterior longitudinal ligament**, the **crura** of the diaphragm and the **aorta** and **inferior vena cava**.

- Laterally, we expect to encounter: the **lumbar arteries** and **veins**, covered by the **psoas major**, which is flanked by the **quadratus lumborum**.

- Posteriorly, we expect to encounter: the **dural sac** and its contents, enclosed by the **posterior elements** of the lumbar vertebra, which in turn are covered by the branches of the **dorsal rami**, which innervate the three major, posterior **back muscles**.

For each structure, certain pertinent details can be applied, in order to perfect the reconstruction.

- The anterior longitudinal ligament is found throughout the lumbar region.
- The crura occur only at upper lumbar levels, as far as L2 for the right crus, and L3 for the left crus.
- The aorta starts between the two crura, and ends at L4.
- The inferior vena cava starts at L5, and is pushed forwards by the right crus.
- The lumbar arteries and veins are clamped against the vertebral bodies by the psoas major.
- The psoas major is narrow at upper lumbar levels but expands to be massive at lower lumbar levels.
- The quadratus lumborum is broad but flat, and is found only above L5, because it arises from the iliolumbar ligament and transverse process of L5.
- The dural sac contains the spinal cord, cauda equina, and lumbar nerve roots.
- The lumbar nerve roots curve around the inferomedial margins of the pedicles, taking a sleeve of dura mater with them.
- The posterior elements are the pedicles, transverse processes, superior and inferior articular processes, and the spinous processes.
- The boundaries of the intervertebral foramina are the vertebral body and disc, the two pedicles, and the ligamentum flavum and zygapophysial joint.
- The multifidus covers the laminae of the lumbar vertebrae, but expands to cover the back of the sacrum.
- The longissimus thoracis pars lumborum is centred over the lumbar accessory processes and proximal transverse processes.
- The iliocostalis lumborum pars lumborum, aims for the tips of the lumbar transverse processes cephalad of L5.

This list and these details constitute what practitioners should *expect* to encounter in the lumbar spine. That expectation is particularly critical when particular structures are not necessarily visible or palpable. Even though they may not be evident, practitioners should be able expect where they should be. This skill – known as **anatomy by expectation** – becomes paramount in the recognition and appreciation of radiographs and magnetic resonance images of the lumbar spine, which is what the concluding chapters address.

Radiographic anatomy

Plain radiographs do not show soft tissues, such as ligaments, muscles and blood vessels. They show only bones. However, the bones behave as if they are transparent. Therefore, if two or more bones are superimposed, their respective images will also be superimposed. The same applies to bones with multiple parts, such as the lumbar vertebrae. If multiple parts are aligned along the X-ray beam, their images will be superimposed. This phenomenon complicates the interpretation of plain radiographs of the lumbar spine.

Lateral views of the lumbar spine are relatively simple; few parts are superimposed, but anteroposterior (AP) views are complicated by multiple parts being superimposed. Under those conditions, interpretation is assisted by the use of *anatomy by expectation* (see Ch. 17). The reader should expect what should be present, and then determine if what they expect is, indeed, evident on the image.

LATERAL VIEWS

When viewing a lateral radiograph of the lumbar spine (Fig. 18.1), the reader should expect to see the osseous anatomy evident in a lateral view of an anatomical specimen (as described in Ch. 17) (Fig. 18.2). Soft tissues, such as the ligamentum flavum and spinal nerves will not be evident, but the vertebral bodies and posterior elements will be evident. The intervertebral discs will not be evident; they will appear as spaces between the vertebral bodies.

For readers to whom the various parts of the vertebrae are not immediately apparent on a lateral radiograph, a systematic approach can be applied, in which the parts of a single vertebra are identified, and subsequently the same process is repeated until the parts of all the vertebrae have been identified.

On the radiograph, select a vertebra image that is the least obscure: typically that of L3. The superior, anterior and inferior margins of the vertebral body should be evident, as they are not obscured by any overlying shadows. Trace those margins (Fig. 18.3). Continue the tracing onto the posterior margin until that margin meets the root of the pedicle. Continue the tracing onto the pedicle. Thereafter, the tracing may become difficult, but the reader is helped by looking for what they *expect* to see. Based on what they know to be the anatomy of the superior articular process (Fig. 18.2), the reader should expect that, from the posterior superior corner of the pedicle, the superior articular process would project dorsally and cephalad, like the rounded head of a small mushroom. Therefore, regardless of any other lines that might be evident, the reader should look to see if any lines correspond with such a rounded projection. From the superior border of the pedicle, the tracing should continue to circumscribe this rounded projection (Fig. 18.3).

Similarly, the reader should expect that, from the posterior inferior corner of the pedicle, a narrow lamina would project caudally and slightly dorsally, and eventually expand into a rounded mass that is the inferior articular process. As before, other lines should be disregarded, and only those that conform to this expectation should be traced to complete the inferior articular process (Fig. 18.3).

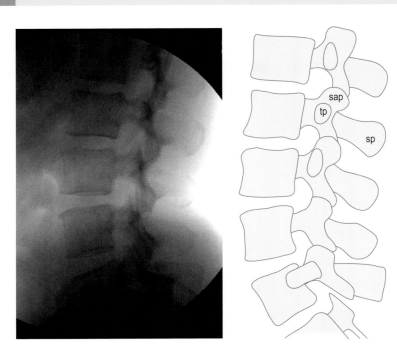

Figure 18.1 A lateral radiograph of the lumbar spine.

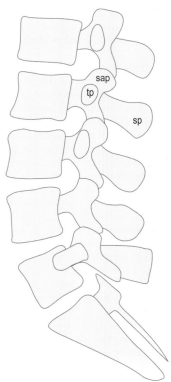

Figure 18.2 A lateral view of the lumbar spine. tp, transverse process; sap, superior articular process; sp, spinous process.

The reader should expect that the transverse process projects as an elliptical shadow at the junction between the pedicle and the superior articular process. Finding such an elliptical shadow locates the transverse process (Fig. 18.3).

For the spinous process, the reader should expect a projection, with the profile of the blade of an axe, arising from the back of the lamina. Finding and tracing the margin of the spinous process completes the identification of the posterior elements (Fig. 18.3).

Having accomplished this tracing of the L3 vertebra, the reader can repeat the process for all other vertebrae, until all lumbar vertebrae have been traced (Fig. 18.4). In this process, two details arise. Firstly, unlike those of typical lumbar levels, the transverse process of L5 has a large base that flows onto the pedicle and vertebral body of L5. Secondly, at all segmental levels, the superior articular processes cover the inferior articular processes of the vertebra above. The latter introduces a complexity.

Because bones behave as if they are transparent under X-ray, multiple markings can appear in the zygapophysial joints. These markings may create the illusion that the joint space projects laterally (Fig. 18.5). This appearance arises when C-shaped or J-shaped joints are viewed from the side. What appear to be the joint margins in a radiograph (lines 1 and 2 in Fig. 18.5) are only the articular margins of the ventral portion of the joint (Fig. 18.6A); but this is not the entire joint. The inferior articular process also presents the remainder of its joint surface laterally (Fig. 18.6B). This surface will be covered laterally by the remainder of the superior articular process (Fig. 18.6C),

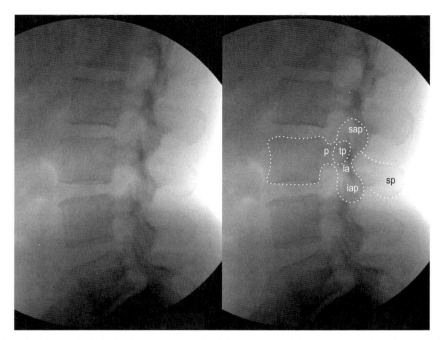

Figure 18.3 A lateral radiograph of the lumbar spine, in which the margins of the L3 vertebra have been outlined. p, pedicle; sap, superior articular process; la, lamina; iap, inferior articular process; sp, spinous process; tp, transverse process.

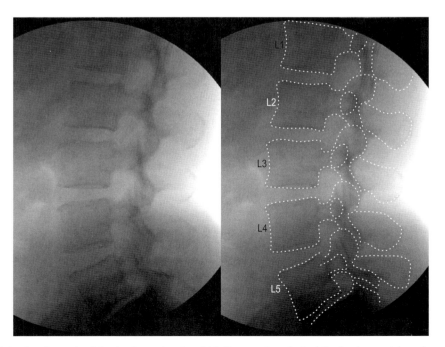

Figure 18.4 A lateral radiograph of the lumbar spine, in which the margins of all of the lumbar vertebrae have been outlined.

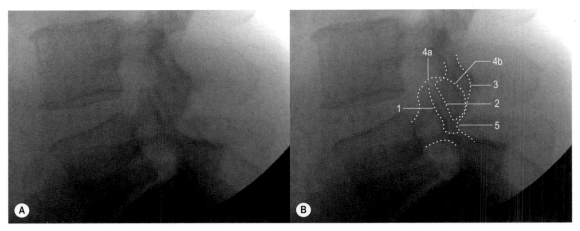

Figure 18.5 Close-up lateral radiographs of an L4–5 zygapophysial joint. (A) Multiple lines are evident in the region of the joint. (B) The multiple lines in the region of the joint have been marked and labelled. Lines 1 and 2 are the articular margins of the ventral compartment of the joint. Line 2 is continuous with line 3, which is the outline of the inferior articular process of L4. Line 4a is the cephalad margin of the superior articular process of L5, and is continuous with line 4b which is the dorsal margin of the superior articular process, and which becomes continuous with the lamina at line 5.

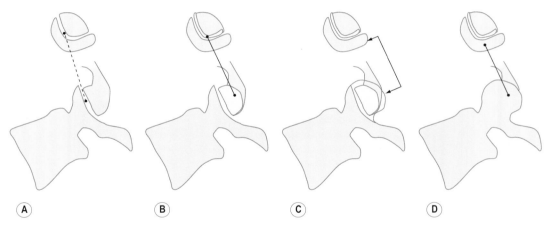

Figure 18.6 Correlations between the cross-sectional structure of a C-shaped zygapophysial joint and its appearance in lateral radiographs. (A) The joint space evident on the lateral view corresponds with only the ventral compartment of the joint in cross-sectional view. (B) The inferior articular process presents a further articular surface laterally. (C) This lateral surface is encompassed by the margin of the superior articular process. (D) The superior articular process obscures the inferior articular process and, therefore, the posterior compartment of the joint.

and in an intact anatomical specimen the inferior articular process will no longer be visible (Fig. 18.6D). As a result of this arrangement, line 2 in Figure 18.5B is continuous with the rest of the inferior articular process (line 3); and lines 4a and 4b form the outer margin of the superior articular process, which becomes continuous with the lamina as line 5. Having identified the silhouettes of all the parts of the lumbar vertebrae, the reader should then be able to imagine the location of related structures that are not visible with X-rays.

In the region of the vertebral bodies, the reader should expect: the **dural sac** behind the vertebral bodies; the **spinal nerves** in the intervertebral foramina; and the **psoas major** clamping the **lumbar arteries** and **lumbar veins** against the vertebral bodies (Fig. 18.7A). Anterior, towards the right, the reader should expect the **right crus** and the **inferior vena cava** (Fig. 18.7A). Posteriorly, behind the laminae and against the spinous processes, they should expect the **multifidus** muscle, with its fibres passing dorsally and cephalad (Fig. 18.7A). Superimposed

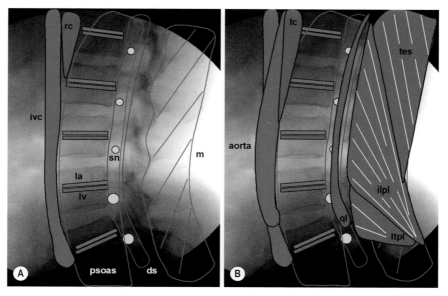

Figure 18.7 A lateral radiograph of the lumbar spine onto which certain related structures have been superimposed. (A) Centrally, dural sac (ds), the spinal nerves (sn), the lumbar arteries (la), lumbar veins (lv) and the psoas major (psoas); anteriorly, the right crus (rc) and inferior vena cava (ivc); posteriorly, the multifidus muscle (m). (B) centrally, the quadratus lumborum (ql); anteriorly, the aorta and left crus (lc); and posteriorly, the lumbar erector spinae, formed by longissimus thoracis pars lumborum (ltpl) and iliocostalis lumborum pars lumborum (ilpl), and the lower fibres of the thoracic erector spinae (tes).

on these structures the reader should expect various additional structures (Fig. 18.7B). Anteriorly, to the left of the inferior vena cava, they should expect the **aorta** and **left crus**. Centrally, they should expect the **quadratus lumborum** behind and lateral to the psoas. Posteriorly, they should expect the fibres of the lumbar and lower thoracic **erector spinae**, lateral to the multifidus. The fibres of these muscles would run cephalad and ventrally.

ANTERIOR (OR POSTERIOR) VIEW

Because of the transparency of bones to X-rays, anterior views and posterior views of the lumbar spine are identical. The transparency, however, complicates the images in two ways. The first is due to the tilting of the vertebrae in the lumbar lordosis. The second is due to the superimposition of posterior elements on the anterior elements.

In anterior or posterior views, because of the lumbar lordosis, not every vertebral body will be seen as horizontal. Upper vertebrae will be tilted to face cephalad and forwards, while lower vertebrae will be tilted caudad and forwards. As a result, whereas the superior and inferior borders of middle lumbar vertebral bodies will present as transverse lines, those of upper and lower vertebrae will present as ellipses (Fig. 18.8). Because upper lumbar vertebrae are tilted upwards, the anterior margins of their

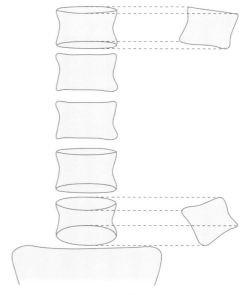

Figure 18.8 An anterior view of the lumbar vertebral bodies, showing how the upper and lower vertebrae present ellipses for their superior and inferior surfaces, because they are tilted in the lumbar lordosis. The insets show the tilt of the vertebrae in lateral appearance, and how the anterior and posterior margins of the vertebral body correspond to respective margins of the ellipses.

superior and inferior surfaces lie higher than the posterior margins. Therefore, the more cephalad margin of the ellipse corresponds with the anterior margin of the body, while the more caudad margin corresponds with the posterior margin (Fig. 18.8). For lower vertebral bodies, the opposite applies. These vertebrae are tilted downwards, and the anterior margins of their superior and inferior surfaces are lower than the respective posterior margins. Therefore, the more cephalad margin of the ellipse corresponds with the posterior margin of the vertebral body, while the more caudad margin corresponds with the anterior margin (Fig. 18.8).

Notwithstanding the tilt of the lumbar vertebrae, because of their transparency to X-rays, their anterior and posterior elements will be superimposed. Consequently, each vertebra will present a mass of overlapping lines and shadows. These can be resolved using *anatomy by expectation*. Readers should disregard any distracting lines, and look for what they expect should be there.

Readers should expect a rectangular shadow, with a scalloped waist, that corresponds to the vertebral body (Fig. 18.9). They should expect a pair of vertical ellipses that correspond to the pedicles, from which the transverse processes project laterally (Fig. 18.9). Finally, they should expect the rectangular plates of the laminae, from whose corners project the superior articular processes and inferior articular processes, and from the centre of which projects the spinous process (Fig. 18.9). Reading an anterior view

then becomes an exercise of identifying these various lines for each vertebra, and adjusting for the tilt of the vertebrae in the lumbar lordosis. An efficient protocol follows.

It is perhaps easiest to recognise first the pedicles and transverse processes, for these are least affected by tilt. Common radiologic teaching is to look for pedicles as if they were the 'eyes' of five vertebra looking forwards (Fig. 18.10). The transverse processes should be evident as rectangular bars projecting laterally from the pedicles.

At some segmental levels, the transverse processes may be hard to discern. When the strength of the X-rays is large, the thin transverse processes may absorb only a small fraction of the rays and, therefore, leave little shadow. At L5, the vertebra may be steeply tilted and the transverse process may look narrower than expected, and appear like a triangle rather than a rectangle. In such cases, when the transverse process is not readily apparent, it may be located by estimating where it should be, and what its profile might look like, by projecting the locations of the transverse processes above and copying the opposite transverse process at the segment in question.

Next, the bodies of the typical lumbar vertebrae can be found and traced. Adjustments will need to be made for superior and inferior surfaces appearing as ellipses (Fig. 18.11). In some cases, the ellipses of superior surfaces may assume the appearance of muffin tops. In tracing a given vertebral body, it is perhaps best to find the inferior corners, and join them with the inferior surface or its

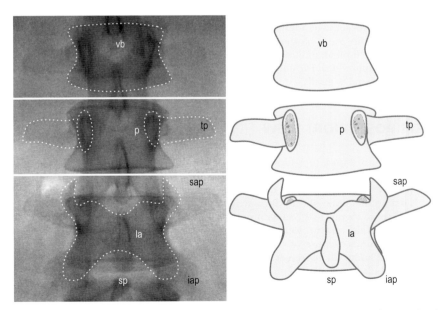

Figure 18.9 A key to the identification of lines seen on anterior views of the lumbar vertebrae. The margin of the vertebral body (vb) is a rectangle with a scalloped waist. The pedicels (p) are vertical ellipses, from which the transverse processes (tp) project laterally. The laminae (la) form a rectangular plate, from whose upper corners project the superior articular processes (sap), and from whose lower corners project the inferior articular processes (iap). sp, spinous process.

Figure 18.10 A pair of anteroposterior radiographs of the lumbar spine. On the right, the pedicles and transverse processes have been outlined.

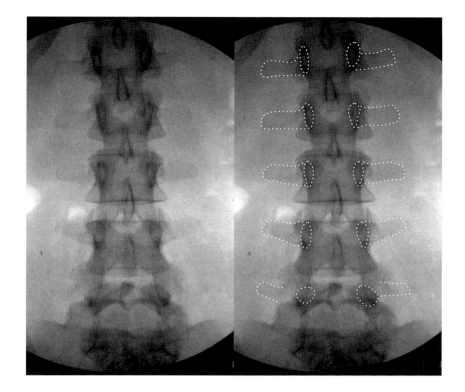

Figure 18.11 A pair of anteroposterior radiographs of the lumbar spine. On the right, the vertebral bodies of L1, L2, L3, and L4 have been outlined.

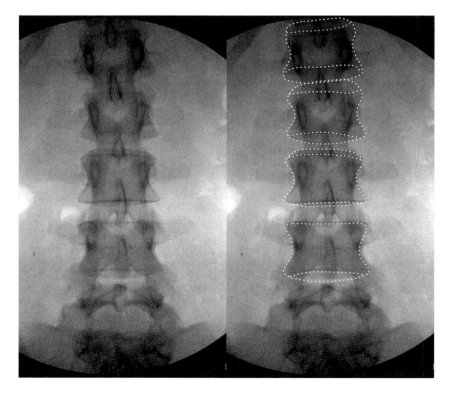

ellipse. From each corner, trace the lateral margin cephalad, expecting that it will assume the shape of the scalloped waist of the vertebral body; and in most instances the lateral margin will run tangential, or near, to the lateral margin of the pedicle. The superior corners may be difficult to discern amongst the shadows of the pedicle and superior articular process. The distinguishing features of a superior corner are that it is the only marking, in that region, that assumes a curved, right-angle bend, and which is simultaneously continuous with the lateral margin and with the superior margin. The latter will be the only transversely running line, or ellipse, that passes medially.

In the example shown in Figure 18.11, the vertebral body of L5 is difficult to discern. This arises because the vertebra is severely tilted into lordosis, so much so that its vertebral body is below the level of most of its posterior elements. Also, the vertebral body itself is wedge-shaped. As a result, it does not present a rectangular outline. Largely, the vertebral body presents its inferior surface. Consequently, inferior corners are not evident. However, on the right of the radiograph, a superior corner is evident, and to a lesser extent a superior corner is evident, symmetrically, on the left (Fig. 18.12). From each of these corners, a scalloped margin of the lateral surface of the vertebral body is evident. Between the lower ends of these lateral margins, a broad ellipse is faintly present, which represents the inferior surface (Fig. 18.12). Between the

superior corners, a dark transverse line is evident, joining the two corners, which corresponds to part of the superior surface. Otherwise, the remainder of the superior surface is faintly evident as a muffin top projecting cephalad, in a curve parallel to the posterior curvature of the inferior surface of L4 (Fig. 18.12). Once the vertebral body has been outlined, its steep inclination becomes evident.

The final step in recognising the radiograph is to trace the posterior elements. A suitable starting point can be the articular margins of a zygapophysial joint where one is evident. Straight, vertical lines will correspond to the articular surfaces (Fig. 18.13). From these straight lines, the respective curvatures of the superior and inferior articular processes can be traced. The convexity of the outer margin of the superior articular process will curve medially and inferiorly, across the pedicle, to become continuous with the lateral margin of the lamina (Fig. 18.13). A confirmatory feature is that, typically, the inferior margin of the transverse process flows seamlessly into the lateral margin of the lamina, opposite the inferolateral corner of the pedicle. The curvature of the inferior articular process continues upwards to become the inferior margin of the lamina (Fig. 18.13). The superior margin of the lamina is usually clearly evident towards the midline. Laterally, however, the superior margin is obscured by the inferior articular process, and its continuity with the superior articular process cannot be defined with certainty.

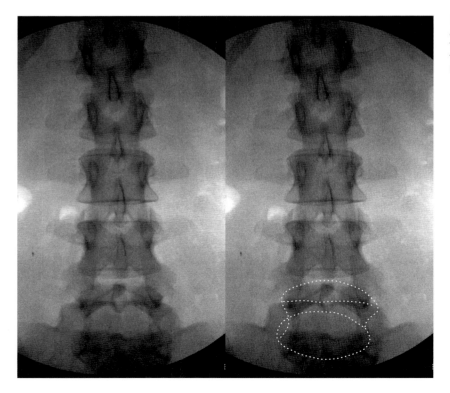

Figure 18.12 A pair of anteroposterior radiographs of the lumbar spine. On the right, the vertebral body of L5 has been outlined.

Figure 18.13 A pair of anteroposterior radiographs of the lumbar spine. On the right, the posterior elements of the lumbar vertebrae have been outlined.

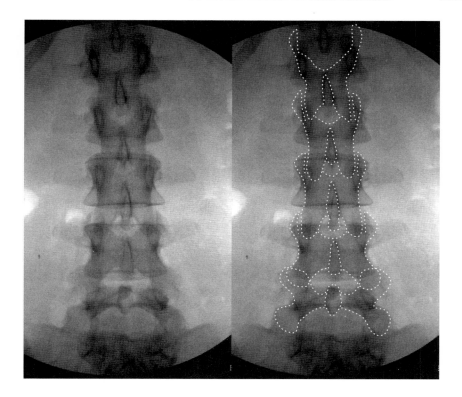

At segments where joint spaces and articular margins are not evident, the reader should recognise that they are looking at zygapophysial joints that face coronally. At these sites, the opposing – and, therefore, overlapping – inferior and superior articular processes will take on a rounded appearance, instead of presenting sharp corners at the superior or inferior end of the joint (Fig. 18.13).

Having established the osseous anatomy of the lumbar spine, readers should then be prepared to imagine the location of the related soft tissues. Behind the lumbar vertebral bodies will run the **dural sac** and its contents, with the lumbar **spinal nerves** and their dural sleeves curving around the pedicles (Fig. 18.14).

Anterior to the vertebral column, the reader should expect the **left crus** and **right crus**, at upper lumbar levels, and the lumbar **sympathetic trunks** throughout the length of the column (Fig. 18.15A). Lateral to the vertebral column they should expect the **quadratus lumborum** covered by the **psoas major** (Fig. 18.15A). Subsequently, the reader should expect the **inferior vena cava** and **aorta** to cover the vertebral bodies, as far as L5 and L4, respectively (Fig. 18.15B).

Posterior to the vertebral column, the reader should expect the **multifidus** covering the laminae, the longissimus thoracic pars lumborum aiming for the accessory processes, and the **iliocostalis lumborum pars lumborum** aiming for the tips of the transverse processes (Fig. 18.16).

DISCUSSION

In clinical practice, plain radiographs are being increasingly less often used, for they provide little diagnostic value; they are being replaced by CT scanning and magnetic resonance imaging (MRI). So, it might appear to students that learning how to read a plain radiograph of the lumbar spine is a pointless exercise. However, there are two virtues.

Firstly, reading a plain radiograph of the lumbar spine provides a suitable exercise and skill that practises the application of *anatomy by expectation*. Secondly, but more significantly for clinical practice, it constitutes a preparation, or rehearsal, for the more demanding exercise of reading MRI scans. Students who master reading plain radiographs will find it easy to anticipate, predict, and therefore read, MRI scans.

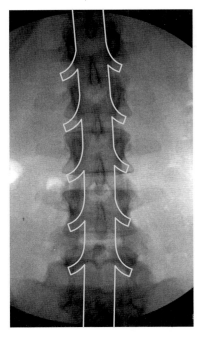

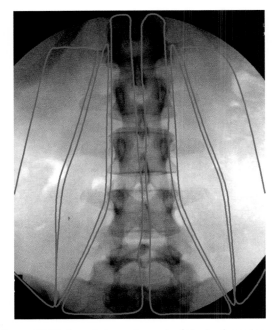

Figure 18.14 An anterior radiograph of the lumbar spine, onto which the location of the dural sac and the sleeves of the roots of the lumbar spinal nerves have been superimposed.

Figure 18.16 An anterior radiograph of the lumbar spine, onto which the locations of the **multifidus, longissimus thoracic pars lumborum** and **iliocostalis lumborum pars lumborum** have been superimposed.

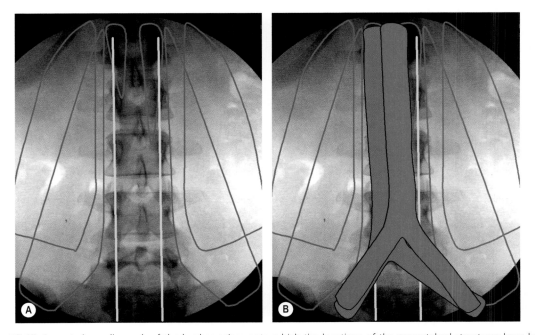

Figure 18.15 An anterior radiograph of the lumbar spine, onto which the locations of the prevertebral structures have been superimposed. (A) The **left crus** and **right crus**, the lumbar **sympathetic trunks, quadratus lumborum** and **psoas major**. (B) **Inferior vena cava** and **aorta**.

Chapter | **19** |

Sagittal magnetic resonance scans

CHAPTER CONTENTS

Anyone who has undertaken the exercises described in Chapters 17 and 18, should find it straightforward to read sagittal, magnetic resonance image (MRI) scans of the lumbar spine. Those exercises asked the reader to *expect* the structures that lie anterior, lateral and posterior to the lumbar vertebral column. In plain radiographs, those structures were invisible, but in MRI scans, they are actually evident. Reading sagittal MRI scans, therefore, amounts to no more than matching expectation with what is actually evident.

The expectations of what should be evident in a sagittal scan can be established by answering four questions:

1. Which parts of the vertebral column will be evident?
2. Which elements of the contents of the vertebral canal will be evident?
3. Which structures anterior to the vertebral column will be evident?
4. Which structures posterior to the vertebral column will be evident?

Sagittal MRI scans are typically taken across five standard planes (Fig. 19.1). Additional scans might be taken between these standard planes, or slightly displaced left or right from them; but the principles of analysis remain the same.

With respect to the vertebral column, a median scan will intersect the vertebral bodies and intervertebral discs anteriorly and the spinous processes posteriorly. Other parts of the vertebral column are not intersected and so will not be seen in the scan. A paramedian scan will intersect the vertebral bodies and intervertebral discs anteriorly, and the laminae posteriorly.

A particular facility of MRI scans is that they can distinguish between the nucleus pulposus of the intervertebral disc and the anulus fibrosus. The nucleus will appear white or grey, reflecting its content of water. The anulus will appear black. Median and paramedian scans will intersect the nucleus pulposus of each disc and the anterior and posterior anulus. Transpedicular scans will do otherwise.

Anteriorly, transpedicular scans will intersect the lateral sectors of the vertebral bodies and the lateral sectors of the intervertebral discs. The latter will be intersected either through the anulus fibrosus or through the most peripheral segments of the nucleus pulposus. Posteriorly, transpedicular scans will intersect the pedicles of the lumbar vertebrae and some portions of the zygapophysial joints. Slightly more lateral transpedicular scans will intersect the superior articular processes. Slightly more medial transpedicular scans will intersect the inferior articular processes.

Tangential scans will intersect the most lateral margins of the vertebral bodies and the anulus fibrosus at each segmental level, or the concavity of the vertebral body. Peripheral scans will intersect only the transverse processes.

With respect to the contents of the vertebral canal, median, paramedian and transpedicular scans will intersect different components of the dural sac and its contents (Fig. 19.2). A median scan will intersect the conus

P T TP PM M

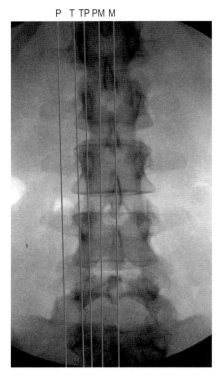

Figure 19.1 An anteroposterior radiograph of the lumbar spine showing the location of standard sagittal magnetic resonance scans. M, median scan; PM, paramedian scan; TP, transpedicular scan; T, tangential scan; P, peripheral scan.

TP PM M

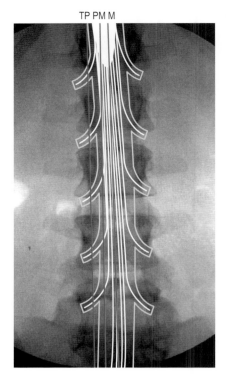

Figure 19.2 An anteroposterior radiograph of the lumbar spine showing the location of the dural sac, the conus medullaris of the spinal cord, the cauda equina, and the lumbar nerve roots, and how they are various intersected by median (M), paramedian (PM), and transpedicular (TP) sagittal magnetic resonance imaging scans.

medullaris of the spinal cord at upper segmental levels, and the cauda equina at lower levels. A paramedian scan may miss the spinal cord and show only the cauda equina. A transpedicular scan will intersect the spinal nerves and their dural sleeves, as they pass under the pedicles. Tangential and peripheral scans will not intersect the contents of the vertebral canal.

In a lateral view, the reader should, therefore, expect a median scan to show the dural sac, the conus medullaris of the spinal cord and the cauda equina (Fig. 19.3A). A paramedian scan would show only the cauda equina (Fig. 19.3B). A transpedicular scan would show only the spinal nerve roots and their sleeves (Fig. 19.3C).

Anteriorly, different scans will variously intersect the crura of the diaphragm and the great vessels, or the psoas major and quadratus lumborum (Fig. 19.4). Posteriorly, the scans will pass through multifidus, longissimus thoracis, or iliocostalis lumborum (Fig. 19.5).

The actual appearance of individual structures: their longitudinal extent and their shape that should be expected on sagittal scans, can be derived from what the reader would expect to see on lateral radiographs. Across the concavities of the vertebral bodies, the reader would expect

to encounter the lumbar arteries and lumbar veins, covered by psoas. (Fig. 19.6A). In front of the vertebral bodies, but to the right-hand side, they would expect the right crus and the inferior vena cava (Fig. 19.6A). Posteriorly, but behind the laminae, they would expect the multifidus (Fig. 19.6A). In front of the vertebral bodies, but more to the centre and to the left, the reader would expect the left crus and the aorta (Fig. 19.6B). Laterally, in front of the transverse processes they would expect the psoas major and the quadratus lumborum (Fig. 19.6B). Posteriorly, behind the transverse processes they would expect the various elements of the erector spinae (Fig. 19.6B).

MEDIAN SCAN

From Figure 19.1, the reader would expect that a median scan should intersect the vertebral bodies and intervertebral discs anteriorly, and the spinous processes posteriorly. Since it is a median scan, it should show the nucleus

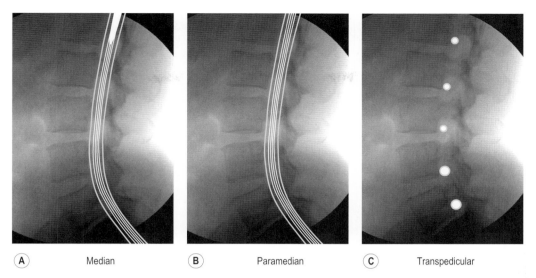

A   Median   B   Paramedian   C   Transpedicular

Figure 19.3 A lateral radiograph of the lumbar spine showing the contents of the vertebral canal that would be intersected and shown by various sagittal magnetic resonance imaging scans.

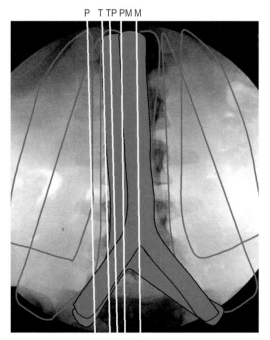

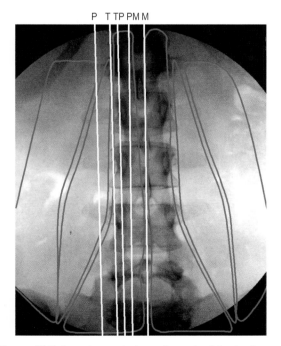

Figure 19.4 An anteroposterior radiograph of the lumbar spine on which the anterior relations of the lumbar vertebral column have been superimposed, and showing how these structures are intersected by standard sagittal magnetic resonance scans. M, median scan; PM, paramedian scan; TP, transpedicular scan; T, tangential scan; P, peripheral scan.

Figure 19.5 An anteroposterior radiograph of the lumbar spine on which the posterior relations of the lumbar vertebral column have been superimposed, and showing how these structures are intersected by standard sagittal magnetic resonance scans. M, median scan; PM, paramedian scan; TP, transpedicular scan; T, tangential scan; P, peripheral scan.

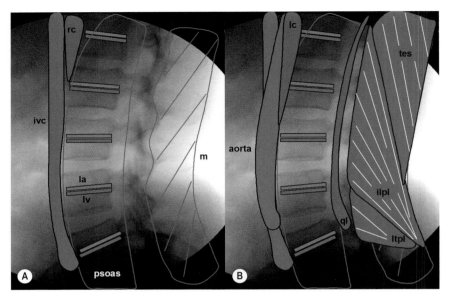

Figure 19.6 Lateral radiographs of the lumbar spine on which the external relations of the lumbar vertebral column have been superimposed. (A) The right crus (rc), inferior vena cava (ivc), lumbar arteries (la), lumbar veins (lv) psoas major (psoas) and multifidus (m). (B) The left crus (lc), aorta, quadratus lumborum (ql), longissimus thoracis pars lumborum (ltpl), iliocostalis lumborum pars lumborum, (ilpl) and the lower thoracic fibres of erector spinae (tes).

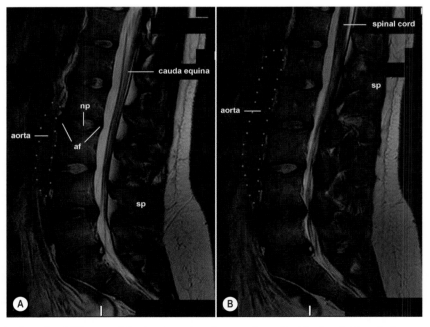

Figure 19.7 A pair of median MRI scans of the lumbar spine. Because the patient had a slight scoliosis, scan A is median at L4 but slightly to the right of midline at upper lumbar levels. Scan B is median at upper lumbar levels, but slightly to the left of midline at lower lumbar levels. Where the scan is in the median plane spinous processes (sp) are clearly evident. The roots of the cauda equina appear as black strings against a background of intensely white signal that is generated by the cerebrospinal fluid in the dural sac. The nucleus pulposus (np) appears white or grey, consistent with its fluid-content. The surrounding anulus fibrosus (af) is black.

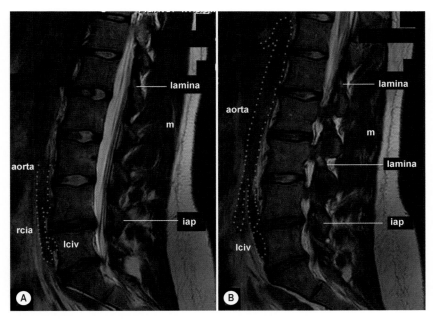

Figure 19.8 A pair of paramedian MRI scans of the lumbar spine. Scan A is to the right of the midline. At most segmental levels, scan (A) passes through the laminae, but at lower levels it intersects the medial edge of the inferior articular processes (iap). Anteriorly, the lower end of the aorta is evident, and the right common iliac artery (rcia) crossing the left common iliac vein (lciv) in front of L5. Scan (B) is to the left of the midline. Posteriorly, it shows the same structures as does scan (A). Anteriorly, the aorta is evident along its entire length, as far as its bifurcation. The left common iliac vein continues across the front of L5. Posteriorly, the multifidus (m) is evident in both scans.

pulposus at the centre of each disc, and the anulus fibrosus anterior and posteriorly. From Figures 19.2 and 19.3, the reader would expect a median scan to intersect the conus medullaris and the cauda equina. From Figure 19.4, the reader would expect that a median scan should intersect the aorta. From Figure 19.6, the reader would expect the aorta to terminate opposite L4. It thus transpires that this is what a median MRI scan shows (Fig. 19.7).

PARAMEDIAN SCAN

From Figure 19.1, the reader would expect that a paramedian scan should intersect the vertebral bodies and intervertebral discs anteriorly, and the laminae posteriorly (or the more medial elements of the zygapophysial joints). It should show the nucleus pulposus at the centre of each disc, and the anulus fibrosus anteriorly and posteriorly. From Figures 19.2 and 19.3, the reader would expect a paramedian scan to intersect the cauda equina. Paramedian scans that are to the right of the midline should pass near or through the right-side edge of the aorta, and in front of L5 they should pass through the right common iliac artery passing to the right, and covering the

left common iliac vein passing to the left (Fig. 19.4). Paramedian scans to the left of the midline should substantially intersect the aorta. Posteriorly, the scan should pass through the multifidus. It thus transpires that this is what paramedian MRI scans show (Fig. 19.8).

TRANSPEDICULAR SCANS

From Figure 19.1, the reader would expect that a transpedicular scan should intersect the vertebral bodies and intervertebral discs anteriorly, and the pedicles and zygapophysial joints posteriorly. From Figures 19.2 and 19.3, the reader would expect a transpedicular scan to intersect the lumbar spinal nerve in their intervertebral foramina. Transpedicular scans on the left most likely will pass lateral to the aorta, although they might intersect the more lateral segments of the aorta. On the right, transpedicular scans should intersect the inferior vena cava (Fig. 19.4). In front of L5 they should pass through the right common iliac artery (Fig. 19.4). Posteriorly, the scan should pass through the multifidus. It thus transpires that this is what paramedian MRI scans show (Fig. 19.9).

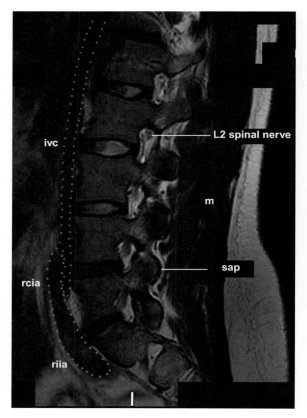

Figure 19.9 A right transpedicular MRI scan of the lumbar spine. The spinal nerves are evident below the pedicles. Posteriorly, the pedicles expand into the superior articular processes (sap), behind which the fibres of multifidus (m) pass dorsally and cephalad. Anteriorly, the scan passes through the left-hand edge of the inferior vena cava (ivc). The right common iliac artery (rcia) and the right internal iliac artery (riia) are evident.

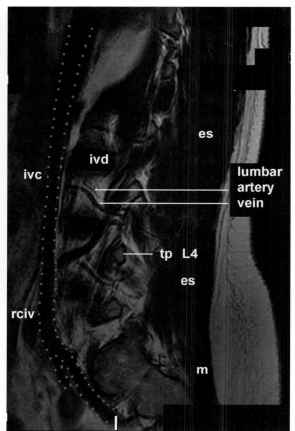

Figure 19.10 A right tangential MRI scan of the lumbar spine. The scan passes through the vertebral bodies and outer margins of the intervertebral discs (ivd). On the lateral surface of the vertebral bodies, the scan reveals the lumbar arteries and veins. Anteriorly, the inferior vena cava (ivc) is seen along its entire length, continuing caudally (in front of L5) as the right common iliac vein (rciv). The scan intersects the roots of the transverse processes (tp). Posteriorly, the fibres of the erector spinae (es) are seen running ventrally and cephalad; behind the sacrum lies multifidus (m).

TANGENTIAL SCANS

From Figure 19.1, the reader would expect that a tangential scan should pass through the edges of the vertebral bodies and intervertebral discs, and across the concavities of the vertebral bodies. From Figure 19.6, the reader would expect a transpedicular scan to intersect the lumbar arteries and veins. Transpedicular scans on the left most likely will pass lateral to the aorta, although they might intersect the more lateral segments of the aorta (Fig. 19.4). On the right, transpedicular scans should intersect the inferior vena cava (Fig. 19.4). In front of L5 they should pass through the right common iliac artery (Figs 19.4, 19.6). Posteriorly, from Figure 19.5, the reader would expect

tangential scans to intersect the erector spinae at most levels, and the multifidus at lumbosacral levels. It thus transpires that this is what paramedian MRI scans show (Fig. 19.10).

PERIPHERAL SCANS

From Figure 19.1, the reader would expect that a peripheral scan should pass through the transverse process. From Figures 19.4, 19.5 and 19.6, the reader would expect a peripheral scan to intersect the psoas major and quadratus lumborum anteriorly, and the erector spinae posteriorly. It thus transpires that this is what peripheral MRI scans do (Fig. 19.11).

CONVERSE READING

The exercise described in this chapter asked readers what they expect to see in sagittal scans. In clinical practice, however, readers are presented with scans, which can be intimidating. Under those circumstances, the same exercise can be applied, once certain landmarks are identified.

Based on what they can discern of the osseous elements: vertebral bodies, spinous processes, laminae, zygapophysial joints, pedicles or transverse processes, the reader can make an initial estimate of whether the scan is median, paramedian, transpedicular, tangential or peripheral. Based on that initial estimate, they should determine what else they expect to see, if that estimate is correct. If the scan displays the expected structures, the estimate proves to be correct. If the scan fails to display the expected structures, the estimate can be revised, and the process repeated until expectations are confirmed. If an algorithm such as this is applied, the scan should no longer be intimidating. It amounts to no more than an invitation to apply '*anatomy by expectation*'.

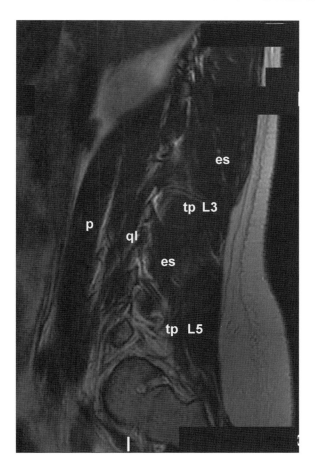

Figure 19.11 A right peripheral MRI scan of the lumbar spine. The scan passes through psoas major (p) and quadratus lumborum (ql) anteriorly, and the erectors spinae (es) posteriorly. Between the anterior and posterior muscles project the transverse processes (tp).

Chapter | 20 |

Axial magnetic resonance imaging

Some practitioners find axial scans of the body difficult to understand and, therefore, to be oppressive. For them, it is as if axial anatomy constitutes yet another subject in anatomy that needs to be separately and additionally studied and mastered. This need not be so.

It can be shown that the appearance of axial scans can be derived from prior knowledge of anatomy. All that is required is that that prior knowledge be rotated 90°, and systematically reassembled. This chapter describes that process.

PRINCIPLES

The prediction of the appearance of an axial scan of the lumbar spine can be reduced to two major steps. The first involves considering what the internal, i.e. neural, relations will be. The second step involves considering what the external relations will be.

INTERNAL NEURAL RELATIONS

Axial magnetic resonance imaging (MRI) scans of the lumbar spine are typical taken through three standard locations at any given segment. The scans can be through the pedicles (transpedicular), below the pedicles (subpedicular) or through the intervertebral disc and zygapophysial joints (transarticular) (Fig. 20.1).

Each of these scans intersects slightly different elements contained within the vertebral canal. Transpedicular scans will intersect the dural sac and the nerve roots of the cauda equina (Fig. 20.2). In these scans, the pedicles will be evident projecting from the posterior surface of the vertebral body. These bones present as a grey signal. Posteriorly, various parts of the laminae and spinous process will complete the vertebral canal. Within the vertebral canal, the dural sac will appear as a black circle or oval, enclosing a white signal generated by the cerebrospinal fluid within the sac. Inside the sac, the nerve roots of the cauda equina appear as block dots, because the nerves appear as if they have been transected and looked at end-on. The nerve roots typically appear towards the posterior surface of the dural sac because patients typically lie supine when the scan is taken, and the nerve roots 'fall' to the rear.

Subpedicular scans will intersect the nerve roots of the cauda equina but also the spinal nerves of the segment, as they run through the intervertebral foramen of the segment (Fig. 20.3). The scan will show the vertebral body anteriorly, and the lamina on each side posteriorly. Behind the centre of the vertebral body, the dural sac will appear as a dark ring, with the nerve roots of the cauda equina appearing as black dots lying in a sea of white signal formed by the cerebrospinal fluid. Lateral to the dural sac a dark signal will appear, behind the vertebral body, created by the spinal nerve. Depending on exactly where the scan is taken, the spinal nerve may be accompanied by a sleeve of dura mater, which in turn may contain a sliver of cerebrospinal fluid surrounding the nerve.

Transarticular scans will intersect the dural sac and cauda equina centrally, but will also show the spinal nerve or ventral ramus leaving the vertebral column and entering the psoas major muscle (Fig. 20.4). Anteriorly, the scan will show the intervertebral disc. Unlike the vertebral body, which appeared grey, the disc will largely appear black. The centre of the disc may appear grey if the scan

is taken close to the vertebral endplate. Posteriorly, the zygapophysial joints will be evident. Centrally, the dural sac will enclose the nerve roots of the cauda equina, as in transpedicular scans. Laterally, near the posterolateral corner of the disc, a dark rounded signal is produced by the spinal nerve becoming the ventral ramus. Because the spinal nerve passes obliquely and caudally through the intervertebral foramen, it will be located further laterally, i.e. peripherally, in transarticular scans than in subpedicular scans, and will be distinctly dissociated from the dural sac.

Irrespective of which segment is scanned, these three, basic alternatives apply. Consequently, by just looking at the neural relations a reader will have great difficulty ascertaining which segment they are studying – because the neural relations will look basically the same at all segments. Identifying the segment relies on knowing the external relations.

EXTERNAL RELATIONS

The external relations that will be seen on an axial scan will differ at different segmental levels. Figure 20.5 summarises what structure the reader should expect at different segments, and what each structure should look like.

At upper lumbar levels, the reader should expect to encounter the left crus and right crus of the diaphragm, arising from the front of the vertebral bodies (Fig. 20.5A). In particular, the crura will be large in front of L1 but tapering and dissipating in front of L2. The crura intervene between the vertebral column and the inferior vena cava and the aorta.

The inferior vena cava lies to the right, and the reader should expect to encounter it at all segmental levels as far

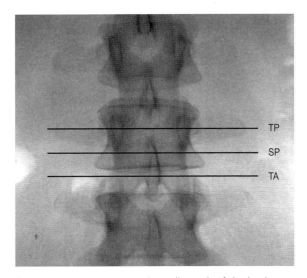

Figure 20.1 An anteroposterior radiograph of the lumbar spine showing the location of typical, axial MRI scans. TP, transpedicular; SP, subpedicular; TA, transarticular.

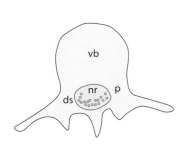
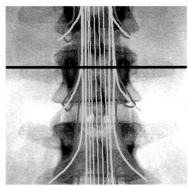
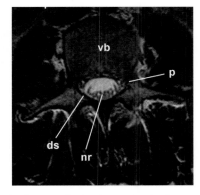

Figure 20.2 The central figure illustrates where a transpedicular scan intersects the lumbar vertebral column, the dural sac and the cauda equina. The figure on the left is a diagram of the vertebral elements and neural elements that would be seen in the scan. The figure on the right depicts an actual transpedicular scan, MRI scan. vb, vertebral body; p, pedicle; ds, dural sac; nr, nerve roots of the cauda equina.

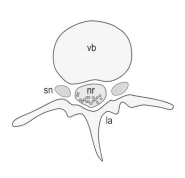

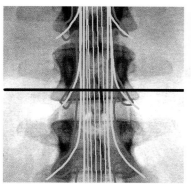

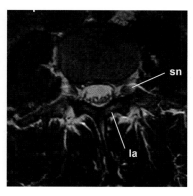

Figure 20.3 The central figure illustrates where a subpedicular scan intersects the lumbar vertebral column, the dural sac and the segmental spinal nerve. The figure on the left is a diagram of the vertebral elements and neural elements that would be seen in the scan. The figure on the right depicts an actual subpedicular scan, MRI scan. vb, vertebral body; la, lamina; nr, nerve roots of the cauda equina; sn, spinal nerve.

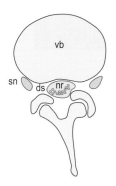

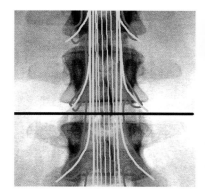

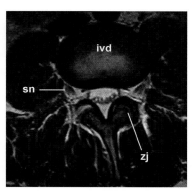

Figure 20.4 The central figure illustrates where a transarticular scan intersects the lumbar vertebral column, the dural sac and the cauda equina. The figure on the left is a diagram of the vertebral elements and neural elements that would be seen in the scan. The figure on the right depicts an actual transarticular scan, MRI scan. ivd, intervertebral disc; zj, zygapophysial joint; ds, dural sac; nr, nerve roots of the cauda equina; sn, spinal nerve.

as L5 (Fig. 20.5A). The aorta lies towards the midline at upper lumbar levels, but deviates somewhat to the left, until it divides at L4 (Fig. 20.5A). At the L1, L2 and L3 levels, the reader should expect to encounter two large vessels: the inferior vena cava and the aorta. At L4, the reader should expect to encounter three vessels: the inferior vena cava and the aorta having divided into the two common iliac arteries. At L5, the reader should expect four vessels: the two common iliac arteries and the two common iliac veins. The number of great vessels in front the vertebra column is the most obvious indication of whether the scan is at L5 or at L4, or at L1, 2 or 3.

Laterally, the reader should expect to encounter quadratus lumborum as a broad, flat mass overlying the transverse processes (Fig. 20.5A); but not at L5, for the quadratus lumborum arises from the iliolumbar ligament and, therefore, above L5. The absence of quadratus

lumborum is one of the features that characterise scans at L5.

The psoas major covers the quadratus lumborum, but progressively enlarges from L1 to L5 (Fig. 20.5A). Therefore, in axial scans, the reader should expect psoas to be narrow at upper lumbar levels, and progressively thicker at lower levels. Indeed, compared to other structures, psoas becomes enormous at lower lumbar levels.

Posteriorly, the reader should expect to encounter the three major posterior back muscles. They should expect multifidus to be confined to the region over the lamina at upper lumbar levels, but to expand progressively widely from L3 to the sacrum (Fig. 20.5B). Lateral to multifidus, the reader should expect the longissimus thoracis to be centred over the roots of the transverse processes; and the iliocostalis lumborum to be centred over the tips of the transverse processes.

245

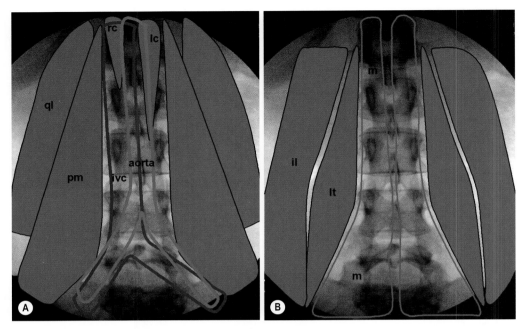

Figure 20.5 Anteroposterior radiographs of the lumbar spine onto which its external relations have been superimposed. (A) Anterior relations. (B) Posterior relations. lc, left crus; rc, right crus; ql, quadratus lumborum; pm, psoas major; ivc, inferior vena cava; il, iliocostalis lumborum; lt, longissimus thoracis; m, multifidus. The inferior vena cava, aorta and multifidus have been drawn as if they were transparent in order to reveal the underlying vertebrae.

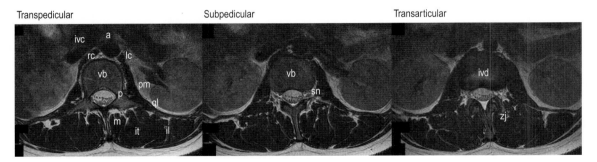

Figure 20.6 Axial MRI scans through L1. vb, vertebral body; p, pedicle; rc, right crus; lc, left crus; ivc, inferior vena cava; a, aorta; pm, psoas major; ql, quadratus lumborum; m, multifidus; lt, longissimus thoracis; il, iliocostalis lumborum; sn, spinal nerve; ivd, intervertebral disc; zj, zygapophysial joint.

AXIAL MRI SCANS AT L1

Using Figure 20.5, the reader should expect to encounter the left crus and right crus in scans at L1, with the inferior vena cava and aorta in front of them. Lateral to the vertebral bodies, the reader should expect a broad, flat quadratus lumborum, but a narrow psoas major, for its fibres will have just arisen from the T12–L1 disc. Posteriorly, the reader should expect a narrow multifidus, flanked by longissimus thoracis and iliocostalis lumborum. This is indeed what scans through L1 show (Fig. 20.6).

AXIAL MRI SCANS AT L2

Using Figure 20.5, the reader should expect modifications at scans through L2. The crura will be attenuated, but the inferior vena cava and aorta will be prominent, anteriorly. The quadratus lumborum should persist, but the psoas major should be larger. Posteriorly, the multifidus, longissimus thoracis, and iliocostalis lumborum should be evident. This is indeed what scans through L2 show (Fig. 20.7).

Scans through L1 and L2 may be quite similar, and may be difficult to distinguish. The immediate differences are only relative: the crura are small, or absent, at L2; and the psoas is only relatively larger. On these grounds alone, readers could be excused for not being able to distinguish absolutely scans through L1 and L2. Further clues appear in the visceral and vascular structures lying anterior to the lumbar spine. For example, the right renal vessels tend to be more caudal than those on the left. Therefore, left renal vessels are likely to be encountered at L1, whereas right renal vessels will be seen at L2 (Fig. 20.7). The anatomy of visceral and vascular structures, however, is outside the scope of this text.

AXIAL MRI SCANS AT L3

Using Figure 20.5, the reader should expect no crura in scans at L3, but the inferior vena cava and aorta will be prominent, anterior to the vertebral column. The quadratus lumborum should be evident, and the psoas major should appear as a substantial mass. Posteriorly, the multifidus should be expanding lateral to the limits of the laminae; but otherwise, it will be flanked by the longissimus thoracis and the iliocostalis lumborum. This is indeed what scans through L3 show (Fig. 20.8). The absence of crura, the prominence of psoas and the expansion of multifidus all characterise scans through L3.

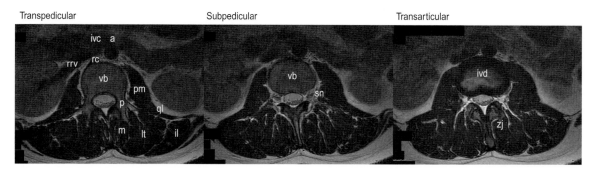

Figure 20.7 Axial MRI scans through L2. vb, vertebral body; p, pedicle; rc, right crus; ivc, inferior vena cava; a, aorta; pm, psoas major; ql, quadratus lumborum; m, multifidus; lt, longissimus thoracis; il, iliocostalis lumborum; sn, spinal nerve; ivd, intervertebral disc; zj, zygapophysial joint. In this scan, the right renal vein (rrv) can be seen draining into the inferior vena cava.

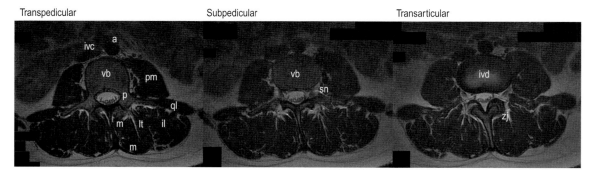

Figure 20.8 Axial MRI scans through L3. vb, vertebral body; p, pedicle; ivc, inferior vena cava; a, aorta; pm, psoas major; ql, quadratus lumborum; m, multifidus; lt, longissimus thoracis; il, iliocostalis lumborum; sn, spinal nerve; ivd, intervertebral disc; zj, zygapophysial joint.

AXIAL MRI SCANS AT L4

Using Figure 20.5, the reader should expect to see three great vessels in front of the vertebral column in scans through L4. Laterally, the psoas should be large. Posteriorly, the multifidus should be wide, and the erector spinae should be correspondingly small. This is indeed what scans through L4 show (Fig. 20.9).

AXIAL MRI SCANS AT L5

Using Figure 20.5, the reader should expect to see four great vessels in front of the vertebral column in scans through L5. Laterally, the psoas should be huge, but the quadratus lumborum should be absent. If the scan passes through the appropriate level, the iliolumbar ligament might be evident. Posteriorly, the multifidus will be very wide. The iliocostalis will be lacking, because its insertion – into the iliac crest – lies above L5. Only a small portion of longissimus thoracis should be evident. This is indeed what scans through L5 show (Fig. 20.10).

CONVERSE APPLICATIONS

Rarely would practitioners be required to predict the appearance of an axial MRI scan. Instead, they are more likely to be confronted with a particular scan, and would be required to interpret across which segmental level that scan was taken. For this problem, the principles outlined in this chapter, nevertheless apply, with few adjustments.

The first step pertains to the internal relations. Determine if the scan is transpedicular, subpedicular or transarticular. Upon doing so, the reader should be able to identify the dural sac, the nerve roots of the cauda equina and the spinal nerve (if evident).

The second step is to estimate the segmental level. This is achieved by examining the external relations in each of the surrounding sectors.

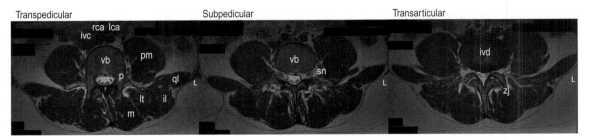

Figure 20.9 Axial MRI scans through L4. vb, vertebral body; p, pedicle; pm, psoas major; ql, quadratus lumborum; m, multifidus; lt, longissimus thoracis; il, iliocostalis lumborum; sn, spinal nerve; ivd, intervertebral disc; zj, zygapophysial joint; ivc, inferior vena cava; rca, right common artery; lca, left common artery.

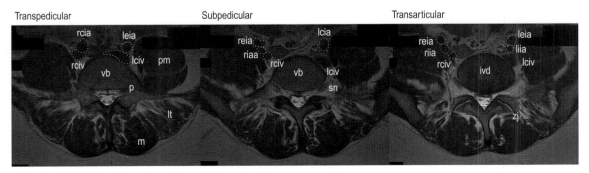

Figure 20.10 Axial MRI scans through L5. vb, vertebral body; p, pedicle; pm, psoas major; m, multifidus; lt, longissimus thoracis; sn, spinal nerve; ivd, intervertebral disc; zj, zygapophysial joint; rcia, right common iliac artery; lcia, left common iliac artery; rciv, right common iliac vein; lciv, left common iliac vein; reia, right external iliac artery; riia, right internal iliac artery; leia, left external iliac artery; liia, left internal iliac artery.

In the anterior sector, two great vessels together with distinctive crura, place the scan at L1. This should be corroborated by finding a narrow psoas major in the lateral sector, and a narrow multifidus in the posterior sector.

Two great vessels in the anterior sector but with dissipating crura, place the scan at L2. This should be corroborated by a less than narrow psoas major in the lateral sector; and confirmed by the presence of right renal vessels.

The presence of two great vessels in the anterior sector but with no crura suggests that the scan is through L3. This should be corroborated by finding a substantial psoas major in the lateral sector, and a multifidus that is starting to expand beyond the lateral margins of the laminae in the posterior sector.

Three great vessels in the anterior sector place the scan at L4. This should be corroborated by a large psoas major in the lateral sector, and a wide multifidus in the posterior sector.

Four great vessels in the anterior sector indicate that the scan is at L5. This should be corroborated by the presence of a large psoas major in the lateral sector, together with an absence of quadratus lumborum. In the posterior sector, the multifidus will be large.

Appendix

IDENTIFICATION OF THE LUMBAR VERTEBRAE

A skill practised by some anatomists is the ability to identify individual bones; students of anatomy are sometimes asked to do this in examinations. While the identification of large bones like the femur and humerus may be easy, to identify the individual lumbar vertebrae seems a daunting challenge. Specifically, the vertebrae seem so alike.

The ability to identify bones has little intrinsic value, except in forensic osteology. Therefore, it may seem pointless to expect students to learn how to identify individual lumbar vertebrae. However, the practice (and examination) of this skill has a certain implicit value. It determines if the student understands the functions of the bone in question and how it is designed to subserve these functions. The exercise of identifying bones is made pointless only if some routine is mindlessly memorised simply to pass a possible examination question. However, if the bone is used to prompt a revision of its functions, then the exercise can be done with insight and purpose, and consequently becomes rewarding and easier. Moreover, if superficially similar bones have different functions or biomechanical needs, then subtle differences in structure can be sought and discovered, whereby individual bones can be recognised.

Having studied the structure of the lumbar vertebrae (Ch. 1), the nature of their joints and ligaments (Chs 2–4) and the form of the intact lumbar spine (Ch. 5), it is possible to review the detailed structure of the lumbar vertebrae and highlight the differences that correlate with the different functions of individual vertebrae. Some of the differences are present in only one vertebra. Others are part of a series of differences seen throughout the lumbar spine. Accordingly, both the structure of individual vertebrae and the structure of the entire lumbar spine should be considered.

The most individual lumbar vertebra is the fifth. Its characteristic feature is the thickness of its transverse processes and their attachment along the whole length of the pedicles as far as the vertebral body. Examining this feature serves to remind the student of the attachment of the powerful iliolumbar ligaments to the L5 transverse processes and their role in restraining the L5 vertebra. In turn, this is a reminder of the problem that L5 faces in staying in place on top of the sloping sacrum.

There are no absolute features that enable the other four lumbar vertebrae to be distinguished but there are relative differences that reflect trends evident along the lumbar spine. First, as a general rule, the lengths of the upper four transverse processes vary in a reasonably constant pattern. From above downwards, they increase in length and then decrease such that the L3 transverse process is usually the longest, and the transverse processes of L1 and L4 are usually the shortest. The reason for this difference is still obscure but the long length of the L3 transverse processes seems to correlate with the central location of the L3 vertebra in the lumbar lordosis, and its long transverse processes probably provide a necessary extra mechanical advantage for the muscles that act on them.

The other serial change in the lumbar spine is the orientation of the zygapophysial joints. Sagittally orientated joints are a feature of upper lumbar levels, while joints

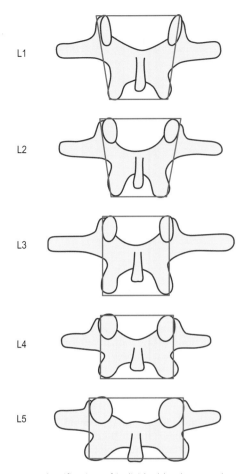

L1

L2

L3

L4

L5

Figure A.1 Identification of individual lumbar vertebrae. By constructing four-sided figures around the tips of the articular processes of the lumbar vertebrae, distinguishing features are revealed. The figures formed around the upper two lumbar vertebrae are trapezia; that around L3 is an upright rectangle; that around L4 is a square; and that around L5 is a horizontal rectangle.

orientated closer to 45° are more characteristic of lower levels. Examining this feature serves as a reminder of the compound role of the zygapophysial joints in resisting forward displacement and rotation, and the need at lower lumbar levels for stabilisation against forward displacement.

From above downwards, the vertebral bodies tend to be slightly larger, and their transverse dimension tends to be relatively longer in proportion to their anteroposterior dimension. This correlates with the increasing load that lower vertebrae have to bear.

A structural idiosyncrasy of the lumbar vertebrae is that if four-sided figures are constructed to include in their angles the four articular processes of each vertebra, different shapes are revealed.[1] For the upper two lumbar vertebrae, a trapezium is constructed. The L3 vertebra forms an upright rectangle. The L4 vertebra forms a square, and the L5 vertebra forms a parallelogram with its longer sides aligned horizontally (Fig. A.1). Although these rules were developed some years ago, based largely on anatomical experience and good observation,[1] quantitative studies have confirmed their validity.[2]

By examining these various features, a student should be able to identify individual lumbar vertebrae to within at least one segment. The L5 vertebra is readily recognised. L4 will tend to have inferior articular processes orientated towards 45°, and will have short transverse processes and a relatively wider body. Its four articular processes will fall inside a square. L3 should have inferior articular processes with intermediate orientations but most often close to 45°. Its transverse processes will be long and its articular processes will fall inside a rectangle. The L1 and L2 vertebrae remain with more sagittally orientated articular facets and articular processes that fall within trapezia. The only feature that may distinguish L1 from L2 is a better development of the mamillary and accessory processes on L1 and its shorter transverse processes. Apart from this, however, the upper two lumbar vertebrae may be indistinguishable.

REFERENCES

1. Fawcett E. A note on the identification of the lumbar vertebrae of man. *J Anat.* 1932;66:384–386.

2. Panjabi MM, Oxland T, Takata K, et al. Articular facets of the human spine: quantitative three-dimensional anatomy. *Spine.* 1993;18:1298–1310.

Index

Illustrations are comprehensively referred to from the text. Therefore, significant material in illustrations and tables have only been given a page reference in the absence of their concomitant mention in the text referring to that figure. Page numbers followed by f indicate figures; t, tables.